EXERCISE

PHYSIOLOGY

ROY J. SHEPHARD, M.D. (Lond), Ph.D.

Director
School of Physical and Health Education

Professor of Applied Physiology
Faculty of Medicine
University of Toronto
Toronto, Ontario

1987
B.C. DECKER INC • Toronto • Philadelphia

Publisher

B.C. Decker Inc
3228 South Service Road
Burlington, Ontario   L7N 3H8

B.C. Decker Inc
P.O. Box 30246
Philadelphia, Pennsylvania   19103

Sales and Distribution

United States
and Possessions

The C.V. Mosby Company
11830 Westline Industrial Drive
Saint Louis, Missouri   63146

Canada

The C.V. Mosby Company, Ltd.
5240 Finch Avenue East, Unit No. 1
Scarborough, Ontario   M1S 4P2

United Kingdom, Europe
and the Middle East

Blackwell Scientific Publications, Ltd.
Osney Mead, Oxford OX2 OEL, England

Australia

Harcourt Brace Jovanovich
30–52 Smidmore Street
Marrickville, N.S.W. 2204
Australia

Japan

Igaku-Shoin Ltd.
Tokyo International P.O. Box 5063
1-28-36 Hongo, Bunkyo-ku, Tokyo 113, Japan

Asia

Infomed
1932, Fei Ngo Shan
Kowloon, Hong Kong

Exercise Physiology

ISBN 0–941158–90–X

Library of Congress catalog card number: 86-073082

10   9   8   7   6   5   4   3   2   1

PREFACE

Exercise physiology might be thought a crowded market for another textbook. When B. C. Decker first proposed that I write such a volume, I shared this opinion. However, after some discussion, I agreed that the majority of currently available offerings were in reality low level physiology texts. Moreover, by attempting to treat both physiology and exercise physiology within a limit of 300 to 400 pages, the available texts failed to do even elementary justice to the exciting progress that has been made in this latter topic over the past decade.

The present text, although written with the undergraduate in mind, is unashamedly directed to exercise physiology. It is based upon nearly 20 years of experience in a third year honors course at the University of Toronto, and it assumes that students have already completed university level courses in the basics of anatomy and physiology. The starting point is thus motion, which is a central characteristic of the animal kingdom. The demand for energy to induce the various forms of human movement is discussed, and identified are the prime bottlenecks in the translation of food stores into external work. Methods of measuring human activity in the laboratory and in the field are compared, and the optimum choice of fuel for physical activity is debated. Chapters 4 through 7 examine the hormonal and neural regulation of the various body systems under the stress of physical exercise. Consideration is then given to methods of measuring fitness, the modification of physical condition by various types of training regimens, and the influences of age and sex upon human working capacity. The following two chapters look at physical performance under conditions of environmental stress—extremes of ambient pressure and temperature. The last two chapters review such important topics as the interactions between exercise and cardiovascular health and potential modification of physical performance by various drugs (ergogenic aids, air pollutants, cigarette smoke, and alcohol).

Although it is often undertaken lightly, in many respects, exercise is a matter of life and death. When prescribed judiciously, an increase of physical activity can add much to the quality of daily life, and in some instances, it may even extend lifespan. On the other hand, sudden bursts of exercise for which an individual is ill-prepared can be life-threatening, and such dangers are substantially increased when the exercise must be carried out under harsh environmental conditions. This book is perhaps the first to acknowledge that physical educators face vital decisions about such issues in their daily practice, and it offers sound physiological reasoning for the recommendations which must be made.

Specific references have been avoided because they date quickly and add unnecessarily to the cost of a text. Those wishing to read further may pursue selected topics via the Cumulative Index Medicus and recent issues of the various international journals of sports science. A detailed bibliography of some 5,000 entries is also available in the author's graduate level text *Physiology and Biochemistry of Exercise* (New York: Praeger, 1982).

Although this book has been written primarily for the undergraduate in physical and health education, the author has deliberately avoided unnecessary and unexplained technical jargon. It is thus hoped that the material presented will appeal to sports physicians, exercise physiotherapists, coaches, trainers, and the growing group of professionals who advise either athletes or the general public on programs of training and physical activity.

R. J. Shephard

CONTENTS

BASIC CONCEPTS

APPLIED EXERCISE PHYSIOLOGY

PERFORMANCE AND TRAINING

ENVIRONMENT AND HEALTH

BASIC CONCEPTS

HUMAN MOTION AND ENVIRONMENTAL CHALLENGE

CHAPTER *1*

Movement as a Characteristic of Life

What is the academic importance of exercise science? Whereas classical physiology describes the characteristics of body function in a person who is living under resting or basal conditions, the exercise scientist is concerned with the woman or man on the move. The resting state has traditionally been considered a convenient frame of reference, both for reporting the functional behavior of the various body systems and for observing their responses to various types of experimental intervention. However, motion is such a fundamental feature of life that classical physiology provides a very incomplete description of human phenomena; a complementary study of reactions to vigorous exercise in average and in athletic subjects is necessary to understand the full range of human responses.

Principle of Homeostasis

One interesting aspect of human functional design noted by the French physiologist Claude Bernard was the principle of homeostasis—an innate ability to maintain the constancy of the body's internal environment or milieu interieur in the face of various challenges. While it is quite remarkable how the concentrations of cellular constituents, acidity, oxygen pressure, and temperature are held within closely specified limits under resting conditions, the process of self-regulation or Selbsteuerung becomes yet more fascinating when the constancy of these same variables is challenged by a 10- to 20-fold increase of metabolic rate, as an athlete moves at high speed through such challenging environments as extremes of heat, cold, or high or low ambient pressures.

Contribution of Movement to Homeostasis

Except in the most artificial of laboratory situations, movement makes an essential contribution to the process of homeostasis. As body food reserves are depleted, the individual must move in search of fresh nutrients to replenish internal stores. Likewise, by moving from a challenging to a more comfortable environment, the cost of maintaining the constancy of internal conditions can be greatly reduced, and if a person is confronted by an excessive environmental challenge, movement away from the problem may be essential to survival.

The central theme of this book is thus the way in which the milieu interieur is held constant in the face of dual challenges from vigorous exercise and an adverse environment. In the present chapter, we shall look briefly at the value of animal versus human studies. We shall then examine the energy needs of motion, the available energy resources, and the efficiency of their translation into external work.

Value of Animal Research

Although the most striking characteristic of the classical physiologist is a preoccupation with descriptions of the basal state, many classical physiologists also show a preference for animal rather than human experimentation. The classical physiologist has argued that the mind has a striking power over human responses and that such problems can be circumvented by studies of the anesthetized or the decerebrate animal.

In fact, the advantages of such preparations are somewhat illusory, particularly in the context of physical activity. Anesthetics often modify systemic blood pressure and various autonomic reflexes. The level of decerebration may vary through continued bleeding or recovery of traumatized brain tissue, and usually the decerebrate animal shows an abnormal increase of muscle tone. Moreover, the only possible form of exercise in an unconscious preparation is the atypical situation of electrical stimulation of a muscle or a nerve.

The main advantages of animal experiments are that biological specimens of blood and muscle can be collected without concern about causing permanent damage, and aging processes can be studied within a fairly brief lifespan, sometimes only 2 to 3 years.

Exercise in Animals

Exercise is sometimes performed on trained, conscious animals. Horses, sheep, dogs, and rats have all been persuaded to exercise on a treadmill, while rats and mice have been forced to swim to exhaustion in a tank, sometimes with weighted tails. Mice have been put in activity wheels, and various species have been trained to perform isometric exercise (the operation of weighted levers), using food pellets as a reward. In such circumstances it is difficult to be certain that there is less emotional disturbance than in human experiments. A rat which is persuaded to run by a repeated electrical shock or a mouse on the verge of drowning is hardly in a relaxed emotional state! A second problem is that between experiments the animal is usually confined to a small cage. It thus begins exercise in very poor physical condition and bears little resemblance to its free-living namesake. In theory, the daily amount of exercise can be controlled more closely than in humans, but in practice many animals run on the treadmill in a very clumsy fashion. The amount of oxygen consumed by small mammals is also quite limited, and measurements of gas exchange thus becomes subject to substantial experimental error. There are finally difficulties of scaling both immediate results and lifespan to an equivalent human value.

Emotional Disturbances in Humans

The scientist who chooses to examine the phenomenon of exercise nevertheless has several advantages over colleagues who study resting responses. Vigorous exercise is a major physiological disturbance, inducing a 10- to 20-fold increase of metabolism, and equally large changes in many other body systems. Minor disturbances of the resting state induced by the emotions thus pale into insignificance before such a major influence. It has also been argued that emotional disturbances become smaller or even disappear as a person becomes involved in an exercise task. Certainly, the relative importance of an emotional increase in heart rate (tachycardia) of 10 beats per minute is much smaller if vigorous exercise has increased the heart rate to 180 beats per minute than if it has remained at a typical resting value of 60 beats per minute. Nevertheless, emotional factors can still be an important source of error when interpreting data; for example, if the heart rate response to a given work-rate decreases from 180 beats per minute to 170 beats per minute with test repetition, this may be attributed to cardiovascular training, when in reality it reflects no more than a decrease of anxiety.

Several simple techniques minimize the effects of anxiety; (1) all experiments must be fully explained to the subjects, and must be conducted with a minimum of fuss and disturbance; (2) if the resting heart rate remains high despite a prolonged initial rest, or if it is thought important to eliminate emotional overlay, the subject should be allowed several preliminary exposures to both the investigator and the laboratory—such "habituation," or negative conditioning, is an important element of a well-designed human experiment; (3) an alternative approach is to examine exercise responses relative to values for loadless pedalling of a cycle ergometer, rather than relative to data for rest or a hypothetical basal state.

Most of the findings to be discussed in this book have been obtained by human research, with all of its advantages and shortcomings. Recourse made to animal research will be clearly indicated.

ENERGY NEEDS OF MOTION

Range of Energy Expenditures

How much energy is consumed by human movement? An old lady who spends most of her day sitting in an armchair at a nursing home has an energy expenditure of approximately 6.3 megajoules per day (MJ per day).[1] However, this energy expenditure may be doubled for individuals involved in hard physical employment, and in exceptional circumstances, such as a 24-hour road race, energy expenditures of 30 to 40 MJ per day are conceivable.

---

[1] Standard international (SI) units and abbreviations have been adopted throughout this book (Table 1–1). This system of measurement has now been accepted by most international journals. However, older books express energy expenditure in calories (1 calorie = 4.186 joules).

TABLE 1–1   The Standard International (SI) Units of Scientific Measurement, with Conversion Factors for Previously Used Units*

Variable	Dimensions	Current Unit and Abbreviations	Previously Used Units
Mass	kg	kilogram (kg)	pound (= 0.454 kg)
Distance	m	meter(m)	foot (= 0.305m) mile (= 1.606km)
Time	s	second(s)	
Speed	m/s	m/s km/hour	foot/min (= 0.508 cm/s) mile/hour (= 0.446 m/s) (= (1.606 km/h)
Force	kgm/s^2	newton (N)	kg-force (= 9.81N) kilopond (= 9.81N)
Work	kgm^2/s^2	joule (J)	calorie (= 4.186J)
Power	kgm^2/s^3	watt (W)	kgm/min (= 0.164W)
Pressure	kg/m s^2	pascal (Pa)	mm Hg (= 133Pa) torr (= 133Pa)
Molality	mol/kg	mol/kg	g/kg
Concentration	mol/dm^3	mol/dm^3	mol/ℓ (= mol/dm^3) g/ℓ, g/dℓ

* Advanced texts generally use negative exponents, e.g., speed is shown as ms^{-1} rather than m/s; however, to simplify typesetting and the writing of equations, the more familiar format of numerator and denominator has been used here.

Resting Energy Usage

Let us look first at the energy used under resting conditions. A variety of homeostatic processes contribute to resting energy usage (Table 1–2). Continued operation of the respiratory pump maintains the constancy of alveolar and thus arterial gas consumption, but energy is used by the chest muscles. Cellular homeostasis depends in turn on the steady pumping of blood by the heart, again an energy-using process. Within individual cells, other pumps transfer food from the gut to the blood stream, and waste products from the blood to the renal tubules. Cell membranes suffer a steady inward leakage of sodium ions and an outward movement of potassium ions, and this tendency must be corrected by operation of a "sodium pump." Likewise, the cycle of muscular contraction and relaxation depends on the pumping of calcium ions. All of these intracellular pumps also consume energy.

The basic cell constituents—protein, fat, and carbohydrate—seem relatively permanent, but are in fact broken down and reformed every few days, again at the cost of a substantial energy expenditure. The energy demands of synthesizing cell constituents are further increased by such processes as growth, tissue hypertrophy, pregnancy, and lactation.

If the environment is cool, the resting rate of metabolism may be deliberately increased (for example, by an increase of muscle tone or a deliberate breakdown and resynthesis of fat) in order to sustain body temperature. Lastly, unless a subject is lying completely relaxed upon a couch, some energy is expended in maintaining body posture against the force of gravity.

Exercise increases many of the sources of resting energy expenditure noted above. The work of the chest muscles and the heart is greatly augmented by the increase of ventilation and cardiac output, the pumping of sodium and calcium ions is increased to compensate for greater leakage of ions, more food must be absorbed, and more waste products excreted. A substantial hypertrophy of muscle may also be induced by a regular exercise program, and postural demands generally rise as a person moves from sitting or lying to an upright position.

Specific Costs of Movement

Movement adds several new specific sources of energy expenditure as the body is displaced against gravitational acceleration and other opposing forces such as wind and friction. Let us consider a young woman with a 55-kg body mass who is cycling up a 1 percent gradient (Table 1-3). She is very conscious of a stiff headwind, and although she crouches low over the handlebars, the silhouette of cycle plus rider presents an area of perhaps $0.3m^2$ to the wind; at the particular wind-speed, this generates an opposing force

TABLE 1–2   Factors Contributing to Resting Energy Usage

Food turnover of protein, fat, and carbohydrate

Pump mechanisms, e.g., respiratory, cardiac, gastrointestinal, renal, sodium, and calcium

Growth and hypertrophy

Pregnancy and lactation (women only)

Temperature regulation

Maintenance of posture

of 43.3 newtons per square meter (13N).[2] There is always a small amount of friction in the chain and pedal bearings, but assuming that these have been well oiled, the main frictional resistance is between the tires and the road. If the tires are narrow and well inflated, the coefficient of sliding friction is about 0.05; this implies that the force opposing forward movement is one-twentieth of the mass of body plus rider, perhaps 3.75 kg force, or about 37N. There is also some air resistance, but since this is proportional to the third power of speed, it can be neglected when riding up hill. Let us assume that speed drops to 4.4 m per second (10 miles per hour). The rate of working against the wind and ground friction is then (13+37) 4.4 or 220 newton-meters per second (220 watts).[3] At the same time, potential energy is being accumulated by lifting the 55-kg woman and a 20-kg bicycle up the 1 percent gradient. The height climbed is (4.4) 0.01 meters per second; thus this element of energy expenditure amounts to a power output of 9.81 (55+20) 0.044 newton-meters per second or about 32 watts. In some sports, much further energy is lost in accelerating and decelerating the limbs or the entire body mass; however, the constant-speed rotary motion of the legs largely overcomes this particular problem for the cyclist.

In our example of the cyclist, it is instructive to notice the substantial power output demanded by a barely perceptible rise in the road. With a 10 percent gradient, the rate of accumulation of potential energy would in itself impose a load of 320 watts. Most individuals could only sustain this load for a fraction of a minute. When climbing a long hill, it is therefore essential to gear down and adopt a much slower rate of climbing.

Conservation of Energy

One of the important biochemical discoveries of the mid-nineteenth century was that the Newtonian

[2] See Table 1–1 Many older texts and gauges are calibrated in pounds or kilograms. 2.2 pounds = 1 kilogram = 9.81 newtons in a standard gravitational field (981 cm per square second). The older units become completely erroneous if the force of gravity changes (for example, during space exploration).

[3] Notice that calculations are greatly simplified when using SI units of newtons, meters and seconds; for instance, 1 watt = 1 J per second = 1 N·m per second.

TABLE 1–3 Work Involved in Cycling Up Grades of 1 Percent and 10 Percent at a Speed of 4.4 m/sec

Component	Elements	Work Calculation
Headwind	Force × projected area × speed	$43.3 N/m^2 (0.3 m^2) 4.4 = 58$
Ground friction	Mass × gravity × friction × speed	$75 × 9.81(0.05) 4.4 = 162$
Air friction	Constant × projected area × speed^3	Neglected
Vertical ascent	Mass × gravity × speed × slope	$75 × 9.81(0.01) 4.4 = 32$ $75 × 9.81(0.1) 4.4 = 320$

principle of the conservation of energy applied to the human organism. People can neither create nor destroy energy. Whether homeostasis is being maintained or external work is being performed, the impact of these activities upon body reserves of energy can be determined by thermodynamic principles; in the long term, input must match output. Moreover, as with most machines of human invention, the body is mechanically inefficient. At best, some 25 percent of the stored energy is translated into "useful" work, with the remaining 75 percent appearing as heat. In a cool environment, the increase of heat production in an active person contributes to homeostasis, but under warmer conditions, elimination of metabolic heat poses a serious problem to continuing exercise.

SOURCES OF ENERGY

The Role of Adenosine Triphosphate

The immediate source of energy in the body is the chemical adenosine triphosphate (ATP). This molecule contains a terminal high energy phosphate bond. Thus, when it is broken down to adenosine diphosphate (ADP) and phosphate, the reaction is exothermal, i.e., energy is released by rupture of the phosphate bond and this energy can be used to perform the functions discussed above (muscular work, metabolic synthesis, or membrane pumping). The precise energy liberated from a single gram molecule of ATP varies somewhat with local conditions of temperature and pH, but is normally approximately 46 kJ:

$$ATP \rightarrow ADP + 46 \text{ kJ}$$

Unfortunately, the total intracellular stores of ATP are extremely small. For example, skeletal muscle contains only $5 × 10^{-6}$ moles per gram. Thus, even if 20 kg of muscle are called into play by vigorous exercise, the effective store of ATP energy is no more than $(20 × 10^3) (5 × 10^{-6})$, or one-tenth mole. The corresponding energy yield is only 4.5 kJ, and at least in theory this reserve could be exhausted by 0.5 seconds of all-out effort.

The Role of Creatine Phosphate

The next energy resource is a small store of creatine phosphate (Fig. 1–1). Creatine phosphate also has

a terminal high energy phosphate bond, and the energy liberated by rupture of this bond can be applied to the resynthesis of ATP with an efficiency of close to 100 percent. The total reserve of creatine phosphate is approximately $15 × 10^{-6}$ mol per gram of wet muscle, so that in theory, both forms of "phosphagen" (ATP + creatine phosphate) could be depleted by approximately 2 seconds of maximum effort.

The two reactions are biochemically linked in such a way that creatine phosphate is depleted first, and only as exhaustion is approached do reserves of ATP decrease.

The Role of Glycogen

Once phosphagen reserves have been depleted, resynthesis must occur if exercise is to continue. The processes of resynthesis use the energy stored in glycogen and other foods. Glycogen can be broken down to pyruvate in the sarcoplasm of an active muscle. Under anaerobic conditions, pyruvate is converted to lactate, which accumulates in both the muscle and the blood stream. However, if the cardiac pump is bringing an adequate amount of oxygen to the working tissues, pyruvate is further metabolized to carbon dioxide and water within the mitochondria. Each glucose mole that is derived from glycogen[4] provides sufficient energy for resynthesis of 37 moles of ATP (a 63 percent efficiency in the transfer of energy from carbohydrate to ATP). Given that approximately 49 percent of the ATP energy can be applied in turn to the task of muscle contraction, the overall efficiency of energy transformation is $0.63 × 0.49$ or approximately 31 percent, with the remaining 69 percent of the initial energy store being dissipated as heat.

Anaerobic Glycolysis

If oxygen is not available to the working muscle, the glycolytic reaction proceeds from pyruvate to lactate, and the latter accumulates within the sarcoplasm. The yield is then no more than 3 moles of ATP for each mole of glucose derived from glycogen, one-thirteenth of the efficiency calculated for aerobic metabolism.

---

[4] If glucose itself is the fuel, it must first be phosphorylated to glucose-6-phosphate, at the cost of one "priming" mole of ATP.

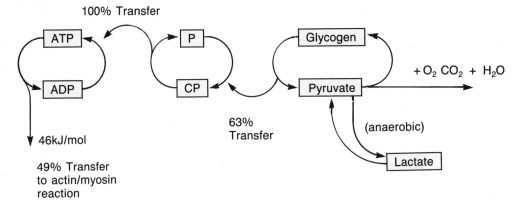

Figure 1–1 Diagram of energy flow in working muscle. ATP = adenosine triphosphate; ADP = adenosine diphosphate; P = phosphate; CP = creatine phosphate.

During the recovery period, a part of the lactate is oxidized to carbon dioxide and water, and the remainder is reconverted to glucose or glycogen, using energy derived from the oxidative reaction. In essence, each mole of glycogen can undergo approximately 10 cycles of anaerobic breakdown and resynthesis before its energy content has been exhausted. From a long-term perspective, the efficiency of anaerobic work may thus rise to ten-thirteenths of that for aerobic exercise.

Anaerobic energy release is limited by the intramuscular accumulation of lactate and associated changes of intracellular pH. When the intramuscular lactate concentration reaches approximately 30 mmol per cubic decimeter, key enzymes needed for the breakdown of glycogen (phosphorylase, phosphofructokinase) are inhibited, and anaerobic metabolism stops. Again assuming an active muscle mass of 20 kg, the total potential build-up of lactate is 600 mmol, equivalent to a yield of 1.8 moles of ATP, or about 87 kJ of energy. The speed of the anaerobic reactions is such (Table 1–4) that phosphagen breakdown may generate a power of more than 9 kilowatts for 2 seconds, while the build-up of lactate over a period of 40 seconds is equivalent to a power output of more than 2 kilowatts. By way of comparison, a sedentary woman with an aerobic power of 40 ml per kilogram per minute and a body mass of 55 kg can probably sustain an aerobic energy release of some 770 watts for 10 minutes (a total yield of 460 kJ); if the intensity of activity is decreased to 50 percent of aerobic power, this level of energy release can be sustained for 4 hours (a total yield of 5.39 MJ).

SUBSTRATE RESERVES

Muscle Glycogen

The main immediate reserve of energy is intramuscular glycogen. Local concentrations vary with diet, habitual activity and type of muscle fiber (fast or slow-twitch), but a typical figure is 15 g per kilogram of wet tissue. With 20 kg of active muscle, the total intramuscular glycogen store is thus 300 g, equivalent to 1.67 moles of glucose. Combustion of any type of carbohydrate in a heat-measuring "bomb calorimeter" shows an energy yield of about 16 kJ per gram or 2.9 MJ per mole of glucose equivalent, so that the total glycogen reserve can contribute approximately 4.8 MJ of energy. Typically, this is depleted over the course of 2 hours of exhausting activity.

Hepatic Resources

The liver also stores approximately 100 g of glycogen. During vigorous exercise, this is released into the blood stream as glucose at a rate of about 1 g per minute (5 to 6 mmol per minute). The total contribution amounts to 1.6 to 2.0 MJ over a bout of sustained exercise.

As physical activity continues, there is also some potential for the hepatic synthesis of glucose ("gluconeogenesis") from circulating glycerol, lactate, and amino acids. Glucose formation does not proceed fast enough to satisfy the full needs of the skeletal muscles once sarcoplasmic glycogen has been exhausted, but it does help to service tissues which can only metabolize carbohydrates (e.g., the brain and the red

TABLE 1–4   Energy Release in the Human Body

Source	Rate of Yield (Watts)	Duration (sec)	Capacity of System (kJ)
Anaerobic power	9200	2*	18.4
Anaerobic capacity	2175	40	87
Aerobic power			
100% loading	770	600	460
50% loading	385	14×10^3	5390

* In practice, ATP, creatine phosphate, and other immediate energy stores are usually depleted less rapidly than the theoretical 2 seconds.

cells). After 40 minutes of exercise, Wahren found that the percentage of freshly synthesized glucose in the hepatic vein was 16 percent at a cycle ergometer loading of 65 watts, 11 percent at a loading of 135 watts and 6 percent at a loading of 200 watts. After 4 hours of moderate activity, however, 45 percent of hepatic glucose output was attributable to gluconeogenesis.

Depot Fat

There are small amounts of fat stored within the muscle fibres. However, if activity is very prolonged, most of the necessary energy is derived from a mobilization of depot fat. The body carries a small amount of essential fat (larger in women than in men), but most sedentary adults have 10 to 15 kg of adipose reserves which can be exploited in any sustained athletic feat. Each gram of fat yields approximately 29 kJ of energy,[5] so that 10 kg of disposable body fat provides a total resource of some 290 MJ, sufficient for 3 to 4 weeks of strenuous exercise. The main drawback to fat as a source of fuel is that it can only be metabolized aerobically. During moderate exercise it provides approximately half of the required energy, but with more intense effort many muscle fibers become short of oxygen, and in such circumstances the limited reserves of glycogen must meet 75 percent or more of total energy needs. One interesting feature of a well-trained athlete is the ability to burn a higher proportion of fat during vigorous submaximal exercise; this conserves glycogen reserves for tasks that can only be performed anaerobically.

Tissue Proteins

If food intake is inadequate (e.g., an athlete attempting to make a specific "weight category," or a ballet dancer who is unduly concerned about her figure), the body may also draw upon protein reserves. The normal process of catabolism (breakdown) continues, or is accelerated, but resynthesis does not occur. The muscle mass is thus steadily depleted. The energy yield from protein is similar to that from carbohydrate, approximately 16 kJ per gram.

Alcohol

Alcohol can serve as an immediate energy source, with a yield of some 27 kJ per gram. A sedentary person who consumes 100 g per day (less than a liter of wine) thus satisfies a substantial proportion of energy needs from alcohol alone. Given that most alcoholic beverages contain few vitamins, a combination of regular drinking and a sedentary lifestyle can lead to the development of serious dietary deficiencies. The most common disorder in a chronic alcoholic is the mental disturbance (psychosis) with peripheral nerve inflammation that is associated with a lack of vitamin B_1.

LIMITATIONS OF GAS TRANSPORT

If all-out physical activity continues for more than 30 to 40 seconds, the build-up of lactate forces a reliance on aerobic metabolism. A further important key to local homeostasis, and thus persistent functioning of the working muscles is therefore the transport of oxygen to and carbon dioxide from the exercising tissues.

Oxygen

The relative barriers to movement of oxygen and carbon dioxide can be gauged from the respective partial pressure gradients between the atmosphere and the working tissues. The total gradient for oxygen is some 20 kilopascals (kPa).[6] During a large muscle task such as treadmill running, approximately one-third of this barrier (or impedance, to think in electrical terms) arises in the ventilatory system, and the remaining two-thirds in the cardiovascular system. The partial pressure in the capillaries of the active muscle drops to near zero. We may thus conclude that the major bottleneck for oxygen flow during this type of exercise is the ability of the heart to pump oxygenated blood from the pulmonary capillaries to the vascular bed of the active muscles. Local tissue factors do not become important until less than 20 percent of the total muscle mass is involved in the exercise.

Carbon Dioxide

The total pressure gradient for carbon dioxide is less than 10 kPa, partly because its effective blood solubility is five times greater than that of oxygen, and partly because CO_2 is more readily transported across the pulmonary membrane. During large muscle work, more than one-half of the barrier of CO_2 elimination arises in the thoracic pump, and in some older individuals performance is limited by an accumulation of carbon dioxide in the blood stream (chronic obstructive lung disease). In younger individuals, the smaller total pressure gradient does not necessarily exonerate carbon dioxide as a factor limiting performance; the key issue is whether the observed tissue pressure of 10 kPa reduces muscle pH to the point that glycolysis is being slowed through an inhibition of phosphorylase and phosphofructokinase. This does not generally seem to be the case.

---

[5] This figure is the energy yield of *body fat*. The heat yielded by dietary fat is somewhat greater (approximately 38 kJ per gram).

[6] Older books have expressed partial pressure gradients in mm Hg. 100 mm Hg is equal to some 13.3 kPa (Table 1–1).

EXTERNAL EFFICIENCY

Measures of Efficiency

The mechanical efficiency of any system can be expressed very simply as the ratio of the output of useful work to the energy expended. The top athlete is commonly marked by not only a large power output, but also an efficient use of energy. The exercise physiologist usually distinguishes gross efficiency (total work output: total energy expenditure) from net efficiency (the latter being the ratio of total work output to total minus basal energy expenditure). Because of considerable difficulties in establishing a true basal reading, the resting energy expenditure is often substituted in the latter calculation. If the intensity of effort is high, the discrepancy between resting and basal values does not have a major influence upon the estimate of net efficiency. Even the resting energy expenditure can be quite variable in an anxious subject. A third possibility is thus to calculate efficiency (the increase of work output for a given increase of energy expenditure).

Typical Net Efficiency

The net efficiency is the most commonly used of these statistics, at least in exercise science. As noted in the section, The Role of Glycogen, there are sound biochemical reasons why efficiency should not exceed 31 percent, even under optimal conditions of aerobic work. In practice, somewhat lower net efficiencies are usually observed because (1) there is an incomplete coupling of biochemical resources to any external machine such as a cycle ergometer, and (2) the body work-rate is boosted above the assumed basal or resting figure by the increased demands on the cardiac and respiratory pumps, together with an increased need for postural activity while the body is moving. Some machines such as a modern cycle ergometer (average efficiency of operation in a young adult approximately 23 percent) come fairly close to the theoretical figure. In other activities such as stepping, the efficiency of upward displacement of the body mass is of a similar order to that seen in cycling. However, in the usual design of step test, the subject not only climbs up, but also descends. The total energy cost of the task is then increased by approximately one-third in assuring a controlled descent from the bench. In some sports, quite low efficiencies have been observed. Thus typical figures for a swimmer are only 1 to 2 percent. In such activities there is substantial opportunity for a coach to improve performance through an increase in the skill of the performer, even if energy output cannot be increased.

Efficiency on the Treadmill

Authors interested in treadmill exercise (particularly Rodolfo Margaria) have quoted mechanical efficiencies ranging from +30 percent to −120 percent, depending upon the slope. When a person is running on the flat, there is no ultimate upward displacement of the body mass. The "useful" work and the mechanical efficiency (at least in the terms of a physicist) are thus both zero. When running downhill the entire potential energy associated with descent of the body mass is lost (an efficiency of −100 percent), and a further 20 percent of energy is expended controlling this descent (a total net efficiency of −120 percent). During uphill running, efficiency reaches or may even exceed the theoretical maximum of 31 percent. A probable reason for this surprisingly satisfactory performance is that some of the potential energy liberated during descent of the leg becomes stored in stretched tendons (see Chapter 2).

FURTHER READING

Knuttgen HG, Vogel JA, Poortmans JR. Biochemistry of exercise. Champaign, Illinois: Human Kinetics Publishers Inc, 1983.

Landry FR, Orban WAR. Third International Symposium on the Biochemistry of Exercise. Miami, Florida: Symposia Specialists, 1978.

Poortmans JR, Nisett G. Biochemistry of exercise IV. Baltimore: University Park Press, 1981.

Shephard RJ. Physiology and biochemistry of exercise. New York: Praeger, 1982.

Shephard RJ. Biochemistry of physical activity. Springfield, Illinois: CC Thomas, 1984.

MEASURING ACTIVITY IN LABORATORY AND FIELD

CHAPTER 2

The exercise physiologist needs well-standardized laboratory forms of exercise in order to determine current levels of fitness, to examine human reactions to graded exercise, and to provide known training stimuli. Field measurements of habitual activity are an important foil to this approach. They can indicate whether the fitness level observed in the laboratory is below the individual's potential, because of a sedentary lifestyle. Moreover, measurement of total daily energy usage provides guidance to nutritional requirements in various situations. Finally, determination of individual costs of selected activities is needed for accurate exercise prescription in work and leisure.

Before delving more deeply into exercise physiology and biochemistry, it is thus important to review how standard exercise is performed in the laboratory, and how energy expenditures are assessed in the field.

EXERCISE IN THE LABORATORY

Cycle Ergometer

The cycle ergometer provides a readily standardized work task. In the mechanical type, subjects crank a flywheel against the friction imposed by a loaded leather belt or the air resistance of a series of vanes, while in the electrical type effort is developed against the impedance of a dynamo or an electro-magnet.

Mechanical Ergometers. The mechanical device of a loaded belt is the simplest type of arrangement, although unfortunately the indicated work-rate ignores a frictional energy loss of 8 to 10 percent in the chain and pedal bearings. The coefficient of friction on the main flywheel decreases as the belt becomes hot, so that a frequent adjustment of tension is needed in order to ensure a constant work-rate. The work performed by the subject also depends on the pedalling rate, so that power output may drop below the intended value as a person becomes fatigued (Table 2–1); it is always important to use a counter to determine the precise number of flywheel revolutions per minute.

Electrical Ergometers. The loading of many electrically-braked ergometers can be modified by adjusting the current flowing through the field coils of the dynamo or electromagnet. Given a suitable type of feedback device, compensation can be made for small variations in the speed of pedalling. Unfortunately, the mechanical efficiency of the subject changes with speed. Thus, if there is any great departure from the optimum 50 to 60 pedal revolutions per minute, the subject must work harder in order to sustain a given output of electrical energy. The main drawbacks of the electrical type of ergometer are a high capital cost and a need for periodic calibration by bolting a known source of power (a torque generator) to the pedal crank shaft.

Advantages and Disadvantages. The main advantages claimed for the cycle ergometer (Table 2–2) are a seated subject (facilitating ancillary measurements of oxygen consumption, cardiac output, and blood pressure) and a relatively constant mechanical efficiency (Table 2-3) of approximately 23 percent (facilitating the conversion of external work-rate into an approximate power demand on the body). The main disadvantages are (1) a need to adjust loadings for inter-individual differences of body mass and thus the likely working capacity of the subject, (2) overloading of the quadriceps muscle at high intensities of effort (so that maximum effort is often halted by local muscular fatigue rather than a general exhaustion of the cardiorespiratory system), and (3) some difficulty in dismounting should an emergency arise.

Maximum Testing. Experienced cyclists sometimes complain that the usually required cadence of 50 to 60 revolutions per minute is less than they adopt in vigorous cycling. By fitting toe clips, drop handlebars, and a very high racing saddle, while allowing the subject to stand for a final "sprint", it is possible to attain the maximum oxygen intake seen on a treadmill. However, with more usual cycle ergometer techniques, the limiting oxygen consumption falls 7 to 8 percent short of a true maximum value, due to local muscular fatigue.

TABLE 2–1   Energy Cost of Three Common Modes of Laboratory Exercise

Measurement Factor	Cycle Ergometer	Treadmill	Step
Force	Pendulum or belt loading (e.g., 20 N)	Weight of body + clothes (e.g., 600 N)	Weight of body + clothes (e.g., 600 N)
Distance	2π (radius of flywheel) (e.g., 2 m)	(e.g., 1 m)	Step height (e.g., 0.45 m)
Work	40 J	600 J	270 J
Speed	2π (radius) pedal revs per second (gear rate) (e.g., (2)1(2.5) = 5 m/s)	Belt speed (slope) (e.g., (2)0.05 = 0.1 m/s)	Ascents per second (e.g., 0.33)
Power output	(20)5 = 100 W	600(0.1) = 60 W	270(0.33) = 90 W

TABLE 2–2 Comparison of the Advantages and Disadvantages of Various Laboratory Forms o.

Cycle Ergometer	Treadmill	Step Test
Advantages		
Seated subject	Effort limited by	Low cost
	central factors	Simplicity
Relatively constant	Effort machine-paced	Portability
mechanical efficiency	Natural exercise	No need for calibration
	(moderate walking)	Familiar exercise
		No need for electricity
Disadvantages		
Inter-individual	Cost	Ancillary measurements
differences of loading	Noise	difficult
Quadriceps overloaded	Need for special wiring	Danger of stumbling
Difficult to dismount	Bulk	(high speeds)
in an emergency	Causes anxiety	Step too tall for
Power output varies	(uphill running)	young children
with pedalling rate	Danger of injury	Self-paced
Cost	Ancillary measurements	
Calibration	difficult	
Peak effort submaximal		

Treadmill

Work Efficiency and Oxygen Cost. Some work is performed while walking or running on the level, since the center of mass of the body is raised and lowered repeatedly. However, the body does not accumulate any potential energy and there is no readily measured external power output; convention thus ascribes a mechanical efficiency of zero to this activity (see Chapter 1). As in cycling (see Chapter 1), the energy cost of moving increases sharply if an uphill gradient is introduced. The vertical component of the total work is calculated quite readily as the product of body weight (expressed in Newtons), the treadmill speed (expressed in m per second) and slope (expressed in decimal format, for example, 5 percent = 0.05). The mechanical efficiency of uphill running (up to 30 percent in terms of vertical work, as much as 40 to 45 percent when account is taken of oscillations in the center of mass) is higher than would be anticipated from the biomechanical reactions involved (see Chapter 1). The explanation is that when the foot hits the track, the tendo-Achilles is stretched and stores some of the potential energy released by descent of the body's center of mass; this resource is used to lift the body when the next stride is taken. At low speeds, walking is more efficient than running, but as the speed of the tread-

mill is increased, the oxygen cost of walking rises more sharply than that of running (Fig. 2–3). Thus, depending somewhat on the individual's leg length, running becomes the more economical mode of progression at a speed of approximately 2 m per second (7.2 km per hour).

Maximum Tests. As the speed of the treadmill is increased, the oxygen cost of running at first shows a proportional rise, but eventually a point is reached where a further increase of speed or slope augments oxygen consumption by less than 2 mℓ per kilogram per minute (1.5 mmol per kilogram per second). This is the generally accepted definition of a "centrally-limited" maximum oxygen intake (Fig. 2–1, also see Chapter 8); it is thought that the maximum cardiac output, and thus the maximum oxygen intake of the individual has been attained.

Because a high proportion (approximately 70 percent) of the body muscles are already involved in uphill treadmill running, it is not possible to increase either cardiac output or oxygen consumption more than marginally by performing simultaneous arm work (for instance, manipulating some form of ski pole while continuing to run on the treadmill).

Downhill Runners. If the treadmill is arranged for downhill walking or running, the body absorbs and releases as heat an amount of potential energy equiva-

TABLE 2–3 The Approximate Oxygen Cost of Common Forms of Laboratory Exercise*

Type of Exercise	Mechanical Efficiency (%)	Oxygen Cost (ℓ/min)	Coefficient of Variation (%)
Cycle ergometer	23	10.5(W) + 300	4–5
Treadmill	25	11.4(W) + 300	5
Step	16	7.3(W) + 300	7

* Assuming a resting oxygen consumption of 300 mℓ/min and a power output of W (watts)

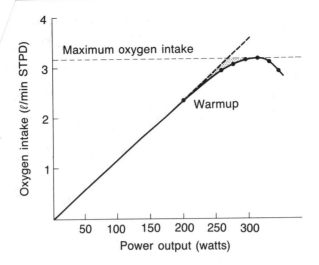

Figure 2–1 Concept of the measurement of maximum oxygen intake. The test begins with a 3-minute warmup at about 70 percent of maximum power output. Loading is then increased to an estimated 95 percent of maximum oxygen intake and is further increased by 5 percent at 2-minute intervals until a plateau has been identified or there are other indications to halt the test. The shaded area indicates a growing component of anaerobic activity. STPD = Standard temperature and pressure, dry gas

lent to the cumulative descent of the body's center of mass. Additional energy must be spent to control the descent (Fig. 2–2). If the cost of control amounts to 20 percent of the lost potential energy, the convention is to express mechanical efficiency as −120 percent (−100 percent, −20 percent). The gastrocnemius muscle must contract vigorously as it is being stretched by the impact of the foot (a process described as "eccentric work"), and the loading can sometimes be sufficient to cause local muscle damage with delayed soreness and a leakage of intramuscular enzymes into the blood stream (see Chapter 9).

Advantages and Disadvantages. The main advantages of treadmill exercise are (1) a central (cardiovascular) rather than a peripheral (muscular) limitation of maximum effort, (2) an exercise task where the subject cannot slow down as fatigue develops, and (3) a fairly natural pattern of activity (most people have some experience of both walking and running, although in practice there is at least a 10 percent inter-individual variation in the oxygen cost of both walking and running (Fig. 2–3) on a treadmill; moreover, many people show a substantial decrease of oxygen cost as they learn the technique of maintaining a constant position

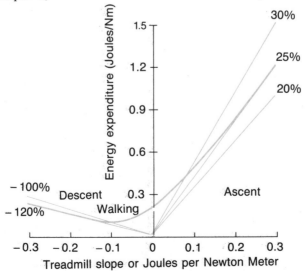

Figure 2–2 Energy cost of treadmill walking in relation to slope, showing isoefficiency lines for ascent (20 to 30 percent efficiency) and descent (−100 to −120 percent). Based on a concept of Margaria.

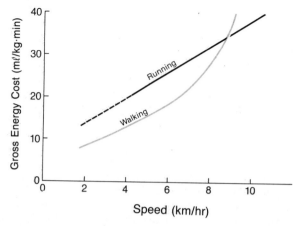

Figure 2–3 A comparison of the oxygen cost of running and walking. Note that at slow speeds walking is more efficient, but that at high speeds running becomes more efficient.

on the sloping belt). Older subjects may be allowed to rest their hands lightly on a hand-rail, but if the arms take an appreciable proportion of the body weight, this again changes the oxygen cost of the activity.

The main disadvantages of the treadmill are (1) a high cost, (2) need for special three-phase electrical wiring, (3) bulk, (4) noise, and (5) anxiety. An older person may be quite nervous about running at high speed on a short belt, with resultant distortion of cardiac and respiratory responses to exercise. However, this problem can generally be overcome by one or more practice sessions (the process of habituation, Chapter 1). Ancillary measurements (including blood sampling) are more difficult to carry out on a treadmill than on a cycle ergometer, and there is some danger of injury if a person stumbles while the belt is moving rapidly.

Step Tests

Power Output. The simplest method of performing a standard amount of physical exercise is to climb a bench repeatedly at a rate set by a metronome, an illuminated signal, or an age- and sex-specific musical rhythm (as in the Canadian Home Fitness Test, Table 2–4). As with treadmill exercise, "useful" work is considered as the cumulative number of ascents of the bench. The power output in watts is thus the product of body weight in newtons, the step height in meters, and the number of ascents per second. For instance, a woman with a weight of 600 N who climbs a 0.4 meter step once every 3 seconds has a power output of $600 \times 0.4 \times 0.333$ or 80 watts. If the exercise is performed on an escalator or a long flight of stairs, the ascent can continue to exhaustion, but the usual laboratory bench has only one or two steps. Unmeasured eccentric work is then performed in controlling descent from the bench. The cost of stepping down is about one-third of that for ascent, so that the apparent efficiency of "useful" work drops to approximately 16 percent. In other words, a power output of 80 watts (as in our example) demands an energy expenditure of some 500 watts by the body.

Submaximal and Maximal Tests. The optimal rate of climbing is 60 to 150 paces per minute. At slower speeds, there is difficulty in following the timing signal, and at faster rates there is a danger of stumbling. A double step with 0.20 to 0.23 meter risers provides a suitable range of activity for submaximal exercise testing, while a single bench of 0.4 to 0.5 meters allows most subjects to reach their maximum oxygen intake.

Advantages and Disadvantages. The step test is plainly suited to field testing. Its main advantages are (1) minimal cost, (2) no need of electricity, and (3) no need of calibration. The power output can be calculated with a precision of 6 to 7 percent provided that subjects keep good time with the metronome, stand erect on the top step, and place both feet flat on the ground at the end of each stepping cycle.

The main disadvantage of a step test is that it is difficult to make ancillary measurements on a subject who is climbing repeatedly. There is also some risk of stumbling as exhaustion is approached, and a hand-

TABLE 2–4   Cadences for Ascent of Double 8-Inch (20.3 cm) Step in the Canadian Home Fitness Test* with Immediate 10-Second Recovery Pulse Counts Corresponding to Undesirable, Minimum, and Recommended Levels of Fitness

Age (yr)	Cadence (paces/min)		Duration of Exercise and 10-Second Recovery Pulse and Fitness Score		
	Women	Men	3 min (undesirable)	6 min (minimum)	6 min (recommended)
15–19	120	144	>30	>27	<26
20–29	144	144	>29	>26	<25
30–39	114	132	>28	>25	<24
40–49	102	114	>26	>24	<23
50–59	84	102	>25	>23	<22
60–69	84	84	>24	>23	<22
Warmup	66	66	≥	≥	≤

* All cadences are intended to approximate 70% of maximum oxygen intake in average subjects

support post should be provided for older individuals. Some learning may occur, particularly when following a six-step rhythm. Young children (less than 10 years of age) may find the step height rather large during maximum testing. Nevertheless, well-motivated subjects can be brought to within 3 to 4 percent of their treadmill maximum oxygen intake by exercising at a progressively faster pace on a 0.45-meter step.

Sport-Specific Devices

When evaluating athletes, it is usually necessary to include a sport-specific test. For example, a swimmer may exercise in a laboratory version of a mill-race (a "flume"), a circular water tank where gas collection apparatus can be wheeled alongside the athlete, or a pool where forward movement is restrained by a weighted waist-harness. Alternatively, the arms may pull upon loaded cords, with a gauge to indicate the total work performed (the product of force and the distance pulled). The average person can develop no more than 80 to 90 percent of the treadmill maximum oxygen intake during these various simulations of swimming, but an international caliber competitor may reach very close to 100 percent of the treadmill figure. Similar sport-specific ergometers have been devised for other sports where a large maximum oxygen intake is an asset, e.g., cycling, rowing, canoeing, and cross-country skiing.

Disabled Subjects

Various ergometers have been developed to assess the aerobic power of the wheelchair-disabled. Current choices include a forearm crank, an ergometer linked to the driving wheels of a wheelchair, and a wide-belted treadmill with guide-rods on which a wheelchair can be safely propelled. Possibly because of energy spent in stabilizing the trunk, the mechanical efficiency of arm exercise is quite low both in normal subjects and in the wheelchair-disabled (14 to 15 percent). Effort is usually limited by local exhaustion of the working muscles, with a peak oxygen consumption which is approximately 70 percent of the treadmill maximum oxygen intake.

One exception to this generalization is the operation of a long arm-crank by an able-bodied person; using such a device, the large muscles of the back can also be brought into play, and the oxygen transport may then reach 100 percent rather than 70 percent of the treadmill figure.

MEASUREMENTS OF HABITUAL ACTIVITY

The wide range of methods currently adopted to assess habitual activity indicate that no one procedure is entirely satisfactory. Various types of dietary records may measure the input of energy over a specified interval, such as a week. Alternatively, the energy output may be estimated from questionnaires, observation by a technician, or direct measurements of mechanical impulses, heart rate, ventilation, oxygen consumption, and biochemical correlates of energy consumption.

Dietary Records

Since the principle of the conservation of energy applies to humans, it might seem a simple matter to assess energy expediture from the amount of food that a person eats. In practice, there are many pitfalls. First, although energy homeostasis is well-maintained over a period measured in months or in years, the body stores of fat are sufficiently large that a substantial deficit can be incurred over the course of 7 days. Moreover, the mere fact of a close monitoring of diet by the subject or an observer often modifies both the quantity and the quality of food that is ingested. An appreciable amount of energy is also lost in the various excrements. In theory, it would be possible to collect the feces, urine, sweat, and expired gas, and determine their energy content, but it is more usual to assume a fixed percentage of energy loss—despite well-recognized interindividual differences in the efficiency of food absorption and excretion. A further problem is that the resting energy expenditure accounts for a substantial proportion of the total food intake, and there is increasing evidence that heavy feeding stimulates resting metabolism (the so-called Luxuskonsumption).

Dietary tables are used to convert "portions" or "servings" of food into their approximate energy equivalents (Table 2–5). The situation is perhaps easiest to control during a military exercise where each soldier is issued with a standard ration pack; but even in such situations, a careful watch must be kept for both wastage and sharing of food. In a free-living situation, both solid and liquid snacks are easily overlooked by a careless subject, and the food that is eaten may differ substantially in its composition from that assumed in standard energy tables.

The most precise assessments of nutrient intake are obtained when a dietician lives with a family and weighs individual food portions. Rather less accurately, subjects can be shown models representing standard food portions, and be asked to record all items that they eat or drink relative to these standards. Much less successfully, subjects are given diary sheets and are asked to recall details of their food consumption on a daily basis.

Questionnaires

Activity questionnaires range from one or two simple, multiple-choice questions, to detailed inventories which are many pages in length, and can only be com-

TABLE 2–5   Approximate Energy Yield of Selected Food Products

Item	Energy Yield (kJ)	Item	Energy Yield (kJ)
1 apple	314	1 tablespoon jam	230
1 serving of apple pie	1,381	85 g of lamb	962
2 slices of bacon	376	1 tablespoon margarine	418
1 cup of lima beans	628	1 cup of whole milk	690
85 g of beef	1,163	85 g of pork	1,192
1 slice of bread	272	1 medium potato	502
1 tablespoon of butter	418	1 serving pumpkin pie	1,109
1 cup of cabbage	167	114 g of pork sausage	1,423
1 slice of angel food cake	460	1 cup of spaghetti	920
28 g of cheddar cheese	481	1 cup of spinach	188
1 cup of chicken soup	314	1 tablespoon sugar	209
1 cup of cornflakes	397	1 cup white sauce	1,799
1 doughnut	565	1 cup wheat flour	1,674
1 egg	314		
1 fillet of haddock	669		

pleted with the help of a skilled interviewer. When designing questions, care must be taken to explore the normal use of both working and leisure ("weekend") days, and particularly in countries with an extreme climate due account must be taken of activity patterns during both winter and summer seasons. As with diet sheets, an activity questionnaire may function as a conscience, modifying both the reported and the actual activity of a subject. There is also a risk that preparation time may be included in the description of an active pursuit, e.g., an hour of tennis may include changing for the game, looking for lost balls, and showering, as well as active play on the court. Likewise, an "hour" of required gymnastics at school may involve pupils in no more than 5 minutes of vigorous exercise. A further difficulty is that the energy cost of most common pursuits varies several fold, depending on the speed, vigor, and skill with which they are pursued.

Very simple questionnaires (Table 2–6) have a fair reliability and validity. Moreover, they can describe 30 to 35 percent of the variation in personal fitness if the intensity of habitual activity is described in both practical and physiological terms—"Do you undertake 20 minutes of vigorous exercise at least 3 times per week—for example, walking a mile or more at a pace sufficient to induce some sweating and leave you a little short of breath?" Much time can be spent on more complicated surveys. The resultant information may provide a helpful picture of the types of pursuit people enjoy at different ages, but it is less clearly established that lengthy questionnaires yield more accurate data on individual daily expenditures.

Direct Observation

A technician may observe the behavior of one or more subjects. The simplest approach is to record the activities observed on a minute-by-minute basis, using a convenient form of shorthand (for example, L = lying, Si = sitting, St = standing, W = walking,

Fig. 2–4). Alternatively, the information can be dictated into a tape-recorder for later analysis, or it can be entered directly into the appropriate memory cell of a portable computer. Less accurately and less objectively, the subject can use a small notepad to record activities on a minute-by-minute basis.

Observational methodology is best suited to the analysis of a relatively stereotyped range of pursuits, followed in a uniform fashion by a small group of people. For instance, it has been applied successfully to examine the typical day of a platoon of soldiers and the

TABLE 2–6   Example of a Simple Activity Questionnaire

Considering a 7-day period (a week) during your leisure time, how many times do you do the following kinds of exercise for more than 15 minutes?

Times per week

1. Strenuous exercise (heart beats rapidly) (i.e., running, jogging, hockey, football, soccer, squash, basketball, cross-country skiing, judo, roller skating, vigorous swimming, vigorous long-distance bicycling)   _____

2. Moderate exercise (not exhausting) (i.e., fast walking, baseball, tennis, easy bicycling, volleyball, badminton, easy swimming, alpine skiing, popular and folk dancing)   _____

3. Mild exercise (minimal effort) (i.e., yoga, archery, fishing from river bank, bowling, horseshoes, golf, snowmobiling, easy walking)   _____

Note: Strenuous exercise is approximately 9 times basal metabolism (9 MET), moderate exercise is approximately 5 MET, and mild exercise is approximately 3 MET. An activity score for the week can thus be calculated by summing MET minutes.

Based on the work of Gaston Godin

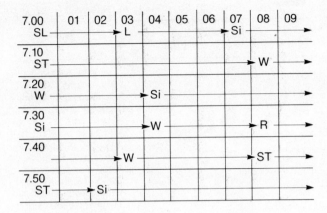

Figure 2–4 Example of a 1-hour segment from an activity diary. SL = Sleeping, L = Lying awake, Si = Sitting, ST = Standing, W = Walking, and R = Running.

energy expenditure of individual postal carriers. By noting also the distances that are covered, estimates can be made of the speed and duration of bursts of activity in games such as football and hockey.

Mechanical Impulses

In the pedometer and related devices, the mechanical impulse generated by a footfall is used to activate a watch escapement or make an electrical contact. Recently, a major footwear manufacturer began producing a track shoe that incorporated a simple electrical impulse detector. In theory, the cumulative count indicated by an instrument of this type is equal to the number of paces that has been taken while it was worn. Thus, if the apparatus has been preset to match the individual's average pace length, the readout reflects the total walking or jogging distance. With electronic shoes, the data can further be used to monitor adherence to a daily training plan.

One problem with all of the impulse counters is that pace-length varies with the speed of movement, so that a consistent individual calibration factor cannot be assumed. More seriously, the impact may be insufficient to operate the counting mechanism during a gentle stroll, while a single pace may initiate a double count with vigorous running. Finally, this group of devices can monitor only the number of foot impacts. A fairly reliable index of daily activity is obtained in occupations where the main source of energy expenditure is walking at a moderate pace, but an alternative approach must be used in other tasks where most of the work is performed by the upper half of the body.

Heart Rate

There is a fairly close linear relationship between heart rate and oxygen consumption over the range 50 to 100 percent of maximum oxygen intake (Fig. 2–5). Accordingly, it has been argued that daily energy ex-

penditures can be monitored by recording the corresponding heart rates.

The average heart rate over a specified time interval can be estimated by applying impulses generated from the electrocardiogram to a suitable counter, which may be a mechanical, electro-chemical or computer integrator. Sophisticated versions of this equipment (Fig. 2–6) now divide the recorded heart rate into several frequency bands (for example, the time periods spent at rates < 80 beats per minute, 80 to 100, 100 to 120, 120 to 140, 140 to 160, 160 to 190, and > 190 beats per minute), thus allowing a measure of the intensity of the daily training stimulus. Erroneous counts owing to loose electrocardiogram (ECG) electrode contacts can be a serious problem. One possible tactic is to discard scores for the lowest and the highest frequency cells. A portable tape recording of the ECG signal (Holter monitor) is an alternative approach. Tapes can be replayed at 60 times the recording speed, generating a minute-by-minute heart rate count. One common difficulty with the Holter monitor is that the vigorous activities of many sports cause a variation in speed of the tape recorder; this problem has been circumvented by recording a time signal on a second channel of the tape. A third possibility, particularly in games played in a confined area, is to transmit the ECG signal to a nearby receiver, using a radiotelemeter.

Heart rate recording is one of the most frequently used methods of assessing human activity; yet it has many limitations. The heart rate–oxygen consumption relationship unfortunately departs somewhat from linearity if effort is less than 50 percent of maximum oxygen intake, but many of the activities of interest to the exercise physiologist require between 10 and 50 percent of maximum oxygen intake. Moreover, the heart rate is often increased by factors other than exercise, e.g., anticipation of effort, anxiety, excitement, and exposure to heat; the heart rate response to a given increment of oxygen consumption is also influenced by the muscle mass involved, the position of the active limb(s)

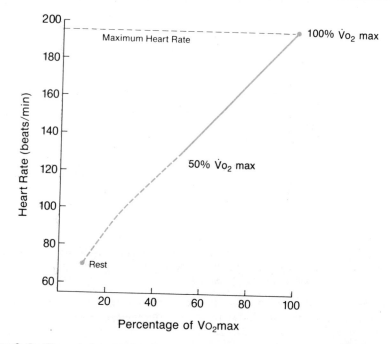

Figure 2–5 The relationship between heart rate and oxygen consumption.

relative to the heart, and overall body posture. Nevertheless, during heavy activities such as running or cycling, the heart rate indicates oxygen consumption as a fraction of the individual's maximum, to within 10 to 15 percent.

Ventilation

In theory, ventilation is more closely related to oxygen consumption than is heart rate, particularly at the lower intensities of exercise. However, the respired volume is also modified by anticipation of effort, anxiety, excitement, and exposure to heat, and when effort exceeds the anaerobic threshold (60 to 75 percent of maximum oxygen intake) there is a disproportionate increase of ventilation (Fig. 2–7). Ventilatory measurements generally suffer because the subject must wear a facemask or use a mouthpiece during testing. Having accepted this inconvenience, it seems logical to undertake the further step of making direct measurements of oxygen consumption.

Oxygen Consumption

Oxygen consumption is rather closely linked to the rate of aerobic energy expenditure. Although there are minor variations of oxygen usage, with changes in the

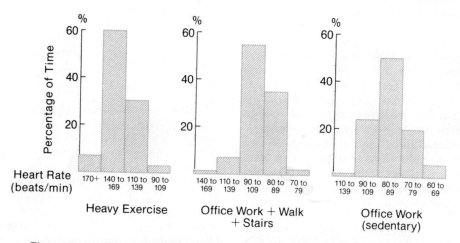

Figure 2–6 Distribution of heart rate counts over an 8 hour work-day in person performing heavy exercise and in two types of office work (based on data of Masironi and Mansourian).

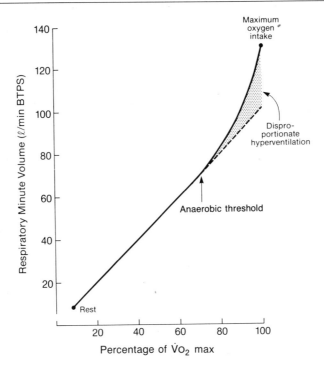

Figure 2–7 The relationship between relative oxygen intake (percent of $\dot{V}O_2$ max) and ventilation. BTPS = Body temperature and pressure, saturated with water vapor.

proportions of the several metabolic fuels (carbohydrate yields 10 percent more energy per liter of oxygen than does fat) to a first approximation, an oxygen consumption of 1 liter implies that there has been an aerobic energy expenditure of 21 kJ.

Some investigators have simply strapped a Douglas bag or a meteorological balloon onto the back of a worker or athlete, collecting expired gas throughout 1 to 2 minutes of "typical" activity. Others have used a similar approach a few seconds after ceasing exercise, making extrapolations to estimate the oxygen consumption during effort. A third approach has been to wear some type of portable respirometer. The Kofranyi Michaelis respirometer is a rugged and well-proved mechanical gasmeter that works well up to flow rates of 50 to 60 ℓ per minute. The respired minute volume is indicated by a mechanical counter, while an aliquot of respired gas (0.3 to 0.6 percent) is pumped to a rubber bladder for later chemical analysis. The bladder is usually filled over 5 to 10 minutes of vigorous exercise. The Wolff IMP uses a screen flowmeter to develop a battery-driven electrical signal (IMP = integrating motor pneumotachygraph); this indicates respired volumes, while a small fraction (0.06 percent) of respired gas is pumped to a bladder stored inside a protective can to prevent loss of gas by diffusion prior to laboratory analysis. Wolff's device can be operated over 50 to 60 minutes of moderate activity, but it is less rugged than the Kofranyi Michaelis respirometer, and there can be annoying breakdowns under field condi-

tions. More recently, the Medilog computer has combined a turbine flowmeter with two oxygen polarographic detectors (inspiratory and expiratory) to provide an instantaneous approximation of oxygen usage. In theory, the transfer of such information to a portable tape recorder allows oxygen consumption to be followed over a long period.

All respirometers have a fair bulk and mass (2 to 3 kg), so that both the pattern of activity and the oxygen cost may be distorted by the measuring device. The problem of distorting normal activity patterns is exacerbated by the need to wear a facemask or mouthpiece. Both methods of coupling the subject to the apparatus are prone to leakage, particularly if measurements are continued for a long time or the subject has a beard.

Biochemical Correlates

It is possible to examine various biochemical correlates of physical activity, such as increases of creatinine or catecholamine excretion, although the collection of 24-hour urine specimens is cumbersome and poorly accepted by most subjects. One method that is currently gaining popularity with many investigators is to administer a small volume of "double-labelled" water to each subject. The subsequent decrease in body stores of an oxygen isotope (^{18}O) indicates metabolic production of carbon dioxide and water, while the decrease of (^2H) indicates the loss of water. The difference thus reflects carbon dioxide output.

Other Measurements

Other methods of measuring human activity which have been suggested but are not widely used, include integration of electrical signals from the brain (electroencephalography) and muscle (electromyography), the recording of eye movements or visually evoked brain potentials, and an integration of the galvanic skin response (a measure of the sweat secreted).

FURTHER READING

Andersen KL, Masirono R, Rutenfranz J, Seliger V. Habitual physical activity and health. Copenhagen: WHO Regional Publications: European Series No. 6, 1978.

Froelicher VF. Exercise testing and training. Chicago: Year Book Publishers, 1983.

Laporte RE, Montoye, HJ, Caspersen CJ. Assessment of physical activity in epidemiological research: problems and prospects. Public Health Rep 1985; 100:131-146.

Larsen LA. Fitness, health and work capacity. New York: MacMillan Publishing, 1974.

Mellerowicz H, Smodlaka VN. Ergometry. Basics of medical exercise testing. Baltimore: Urban & Schwarzenberg, 1981.

Saris WHM. Aerobic power and daily physical activity in children. With special reference to methods and cardiovascular risk indicators. Nijmegen: Krips Repro Meppel, 1982.

Shephard RJ. Endurance fitness (2nd Ed.) Toronto: University of Toronto Press, 1977.

Shephard RJ. Human physiological work capacity. London: Cambridge University Press, 1978.

Weiner JS, Lourie JA. Practical human biology. New York: Academic Press, 1981.

THE FUEL FOR PHYSICAL ACTIVITY

CHAPTER 3

ENERGY YIELD AND ENERGY DEMANDS
Energy Yield of Common Foods
Carbohydrate Reserves
Fat Reserves
Incomplete Metabolism
Energy Demands Other Than External Work
Influence of Energy Intake Upon Energy Output

FUEL FOR PHYSICAL ACTIVITY
Effect of Intensity
Effect of Duration
Effect of Training
Exhaustion and Supercharging of Glycogen Stores
Gluconeogenesis
Protein Metabolism During Exercise
Metabolic Role of Lactate
Interconversion of Metabolic Fuels

EXHAUSTION AND FATIGUE
Psychological and Physiological Fatigue
Role of Central Inhibition
Limitations of Oxygen Transport
Glycogen Depletion
Mineral Ion Depletion
Pathological Fatigue
Overtraining and Fatigue

OBESITY
Ideal Percentage of Body Fat in the Athlete
Ideal Body Mass for the General Public
Epidemiological Indices of Obesity
Skinfold Predictions
Other Estimates of Body Fat
Estimations Based on Lean Tissue Mass
Overfeeding and Obesity
Role of Inactivity
Correction of Obesity

BLOOD LIPID PROFILE
Characteristics of Lipid Profile
Modification of Lipid Profile by Low Cholesterol Diets
and by Exercise

DRASTIC WEIGHT LOSS
Weight Categorization
Anorexia Nervosa
Energy Balance in Female Athletes

This chapter recapitulates the energy yield of various forms of food, and considers the normal choice of fuel for physical activity. Specific consideration is directed to the causes of exhaustion and fatigue, and to problems of energy balance (including obesity, the lipid profile, and drastic "weight loss").

ENERGY YIELD AND ENERGY DEMANDS

Energy Yield of Common Foods

Carbohydrate (Fig. 3-1), fat (Fig. 3-2) and protein can all provide energy needed for the resynthesis of adenosine triphosphate (ATP). The energy content of common foods was indicated briefly in Chapter 1. There is a fair variation in the metabolic yield of "carbohydrate," "fat," and "protein" from one food to another (Table 3-1). McCance and Widdowson have proposed average values slightly higher than the classical estimates of Atwater and Benedict (17.2 kJ per gram for protein, 39 kJ per gram for fat, 15.7 kJ per gram for carbohydrate, and 29.3 kJ per gram for alcohol). The energy yields seen in the body are, nevertheless, smaller than those found by burning the food in a "bomb calorimeter," due to incomplete absorption from the intestines, and an excretion of energy-containing products in the breath, sweat, and urine (e.g., urea, ketones, and alcohol). If fat is lost by dieting, the energy yield again tends to a figure of 29 kJ per gram rather than 38 or 39 kJ per gram. Nevertheless, fat is much more energy-dense than carbohydrate and thus provides the body's main energy store. While a 1- to 2-hour reserve of glycogen is found in muscle, the long-term energy store is neutral fat, which accumulates in subcutaneous, omental, and perirenal adipose tissue.

Carbohydrate Reserves

There are 5 to 6 g of glucose in the blood stream, but no more than 3 g can be metabolized without replenishment if symptoms of low blood sugar (hypoglycemia) are to be avoided. Sources of glucose include (1) absorption during exercise (maximum about 5 g per hour), (2) hepatic synthesis from glycerol, lactate, and amino acids (gluconeogenesis), and (3) the breakdown of glycogen stores (glycolysis). Glycogen provides the main reserve of carbohydrate, with stores of some 400 g in muscle and 100 g in the liver. The energy yield of glycogen per unit of mass is decreased by associated water molecules of hydration. Each gram of stored glycogen has 3 g of water linked to it by hydrophilic bonding. While an increase of glycogen reserves has the disadvantage of increasing total body mass, the potential for liberation of the associated bound water during prolonged exercise can be a useful defence against dehydration in a hot climate. If all of the stored glycogen is metabolized, as much as 1.5 ℓ of water may enter the tissue fluid pool.

Fat Reserves

One serious limitation of fat as an energy reserve is that it can only be metabolized under aerobic conditions. If the blood flow to a muscle becomes inadequate (as is quite likely in vigorous endurance effort), activity

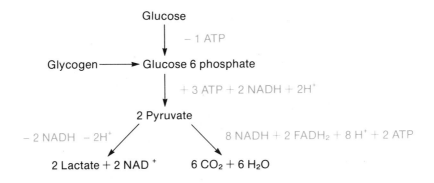

Figure 3-1 Energy yield from carbohydrate metabolism.

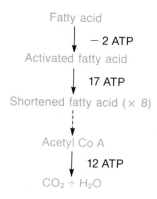

Fatty acid

↓ − 2 ATP

Activated fatty acid

↓ 17 ATP

Shortened fatty acid (× 8)

⋮

Acetyl Co A

↓ 12 ATP

$CO_2 + H_2O$

Total yield = (17 × 8) + 12 − 2 = 146 moles
of ATP for 18 carbon fatty acid.

Figure 3–2   Energy yield from fatty acid metabolism.

can only be sustained if there is a transition to aerobic fuels (stored carbohydrate and glucose formed by gluconeogenesis). A further problem in heavy exercise is that the energy yield per liter of oxygen is 10 percent less for fat than for carbohydrate metabolism. Finally, only very small amounts of fat are stored within the muscle fiber; effort thus becomes limited by the rate of mobilization of free fatty acids from adipose tissue, their carriage in the blood stream, and their further transport from the muscle capillaries to the inner surfaces of the muscle mitochondria where they are metabolized. After analysis of world track records for various distances, Lloyd concluded that there was a dra-

matic drop of performance once tissue glycogen reserves had been exhausted and the runner was obliged to rely upon fat delivery from the adipose depots to the working muscles (Fig. 3–3).

Incomplete Metabolism

Sometimes the energy yield from either carbohydrate or fat is substantially less than that suggested above. The usual reason is an incomplete breakdown of the food product. Under anaerobic conditions, carbohydrate accumulates as lactate. The energy yield (equivalent to the resynthesis of three rather than 39 moles of ATP) is then one-thirteenth of that for complete aerobic metabolism if the starting point is glycogen, or one-ninteenth of the complete aerobic value (two rather than 38 moles of ATP resynthesized) if the starting point is glucose (in the latter case, one mole of ATP is needed to finance an initial conversion of glucose to glucose-6-phosphate before the breakdown to pyruvate and lactate can begin).

If a high proportion of the energy is derived from fat (cold exposure and/or prolonged moderate exercise), there is again incomplete metabolism, with an accumulation of ketone bodies (acetone, acetoacetic acid, and beta-hydroxybutyric acid) in both blood and tissues. In consequence, the energy yield is less than would result if fatty acids were oxidized completely to carbon dioxide and water (Fig. 3–4).

Energy Demands Other Than External Work

Several factors other than physical activity contribute to the total energy demand. Energy is used in pump-

TABLE 3–1   Energy Yield of Protein, Fat, and Carbohydrate from Selected Foodstuffs

Food	Protein			Fat			Carbohydrate		
	Heat of Combustion* (kJ/g)	Digestibility (%)	Yield (kJ/g)	Heat of Combustion (kJ/g)	Digestibility (%)	Yield (kJ/g)	Heat of Combustion (kJ/g)	Digestibility (%)	Yield (kJ/g)
Eggs	18.8	97	18.2	39.8	95	37.7	15.7	98	15.4
Meat	18.4	97	17.9	39.8	95	37.7	--	--	--
Milk	18.4	97	17.9	38.7	95	36.8	16.5	98	16.2
Butter	18.4	97	17.9	38.7	95	36.8	16.5	98	16.2
Fruit	16.5	85	14.1	38.9	90	35.0	16.7	90	15.1
Wheat (97–100% extraction)	19.0	79	15.0	38.9	90	35.0	17.6	90	15.8
Soya beans	18.6	78	14.5	38.9	90	35.0	17.6	97	17.0
Cane sugar	--	--	--	--	--	--	16.5	98	16.2
Potatoes	15.7	74	11.6	38.9	90	35.0	17.6	96	16.9
Vegetables	15.7	65	10.2	38.9	90	35.0	17.6	85	14.9
Chocolate	18.2	42	7.7	38.9	90	35.0	17.4	32	5.6
Average (McCance & Widdowson)			17.2			39.0			15.7

* Heat of combustion adjusted downwards by 5.2 kJ/g to correspond to Atwood's "available protein"; this adjustment reflects the loss of unburnt energy as urea in sweat and urine.
Based in part on data tabulated by K. L. Andersen

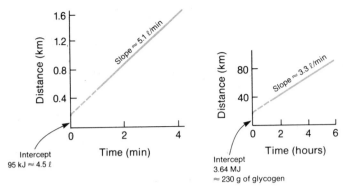

Figure 3–3 Male world records for running, as analyzed by Lloyd. The energy cost of running has been set at 0.27 kJ/m.

ing molecules across various biological membranes. For example, a malate–aspartate shuttle moves carbohydrate residues and associated electrons to the interior of the mitochondrion for final oxidation to CO_2 and water; this transfer process costs the equivalent of 1 mole of ATP for every mole of pyruvate (or 2 moles of ATP for every mole of glucose) that is oxidized (Fig. 3–5).

A further source of energy usage is the regular breakdown and resynthesis of the body constituents. Many apparently stable compounds—protein, fat, and carbohydrate—are in fact regularly destroyed and rebuilt over the course of 1- to 2-day cycles. In a cold environment, such "futile cycles" are deliberately enhanced as a means of sustaining body temperature. There have also been suggestions that humans synthesize a special form of fat ("brown fat") in the cold. Brown fat contains a specific protein that encourages membrane leakage of sodium ions, and thus increases energy usage by the membrane pump.

Pregnancy, lactation, growth, and muscle hypertrophy induced by a training program are other situations where ingested energy is diverted to the needs of tissue synthesis. Naturally, the synthetic process is not

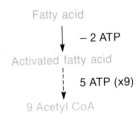

Energy yield = (9x5) − 2 = 43 moles ATP for 18 carbon fatty acid, broken down to 2 carbon fragments.

Figure 3–4 Energy yield during ketosis.

100 percent efficient, and the increased tissue mass is thus less than might be anticipated from the quantity of food energy that is consumed.

Influence of Energy Intake Upon Energy Output

The ingestion of food induces an immediate increase of body metabolism (the so-called specific dynamic action, greatest after a fat-containing meal). There have also been reports of a more long-term autoregulatory interaction between metabolism and food supply; overfed laboratory animals have increased their resting energy consumption by 10 to 15 percent (the so-called Luxuskonsumption), and starved animals have reduced their energy output by a similar amount. Such observations have obvious application to the difficulty that some people find in reducing their body mass by dieting.

FUEL FOR PHYSICAL ACTIVITY

The preferred fuel for physical activity depends on the intensity and duration of exercise, together with the individual's state of training. We shall here consider these issues in relation to glycogen stores, gluconeogenesis, metabolism of protein and lactate, and interconversion of the various fuels.

Effect of Intensity

As the intensity of effort increases, an ever-larger proportion of the active muscle fibers are inadequately perfused. There is thus a progressive shift from aerobic metabolism (which consumes roughly equal proportions of carbohydrate and fat) to anaerobic metabolism. Anaerobic activity relies almost exclusively upon the usage of stored glycogen; this is broken down to pyruvate, with an accumulation of lactic acid in the active muscle fibers.

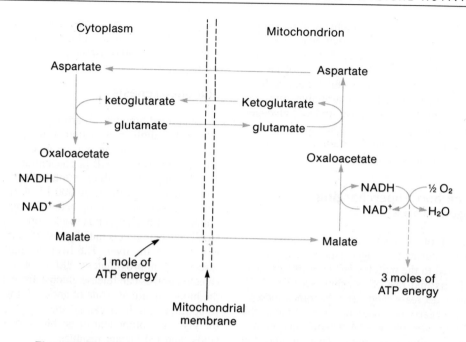

Figure 3–5 The malate/aspartate shuttle which transfers electrons from the muscle cytoplasm to the inner aspect of the mitochondrion.

The relative usage of fat and carbohydrate can be gauged approximately from the respiratory quotient (RQ). Ignoring the small contribution from protein, a pure metabolism of fat would lead to an RQ of 0.70, and a pure metabolism of carbohydrate to an RQ of 1.00. At rest, a figure of 0.80 to 0.85 is seen, implying a slight preponderance of fat usage. At 50 percent of maximum oxygen intake, approximately equal amounts of energy are drawn from fat and carbohydrate, but at larger power outputs the RQ rises sharply. Above 75 percent of maximum oxygen intake, most of the energy is derived from carbohydrate, and a buildup of lactic acid pushes the respiratory gas exchange ratio as high as 1.10 to 1.20 during maximum effort.

The twin considerations of glycogen sparing and avoidance of lactate accumulation explain why average contestants in long-distance events, such as a marathon race, hold their speed to approximately 75 percent of their personal maximum aerobic power; through this tactic, anaerobic metabolism is kept to a minimum. Some well-trained distance runners can exercise to a higher fraction of maximum oxygen intake (e.g., 85 percent) without a build-up of lactate, and this in itself gives them a substantial competitive advantage over less well-conditioned individuals.

Since relatively more fat is consumed in moderate than in vigorous intensity exercise, the person who wishes to lose body fat is better advised to walk a substantial distance on a regular basis than to consume a similar total amount of energy by daily jogging over a shorter course.

Effect of Duration

There is necessarily a shift from carbohydrate to fat metabolism as muscle and liver glycogen reserves become depleted. The glycogen stores of a given muscle can probably be exhausted by 10 to 12 maximal isometric contractions, each lasting no more than 30 seconds. With rhythmic activities, the speed of depletion is much slower. In team games such as ice-hockey and soccer, which involve frequent accelerations and decelerations of the body mass, the more heavily recruited muscles become short of glycogen by the end of a 90 minute game. In a road or ski marathon, the depletion time is about 2 hours; exhaustion of carbohydrate reserves is probably one factor contributing to the "wall" that many competitors report after 30 to 35 km of running. Replenishment of glycogen stores takes place relatively slowly, over 1 to 2 days of rest, so that if the intense or prolonged activity must be repeated within 24 hours, an increased proportion of fat will be used on the second occasion. This finding has application not only to the organization of tournaments, but also to the design of training programs; it is usually best to alternate days of heavy and light physical activity. Such a schedule not only allows recovery from sub-clinical muscle injuries, but also avoids the fatigue of severe glycogen depletion.

Effect of Training

Training increases the activity of intramuscular aerobic enzymes, and for this reason a well-conditioned subject is able to reach a high percentage of maximum oxygen intake before exercise becomes anaerobic. The metabolic corollary of this development is that at any given intensity of exercise, the proportion of fat that is burnt is higher than it is in a sedentary person. Reliance upon fat helps to eke out available glycogen reserves during prolonged exercise. Indeed, glycogen sparing is now thought to be one of the most important athletic gains resulting from the training-induced increase of aerobic enzyme activity.

Exhaustion and Supercharging of Glycogen Stores

Exhaustion of glycogen stores creates two metabolic problems during prolonged exercise: (1) fat cannot be delivered to the muscles fast enough to sustain the desired maximal rate of working (see Fig. 3–3), so that speeds decrease, and (2) it becomes increasingly difficult to carry out anaerobic exercise (since this requires glycogen or glucose). A person can continue sub-maximal running or cycling on level ground, but suffers a major handicap if a slight hill requires more forcible efforts that cut off the blood supply to the working muscles.

A necessary corollary of these findings is that competitive advantage can be gained if the muscles are "supercharged" with glycogen during the days immediately before competition (Fig. 3–6). The usual tactic adopted for this purpose is to deplete the limbs of glycogen by a bout of exhausting work, following a diet rich in fat and protein for 2 to 3 days, and switching to a high-carbohydrate diet for the final 3 days prior to a major competition. With such a regimen, muscle glycogen stores may be brought to about twice the normal resting level. However, it is undesirable to adopt a high-carbohydrate diet on a continuous basis, as this encourages the development of glycolytic enzymes; there is then a preferential use of glycogen rather than fat reserves during actual competition.

Gluconeogenesis

A limited amount of carbohydrate remains available for metabolism even after prolonged exercise has broken down all of the muscle glycogen. The blood store of glucose is small (a concentration of no more than 120 mg per deciliter, a total of approximately 6 g of glucose, equivalent to 100 kJ of energy). If the blood glucose were to drop below 60 mg per deciliter, symptoms of hypoglycemia would appear. However, the blood concentration is initially sustained by glucose that is formed in the liver. The liver normally contains a reserve of approximately 100 g of glycogen, and catecholamines can release glucose from this store into the blood stream at a rate of about 20 mg per second. In addition, the liver can synthesize glucose from (1) the glycerol component of fat breakdown, (2) amino acids, and (3) lactate residues.

Gluconeogenesis is important to normal health and function, since some tissues such as the brain and red cells are unable to metabolize fat. If blood glucose drops below 50 to 60 mg per deciliter, brain function is disturbed, with symptoms such as irritability, poor judgment, and eventually coma. Situations where this can cause a deterioration of athletic performance include orienteering and dinghy sailing. For the latter sport, a high level of mental concentration is needed to plan tactics. At the same time, glucose and glycogen reserves are being depleted by the characteristic "hiking" position of the crew, which requires very sustained isometric contractions of the abdominal and leg muscles.

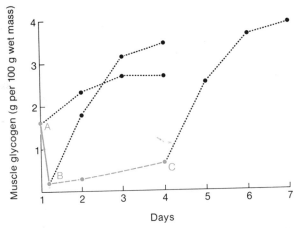

Figure 3–6 To illustrate the principle of glycogen supercompensation. The normal resting state is at point *A*. Hard physical work is performed from *A* to *B*, and a fat/protein diet is fed from *B* to *C*. The light interrupted lines indicate the course of muscle glycogen replenishment if a high carbohydrate diet is initiated at *A*, *B* or *C*. (After Shephard RJ. Physiology and biochemistry of exercise. New York: Praeger, 1982: Figure 2:19. Courtesy of the publisher.)

Protein Metabolism During Exercise

At one time, it was argued that protein did not serve as a fuel for muscular activity. The main evidence for this conclusion was a rather insensitive comparison of 24-hour urinary nitrogen excretion rates for days when light and heavy activity had been undertaken. Since heavy activity did not increase nitrogen output, it was argued that no additional protein had been metabolized during exercise. On the other hand, if blood urea is monitored over an event such as a marathon race, a substantial rise of concentration is seen; the source of urea is a deamination of proteins, and if blood volume has been maintained, the only possible explanation of the increased urea concentration seems a substantial increase in the metabolism of amino acids during exercise, a response equivalent to an energy expenditure of about 800 kJ, 5 to 6 percent of the energy cost of running a marathon race. What are the dietary implications of this protein usage? Nutritionists have argued that 0.7 to 1.0 g of protein per kilogram of body mass provides an adequate allowance for a sedentary person. However, the athlete who is attempting to synthesize new protein-containing tissue and is also breaking down 50 g of protein per day in competition probably needs more; 2 g per kilogram now becomes a reasonable allowance. The dietary requirement can be checked by determinations of nitrogen balance. Some recent studies have suggested that a protein intake of 1.8 to 2.0 g per kilogram is need to achieve a balance between nitrogen intake and excretion during hard physical training.

Metabolic Role of Lactate

Lactate provides a potential source of fuel in well-oxygenated tissues; pyruvate is reformed, and then the normal pathway of carbohydrate metabolism is followed. The limiting intramuscular concentration during anaerobic activity is usually approximately 30 mmol per cubic decimeter, although somewhat higher figures may be tolerated if tissue buffering capacity has been increased by sprint training or bicarbonate doping. The lactate which is formed in hypoxic tissues may be metabolized locally, diffusing to better oxygenated fibers within the same muscle group, or it may escape into the blood stream. With a single bout of steady, exhausting exercise, the peak blood level of lactate is usually 10 to 12 mmol per cubic decimeter, but if greater time is allowed for transfer to the blood stream (repeated short bouts of very intensive exercise), concentrations as high as 25-30 mmol per cubic decimeter may be reached. The blood lactate may be metabolized immediately in other parts of the body (for instance, the heart and resting skeletal muscle), or it may be converted to glucose and glycogen within the liver (the process of hepatic gluconeogenesis).

Interconversion of Metabolic Fuels

It is finally useful to note the potential for interconversion of carbohydrate, fat, and protein (Fig. 3–7). All three metabolites can provide energy for aerobic exercise. If the diet provides an excess of carbohydrate or protein, this excess can be converted to fat; however, the reaction is less easily reversed. Indeed, the only component of the fat that can contribute to maintaining blood glucose is the glycerol moiety released by the breakdown of neutral fat.

EXHAUSTION AND FATIGUE

Is fatigue due to an exhaustion of metabolic reserves? In responding to this question, we must dis-

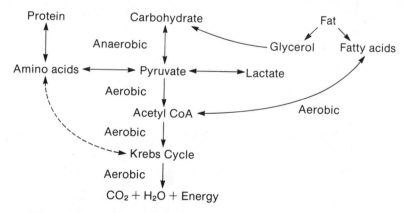

Note: Anaerobic metabolism depends on carbohydrate (glycogen or glucose). The latter can be synthesized from amino acids, lactate, or glycerol. Aerobic metabolism can involve the breakdown of protein, fat, or carbohydrate. Excess energy intake leads to formation of fat. Fatty acids cannot be used in synthesis of carbohydrate.

Figure 3–7   Interconversion of energy sources.

tinguish physiological from psychological fatigue, and must consider other possible explanations (including central inhibition, limitations of oxygen transport, and depletion of mineral ions). Brief comment will also be made on pathological fatigue and over-training. Neuromuscular aspects of fatigue are considered in Chapter 5.

Psychological and Physiological Fatigue

In industry, fatigue often has a psychological rather than a physiological basis; the employee has become bored by carrying out a dull, repetitive task, and although productivity has fallen dramatically, there is a miraculous return of energy with the sprint to the canteen for the coffee break, or the bus for the journey home. Nevertheless, if the work is heavy, there may also be an important physiological component to fatigue. Field studies of self-paced work and laboratory research on the cycle ergometer both suggest that fatigue is likely if the average intensity of effort exceeds 40 percent of the individual's maximum oxygen intake, measured over an 8-hour work day (Table 3–2). Under arduous conditions (high peak rates of working, awkward postures, use of small muscles, activities performed with the arms raised, exposure to high environmental temperatures), the threshold loading for fatigue may be even lower.

Role of Central Inhibition

In theory, fatigue could arise at any link in the process of translating food energy into a muscular impulse. It has been argued that in humans, performance is most commonly limited by cerebral inhibition. For example, an athlete whose pace is slowing from apparent exhaustion can develop a further burst of speed in response to cheering and various forms of hypnotic suggestion, and a relatively weak woman who sees her child trapped under a car can momentarily develop the force needed to lift the vehicle and release the child. Inhibition is certainly a well-recognized phenomenon in neurophysiology, but much of any unexpected feats of physical performance in an apparently exhausted athlete must also be attributed to physiological factors, particularly a change in both the pattern and distribution of neural activity; as a consequence of recruitment of additional motor units and an alteration of discharge patterns in the motor nerves, maximal use is made of muscle fibers which still have adequate glycogen reserves and are able to contribute some contractile force towards the desired movement.

Limitations of Oxygen Transport

With brief bouts of exhausting exercise, the usual problem is that oxygen transport fails to meet local metabolic demands. Intramuscular accumulations of lactic acid are thus sufficient to inhibit the key enzymes of glycolysis, and although glycogen reserves may remain relatively intact, energy is no longer liberated in the amounts needed for the regeneration of creatine phosphate or ATP.

If the activity involves the large muscles of the body and is of an order that can be sustained for several minutes (for instance, running a 1,500 or 5,000 meter race), the problem can usually be traced to a respiratory or central circulatory limitation of performance. A sedentary person who is unaccustomed to vigorous exercise may halt such activity because of severe breathlessness, but the more disciplined athlete has become accustomed to, and accepts unpleasant respiratory sensations; an endurance competitor thus stops running or even collapses because the heart is unable to pump a sufficient flow of blood to sustain the combined needs of muscle, skin, and brain. Circulatory exhaustion is particularly likely to limit endurance effort if the blood volume has been reduced, either by immediate sweating and exudation of fluid into the working muscles, or more chronically by salt depletion. A point is reached where blood pressure begins to fall and coordination deteriorates; if running, the gait becomes unsteady, there are sensations of nausea and dizziness, the competitor becomes confused, and consciousness is lost. Alternatively, blood pressures during the exercise bout may not rise to a high enough level to counter the forces developed by the contracting muscle; this again leads to local hypoxia, accumulation of lactate, and inhibition of glycolysis despite adequate glycogen reserves.

Glycogen Depletion

Fat reserves do not become depleted unless exercise is continued for many weeks (for instance, a cross-Canada run). However, over a period of 1 to 2 hours of vigorous activity, fatigue can reflect a total depletion of glycogen stores in the working muscle fibers. The most vulnerable are fast-twitch white fibers. There may be a change of recruitment pattern (from fast- to slow-twitch fibers) as glycogen depletion develops in the fast-twitch fibers.

TABLE 3–2   The Allowable Work Rate in Relation to the Duration of Effort

Duration of Effort (hours)	Recommended Ceiling (% $\dot{V}O_2$ max)	Voluntary Choice (%)
8	33	40
4	47	--
2	53	--
1	63	76

All values are expressed as percent of maximum oxygen intake.

Training increases the oxidative potential of fast-twitch anaerobic (Type IIb) muscle fibers so that they assume a combination of oxidative and glycolytic properties (fast-twitch oxidative fibers, Type IIa); in consequence, their resistance to fatigue is increased.

Mineral Ion Depletion

Occasionally, fatigue can be traced to a lack of some key mineral ion needed in the process of energy release; e.g., sodium depletion may be caused by a prolonged sweating, or a failure of the "calcium pump" within the active muscle may deprive the basic contractile mechanism (the interaction of actin and myosin) of needed calcium ions. It seems significant that one action of a socially used fatigue-relieving drug (caffeine) is to facilitate calcium flux within muscle.

Pathological Fatigue

Certain clinical disorders predispose to the premature onset of fatigue. Pathological causes of fatigue include myasthenia gravis (where there is a failure of impulse transmission at the neuromuscular junction) and Addison's disease (where a deficiency of secretions from the adrenal cortex leads to problems in the regulation of blood sugar and liver glycogen reserves). Does this type of fatigue ever occur in normal individuals? There is some evidence that cortisol secretion decreases over the course of very prolonged exercise, even in a healthy person, but it is unclear whether this disturbance is sufficient to be the prime cause of fatigue except in disease.

Overtraining and Fatigue

Repeated fatigue merges into the syndrome of "overtraining" (Chapter 9). Again, this is partly situational in its manifestation, with a strong psychological overlay. The athlete may have few complaints of overtraining during a successful season, but problems are likely to arise where much time has been invested in training without substantial gains in performance and competitive standing.

To the extent that overtraining has a physiological or a pathological basis, it may be attributed to one or more of such factors as a progressive depletion of body mineral reserves, an exhaustion of glycogen stores, a disturbance of fluid balance (decrease of blood volume and/or intracellular fluid), and a buildup of subclinical injuries. If there is an accompanying muscle soreness, there are often biochemical correlates of local tissue injury—an alteration of the urinary hydroxyproline-creatine ratio (reflecting a disruption of connective tissue) and increased blood levels of enzymes such as creatine phosphokinase (reflecting a disruption of muscle tissue).

Some authors have also described structural changes such as a swelling of the mitochondria and a destruction of their internal membranes (the mitochondrial cristae) within affected muscle fibers.

OBESITY

Obesity arises because the intake of food is excessive relative to the depletion of body reserves by the various forms of energy usage as discussed. Issues to be reviewed include the ideal body fat for athletes and for the general public, methods of estimating body fat, the respective contributions of over-feeding and inactivity to the development of obesity, and practical regimens for the correction of obesity.

Ideal Percentage of Body Fat in the Athlete

The ideal fat content of the human body depends partly on one's objectives. If a cross-Canada run were to be contemplated, it would be difficult to eat sufficient food to sustain energy balance over the event, and an 8- to 10-kg increase of body fat reserves might be a useful preparation for such an event. Likewise, if an athlete wished to swim across the cold waters of Lake Ontario, a few additional millimeters of subcutaneous fat might provide vital thermal insulation and increase buoyancy. Again, in a contact sport such as Canadian or American football, a moderate (5- to 10-kg) increase of body fat contributes to the development of a large body mass while protecting the bones and joints against injury.

However, in many sports such as running, where body mass must be displaced against gravity, the inert mass of fat is a severe handicap. Among international track competitors, around 10 percent of body fat is common in a female, and values are as low as 4 to 5 percent in a male. Large amounts of subcutaneous fat are a particular disadvantage in events such as figure skating and gymnastics, where scores reflect in part the personal appearance of the competitor; however, many female participants in these activities develop an undesirable negative energy balance in their search for a sylph-like figure.

Ideal Body Mass for the General Public

From the viewpoint of the ordinary person, severe obesity (an additional 20 to 30 kg of fat) leads to an increased risk of various medical problems, including hypertension, atherosclerosis, diabetes, diseases of the gallbladder and urinary tract, and osteoarthritis of the knee, hips, and spine. Surgery also becomes more difficult, and abdominal healing is delayed after an operation (Table 3–3).

TABLE 3–3   Mortality of Grossly Obese Subjects Aged 15 to 69 Years, Classified by Disease, and Expressed as Percent of Standard Values for Subjects of Same Standing Height and Sex

Disease Condition	Women		Men	
	+28 kg (%)	+46 kg (%)	+24 kg (%)	+42 kg (%)
Diabetes	270	250	179	629
Vascular diseases of brain	143	210	136	215
Heart and circulation	175	217	131	185
Pneumonia and influenza	148	*	128	242
Digestive diseases	140	225	147	298
Renal diseases	93	*	146	298

* Insufficient cases
Based on data of Society of Actuaries, 1959

More moderate degrees of obesity (5 to 10 kg of excess fat) have only a small effect upon the incidence of these various conditions. In individuals who are a little "overweight," arguments for a slimmer figure are thus based upon the physical work involved in displacing excess fat, problems of thermoregulation, and the potential for an improvement of physical appearance. Currently, it is fashionable to have the body build of an endurance competitor, and some loss of body fat may thus improve self-image. However, in the time of Rubens, a much more substantial figure was regarded as the epitome of both female and male beauty.

The clinician gauges obesity from weight for height tables (Table 3–4). This is generally an adequate approach in a population sense, but it can be misleading when applied to an individual. For example, a low weight for height in a female office worker may reflect a combination of substantial obesity plus inadequate musculature, while an apparent excess of body mass in a male football player may be due to well-developed muscles rather than to an excessive accumulation of body fat.

There are two types of weight for height table. One presents average values for the North American population. This shows an 8- to 10-kg increase of body mass between 25 and 45 years of age (as fat accumulates), while at later ages the proposed weight for height remains constant or declines (as lean tissue is lost). The second type of table, exemplified by the 1959 "Build and Blood Pressure" Study of the Society of Actuaries, is based on the observed body mass at the time of purchasing life insurance (often around 25 years). It shows values that are optimal in terms of life expectancy for a given standing height. Although the second type of table is often used in the dietary counseling of older subjects, there is no good evidence that what was an ideal mass at the time of buying insurance remains ideal for the same individual when he or she is 20 or 30 years older. In 1983, the Metropolitan Life Assurance Company proposed a small upward revision of the 1959 Society of Actuaries weight for height standards. Critics have suggested that one reason why an adjustment of the tables appeared necessary was that the influence

of smoking habits upon mortality had increased between 1959 and 1983. Heavy smokers tended to have a lower body mass than average, along with a higher risk for various types of cancer. However, if the most recent statistics are adjusted for smoking habits, there remains a need to make a small increase in standards of "ideal weight." It may be that people who take regular exercise conserve lean tissue, and thus weigh a little more than those who are totally sedentary. Both the 1959 and the 1983 tables list acceptable ranges of mass for three types of body frame—"light," "medium," and "heavy." In 1959, the observer had to make a difficult subjective decision on frame type, but the 1983 tables have proposed objective measurements of knee and elbow

TABLE 3–4   Ideal Body Mass in Relation to Height and Gender for Subjects of Medium Body Frame

Height (cm) (No shoes)	Ideal Body Mass (kg) (Indoor Clothing)	
	Female	Male
147.3	48.5	50.5*
149.9	49.9	51.9*
152.4	51.2	53.5*
155.0	52.6	55.3*
157.5	54.2	57.6
160.0	55.8	58.9
162.6	57.8	60.3
165.1	60.0	61.9
167.6	61.7	63.7
170.2	63.5	65.7
172.7	65.3	67.6
175.3	66.8	69.4
177.8	68.5	71.4
180.3	70.6*	73.5
182.9	72.6*	75.5
185.4	74.6*	77.5
188.0	76.9*	79.8
190.5	79.2*	82.1
193.0	81.4*	84.3

* Extrapolated value

diameters as a means of classifying frame size. The main limitation inherent in both early and more recent actuarial tables is a lack of precision in the data base—the information is necessarily restricted to people purchasing life insurance, and in most cases observations have been collected in a busy doctor's office where measurements of height and weight are necessarily rather crude; for instance, the time of day when measurements have been made is never specified, yet both height and body mass show a substantial diurnal variation.

Epidemiological Indices of Obesity

Epidemiologists commonly judge population obesity in terms of weight–height ratios (W/H, W/H², and H/∛W). The most popular is the ratio of body mass to the square of stature (Quetelet's index). Objections to this type of index are similar to those raised in interpreting weight for height tables of ideal body mass. In particular, uncritical interpretation of average W/H² and H/∛W values led a national survey to the erroneous conclusion that the Inuit population of northern Canada was obese, whereas in fact, high W/H² scores and low H/∛W scores at the time of data collection reflected the fact that the Inuit were vigorously active and highly muscular. However, in most samples of the general adult population, high W/H² values reflect overnutrition and obesity.

Skinfold Predictions

A more objective method of examining body fat content is to measure the thickness of a double fold of skin and subcutaneous fat, using a specially designed caliper that exerts a standard pressure (10 g/mm² over a face area of 35 mm³). The fold of fat is supported by the thumb and index finger during measurement. Readings are taken 2 sec after grasping the fold, before compression of the skin has occurred.

Various authors have measured anywhere from one to 10 skinfolds. The precision of body fat estimation is not increased by using more than 3 to 4 folds, although information on fat distribution is obtained. Sometimes the data have been interpreted in their own right, relative to the fat distribution observed in young adults of ideal body mass (Table 3–5), but more commonly the skinfolds have been used to predict body density and thus body fat percentage. For example, Durnin and Womersley recommended the following general formulas* for women and men respectively:

Body density (women 16 to 68 years)=
$$1.1327 - 0.0643 \log_{10} \Sigma$$

Body density (men 17 to 72 years)=
$$1.1704 - 0.0731 \log_{10} \Sigma$$

* Formulas were also calculated for age-specific groups.

where Σ is the sum of triceps, subscapular and suprailiac folds in millimeters. Then, in both sexes, body fat percent = (4.95/density − 4.50) × 100.

The fundamental argument against prediction of body fat is that the mathematical manipulation of the skinfold readings has not increased their information content. Although the Durnin and Womersley equations have proven surprisingly robust when used on a variety of world populations, it is difficult to envisage that such factors as aging, starvation, athletic training, and ethnic differences would not alter the distribution of body fat, both over the body surface and between superficial and deep stores. It is also necessary to make the assumption that the observed body density reflects the presence of two tissues of fixed density (fat, 0.90 and lean, 1.10), whereas in reality the lean compartment comprises varying proportions of muscle and bone, and the density of the bone diminishes with age. Age and sex-specific prediction equations are thus essential. Finally, the literature contains a wide variety of skinfold prediction formulas that yield widely differing estimates of percent fat. The one strong argument in favor of attempting to predict the percentage of body fat is that the lean tissue mass can then be estimated; the age and sex specific equations of Durnin and Womersley seem the best of the currently available procedures for making this calculation.

Other Estimates of Body Fat

There are many alternative methods of examining the extent of body fat stores. The most popular approach, commonly used as a reference method for assessing the accuracy of other procedures, is hydrostatic weighing. The volume of the subject is in essence estimated from the apparent decrease of body mass while submerged. The recorded buoyancy reflects not only tissue volume, but also the volume of any gas in the

TABLE 3–5   Skinfold Readings Corresponding to an Actuarial Ideal Body Mass

Skinfold Site	Skinfold Thickness		
	Female (mm)	Male (mm)	Female/Male (%)
Triceps	15.6	7.8	200
Subscapular	11.3	11.9	94
Suprailiac	14.6	12.7	115
Waist	15.3	14.3	106
Suprapubic	20.5	11.0	186
Medial knee	11.8	8.6	137
Chin	7.1	5.8	122
Chest	8.6	12.0	72

Note: In a relatively thin subject, the female has relatively more fat than the male in the lower half of the trunk. The regional distribution of body fat is susceptible to estrogen levels, and a "female" pattern of distribution is associated with a reduced risk of ischemic heart disease.

intestines (usually ignored) and the lungs (the residual volume is usually measured while submerged, although in healthy young children it may be more satisfactory to assume that it corresponds to a fixed 28 percent of vital capacity). Less commonly, body volume is estimated by water or gas displacement while the subject sits in a rigid container. In either case, density is estimated as mass/volume. Using a two compartment model as for skinfolds, body density can then be converted to an estimate of body fat.

Soft tissue radiographs show the relative proportions of muscle and fat in a limb, but this technique is not very popular because it involves at least a small exposure to radiation, and the information obtained is localized. There is some interest in using ultrasound photographs in a similar fashion, but the main problem with such an approach is again that the resultant pictures are representative of only one part of the body.

Estimations Based On Lean Tissue Mass

A further possibility is to estimate body fat as the difference between total and lean body mass (see further, Chapter 5). Lean mass may be determined from the dilution of markers (for instance, the ingestion of a small volume of deuterated or tritiated water, which it is assumed becomes distributed uniformly through lean tissue containing a consistent 73 percent water). Alternatively, the naturally occurring isotope ^{40}K or whole-body nitrogen may be estimated by enclosing the subject inside a whole-body counter; the apparatus is costly, and is only available at major hospital centers. Moreover, rigid assumptions must be made about the potassium or the nitrogen content of the tissues. Potassium, found mainly in muscle, is 0.21 to 0.23 percent of lean tissue, and nitrogen is 3.0 to 3.5 percent; both figures are influenced strongly by bone mass and tissue hydration.

Overfeeding and Obesity

Obesity arises in essence because the intake of food is excessive relative to the daily energy expenditure. Given the large daily intake (10 to 16 MJ) relative to the size of fat reserves, an overfeeding by only 1 percent of requirements, if repeated on a daily basis, can lead to a large accumulation of fat over the course of a few years (1 percent of 13 MJ per day for 365 days=47.5 MJ, the energy equivalent of some 1.7 kg of fat). Even a skillful nutritionist finds difficulty in estimating the energy content of meals to within 5 to 10 percent, so that the normal precision with which the body systems regulate the amount of food intake is quite remarkable.

It is believed that there are specific centers in the hypothalamus that regulate both blood glucose levels and activity patterns. There may also be satiety signals coming from peripheral adipocytes, and there is some evidence that obese individuals have an above-average number of adipocytes clamoring for further deposition of fat. The high adipocyte count of the obese may reflect inheritance or, possibly, a hyperplasia of the adipocytes induced by overfeeding in the first year of life.

Experiments with constitutionally obese mice suggest that genetic fatness is associated with a below-average metabolic response to overfeeding. In a normal individual, an increased intake of food leads to a substantial increase of metabolic rate (Luxuskonsumption), possibly associated with an increase of proton leakage in the adipocytes. Likewise, severe dietary restriction quickly reduces resting metabolism by 10 to 15 percent. However, this self-regulating mechanism seems much less well developed in the obese.

Role of Inactivity

In general, there seems to be little relationship between newborn fatness and the development of obesity as an adult. During primary school, a proportion of students begin to accumulate an above-average amount of fat. This leads to a negative self-image and a sedentary lifestyle, and the problem is exacerbated by the mental and emotional stresses of adolescence. Time and motion studies suggest that the main problem of the obese adolescent is a lack of physical activity rather than excessive food consumption. A summer camp with a vigorous activity regimen generally corrects the situation at least temporarily, although there is often recidivism on return to the home environment.

The typical older person who has accumulated 8 to 10 kg of fat over the span of adult life has a similar problem of inadequate physical activity. Appetite tends to remain unchanged in middle age, but the balance between food intake and total energy intake is upset, because of a minor (1 percent) reduction in daily physical activity.

Correction of Obesity

Nutritionists sometimes argue that it is impossible for the obese person to undertake sufficient physical activity to correct moderate or severe obesity; the only solution is to insist upon a rigorous diet. If a major fat loss is required over a span of a few weeks, this is certainly true. Obese individuals find difficulty in increasing their daily expenditure by more than 1 to 2 MJ. However, if the excess of body fat has accumulated for 10 to 20 years, it is better to view correction of the problem as a long-term rather than a short-term project. If rapid fat loss is achieved by starvation or near-starvation, there is much associated loss of lean tissue. The leakage of potassium ions from wasting lean tissue gives a substantial risk of death from cardiac arrhythmia, and as soon as treatment has ended it is likely that an excessive amount of fat will be regained.

The optimum regimen for the treatment of moderate obesity involves a modest decrease of energy intake (2 MJ per day) and a corresponding increase of energy expenditure, the latter being based on sustained endurance activities such as walking. Advantages cited for adding physical activity to the treatment plan include: (1) the positive nature of the advice (restriction of eating is viewed as one more medical prohibition), (2) an immediate elevation of mood (food restriction is depressing), (3) an immediate suppression of appetite, (4) a conservation of lean tissue relative to dieting alone, and (5) the development of an improved lifestyle which is attractive enough to persist after close surveillance has ceased.

BLOOD LIPID PROFILE

Overnutrition and obesity are associated with adverse changes in the blood lipid profile, including an increase of serum cholesterol. This section examines the phenomenon and the possibility of correcting it by diet and exercise.

Characteristics of Lipid Profile

In recent years, much attention has been focussed upon the lipid profile of the blood and its relationship to the development of ischemic heart disease. Significant relationships have been demonstrated between the likelihood of developing fatty deposits in the aorta and coronary vessels (the process of atherosclerosis), the onset of clinical manifestations of atherosclerotic disease (such as angina, an abnormal electrocardiogram, a nonfatal or a fatal myocardial infarction, see Chapter 13), and the level of serum cholesterol. Further investigation has clarified that the adverse cardiovascular prognosis is associated specifically with accumulation of cholesterol in the low-density lipoprotein fraction of the serum, and that high-density lipoprotein (HDL)

cholesterol actually protects the body against ischemic heart disease. It has thus been hypothesized that certain of the HDLs function as "scavengers," clearing the blood of cholesterol before it can accumulate in the vessel walls (Table 3-6 and Fig. 3-8).

Modification of Lipid Profile by Low Cholesterol Diets and by Exercise

The early reaction of physicians to the correlation between serum cholesterol and ischemic heart disease was to restrict the dietary intake of cholesterol, insisting that patients with a high serum cholesterol avoid such foods as butter, eggs, and rich meat (Table 3-7). Over the long term, there have been some changes in North American eating patterns, but it has proven very difficult to persuade individual cardiac patients to accept a drastic reorganization of their intake of saturated animal fats, since this usually involves an alteration of menus for the entire family. Moreover, even if the body intake of cholesterol is drastically reduced by a combination of dietary change and drugs such as cholestyramine, a resin which sequesters cholesterol and prevents its intestinal absorption, the decrease of serum cholesterol remains disappointingly small. The Lipid Research Clinics trial took subjects with high initial cholesterol readings, but were nevertheless only able to reduce average values by 19 percent. The explanation is that a major part of the total body cholesterol is synthesized in the liver; the observed blood level thus reflects total energy balance as much as the specific dietary intake of cholesterol.

Can exercise control lipid profile more effectively than diet? Adequate exercise is certainly important to energy balance. Moreover, the ratio of HDL to total cholesterol seems to be substantially increased by a program of endurance running, although the threshold for such a benefit is a weekly jogging distance of approximately 20 km; this is a feasible prescription for a young

TABLE 3-6   Fractions Examined in Lipid Profile

Fraction	Density (g/mℓ)	Molecular Mass (kdal)	Apoprotein	Lipid
Alpha fraction (HDL)	1.06–1.21	180–360	A I (intestine) A II (intestine) CI-III (hydrolysis of prebeta)	Phospholipids, cholesterol
Beta fraction (LDL)	1.01–1.06	2,700–4,800	B	Cholesterol esters, phospholipids
Prebeta fraction (VLDL)	0.95–1.01	5,000–10,000	B CI-III E	Triglyceride
Chylomicrons	<0.95	>0.4 × 10^9	B CI-III	Triglyceride

Note: (1) HDL cholesterol is higher in women than in men, and shows a small increase with long-distance running. (2) HDL cholesterol, especially the HDL$_2$ subfragment, is associated with a reduced risk of ischemic heart disease. (3) The high density α particles are probably formed from the remnants of chylomicrons and prebeta particles under the influence of the enzyme lecithin-cholesterol acyltransferase (LCAT). (4) HDL cholesterol is transported to the liver; this reduces serum cholesterol and also inhibits endogenous formation of cholesterol.

(a) Chylomicrons

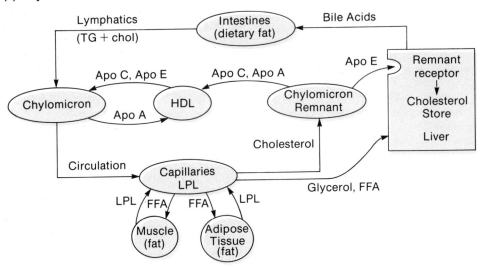

(b) VLDL

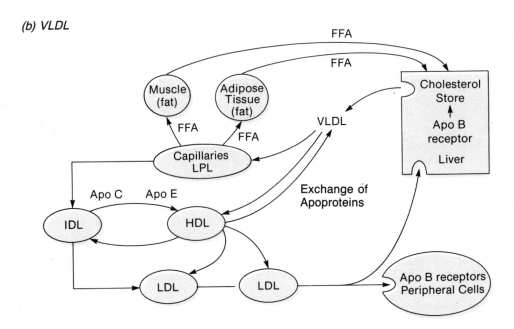

Notes: ApoA transferred from chylomicron to HDL cholesterol in exchange for ApoC and ApoE in thoracic duct ApoC activates lipoprotein lyase (LPL) attached to capillary endothelium.
Chylomicron remnant with high cholesterol content cleared by ApoE receptor in liver VLDL formed in liver—loss of triglycerides yields intermediate density (IDL) and low density lipoprotein (LDL). LDL is removed by liver and peripheral cells, using ApoB receptors. An increased uptake of LDL inhibits cholesterol synthesis and suppresses ApoB receptors; cholesterol is then diverted to the smooth muscles of the arterial wall, favoring the development of atherosclerosis.

Figure 3–8   The metabolism of lipid fractions (based in part on Zonderland).

TABLE 3–7   Cholesterol Content of Average Portion of Some Common Foods (1 mmol = 386 mg)

Food	Cholesterol Content (mmol per average portion)
Beef (raw)	220
Butter (one pat)	100
Cheddar cheese	80
Chicken (raw)	160
Egg (one)	650
Fish	180
Ice-cream	90
Kidney (raw)	100
Lamb (raw)	210
Liver (raw)	850
Margarine (vegetable)	0
Milk (1 cup whole)	70
(skim)	20
Oysters	3,000
Pork	220
Veal	300

adult, but is a substantial load to recommend to a "post-coronary" patient.

DRASTIC WEIGHT LOSS

Weight Categorization

Certain athletes such as wrestlers attempt to induce a drastic "weight loss" in order to enter a weight category inappropriate to their intrinsic body build. The regimen adopted for this purpose may include restriction of food and fluids, use of diuretics, and induction of vigorous sweating in a sauna. Apart from the poor sportsmanship implicit in this deceit, the combination of severe heat and fluid depletion carries some danger of provoking cardiac arrhythmias and other medical problems. Usually the hope of the athlete is that rehydration can be accomplished immediately following a major competition. However, muscle strength remains impaired for some hours following rehydration, presumably because of associated mineral ion disturbances. Methods of preventing this type of abuse include the maintenance of careful weight records on known competitors, and detailed examination of a contestant whose weight category changes downwards. Some guidance can be obtained from weight-for-height tables, while chemical analyses of blood, urine, and body water usually reveals the increased concentrations of body constituents which have been caused by deliberate dehydration.

Anorexia Nervosa

The popular culture of the very thin female causes some adolescents to reduce their food intake to a dangerously low level. In a proportion of such individuals, the condition becomes pathological (the condition of anorexia nervosa). Often there is a history of associated psychological disturbances, including obsessional tendencies; the body mass drops to 35 to 40 kg, and weight loss may be sustained by compulsive exercising or deliberate vomiting after an eating "binge" (bulimia).

A parallel has been drawn between addiction to endurance running (a phenomenon associated with the exercise-induced secretion of beta-endorphins) and anorexia nervosa. Certainly many underweight adolescents exercise obsessively, but it is less certain that exercise addiction and anorexia nervosa are part of the same syndrome; in the true anorectic, the psychological disturbance is primary, while in the endurance exerciser, the addiction is probably secondary to the vigorous activity.

Energy Balance in Female Athletes

Inadequate food intake is common in sports where the current concept of beauty may influence the judges' decision, for example gymnastics, figure skating, and ballet dancing. Formal dietary studies have shown daily food intakes as low as 4 to 5 MJ, despite participation in vigorous activity programs. Debate continues as to whether an energy deficiency is at least one factor contributing to the primary amenorrhea seen in many competitors (Chapter 10).

FURTHER READING

American College of Sports Medicine. Position statement on proper and improper weight loss programs. 1983.

Bazan NG, Paoletti R, Iacono JM, eds. Current topics in nutrition and disease: new trends in nutrition, lipid research and cardiovascular diseases. New York: Allan R. Liss, 1981.

Bjorntorp P. Physiological and clinical aspects of exercise in obese persons. Exerc Sport Sci Rev 1983; 159–180.

Booth FW, Nicholson WF, Watson PA. Influence of muscle use on protein synthesis and degradation. Exerc Sport Sci Rev 1982; 10:27–48.

Brotherhood JR. Nutrition and sports performance. Sports Med 1984; 1:350–389.

Carlson FD, Wilkie DR. Muscle physiology. Englewood Cliffs: Prentice Hall, 1974.

Darby PL, Garfinkel PE, Garner DM, Coscina DV. Anorexia nervosa. Recent developments in research. New York: Alan R. Liss, 1983.

Davidson S, Passmore R, Brock JF. Human nutrition and dietetics. Edinburgh: Churchill Livingstone, 1972.

Durnin JVGA. Protein requirements and physical activity.

In: Pařízková J, Rogozkin VA, eds. Nutrition, physical fitness and health. Baltimore: University Park Press, 1978.

Durnin JVGA, Passmore R. Energy, work and leisure. London: Heinemann, 1967.

Gollnick P. Delivery and uptake of substrates. In: Landry F, Orban WAR, eds. Third international symposium on the biochemistry of exercise. Miami: Symposia Specialists, 1978.

Goodman MN, Ruderman NB. Influence of muscle use on amino acid metabolism. Exerc Sport Sci Rev 1982; 10:1–26.

Gooto AM, Smith LC, Allen B. Atherosclerosis V. Berlin: Springer Verlag, 1980.

Harrison GA. Energy and effort. London: Taylor & Francis, 1982.

Hartung GH. Diet and exercise in the regulation of plasma lipids and lipoproteins in patients at risk of coronary disease. Sports Med 1984; 1:413–418.

Haskell WL. The influence of exercise on the concentrations of triglyceride and cholesterol in human plasma. Exerc Sport Sci Rev 1984; 12:205–244.

Holloszy JO, Winder WW, Filts RH, et al. Energy production during exercise. In: Landry F, Orban WAR, eds. Third international symposium on the biochemistry of exercise. Miami: Symposia Specialists, 1978.

Howald H, Von Glutz G, Billiter R. Energy stores and substrate utilization in muscle during exercise. In: Landry F, Orban WAR, eds. Third international symposium on the biochemistry of exercise. Miami: Symposia Specialists, 1978.

Hultman E. Regulation of carbohydrate metabolism in the liver during rest and exercise, with special reference to diet. In: Landry F, Orban WAR, eds. Third international symposium on the biochemistry of exercise. Miami: Symposia Specialists, 1978.

Karlsson J. Localized muscular fatigue: role of muscle metabolism and substrate depletion. Exerc Sport Sci Rev 1979; 7:1–42.

Lemon PW, Nagle F. Effects of exercise on protein and amino acid metabolism. Med Sci Sports 1981; 13:141–149.

Levine R, Pfeiffer EF, Mahler RJ, Zeigler R. Lipid metabolism, obesity and diabetes mellitus: impact upon atherosclerosis. Stuttgart: Thieme, 1974.

Levy RI, Rifkind BM, Dennis BH, Ernst ND. Nutrition, lipids, and coronary heart disease—a global view. New York: Raven Press, 1979.

Margaria R. Biomechanics and energetics of muscular exercise. Oxford: Clarendon Press, 1976.

McCance RA, Widdowson EM. The composition of foods. Spec. Rep. Series, Med. Res. Counc. London. 297. 1960.

McGarry JD, Foster DW. Regulation of hepatic fatty acid oxidation and ketone body production. Ann Rev Biochem 1980; 49:395–420.

Newsholme EA. Control of energy provision and utilization in muscle in relation to sustained exercise. In: Landry F, Orban WAR, eds. Third international symposium on the biochemistry of exercise. Miami: Symposia Specialists, 1978.

Oscai LB, Palmer WK. Cellular control of triacylgylcerol metabolism. Exerc Sport Sci Rev 1983; 11:1–23.

Oscai LB, McGarr JA, Borensztayn J. Sources of fatty acids for oxidation during exercise. In: Landry F, Orban WAR, eds. Third international symposium on biochemistry of exercise. Miami: Symposia Specialists, 1978.

Pernow B, Saltin B. Muscle metabolism during exercise. New York: Plenum Press, 1971.

Pollitt E, Amante P. Energy intake and activity. New York: Alan R. Liss, 1984.

Poortmans JR. Protein turnover during exercise. In: Landry F, Orban WAR, eds. Third international symposium on biochemistry of exercise. Miami: Symposia Specialists, 1978.

Porter R, Whelan J. Human muscle fatigue: physiological mechanisms. London: Pitman Medical, 1981.

Randle PJ. Molecular mechanisms regulating fuel selection in muscle. In: Poortmans J, Nisset G, eds. Biochemistry of exercise IVa. Baltimore: University Park Press, 1981.

Ricci G, Venerando A. Nutrition, dietetics and sport. Torino: Ed. Minerva Medica, 1978.

Shephard RJ. Biochemistry of physical activity. Springfield, Ill: CC Thomas, 1984.

Smith LC, Pownhall HJ, Gotto AM. The plasma lipoproteins: structure and metabolism. Ann Rev Biochem 1978; 47:751–777.

Wahren J, Bjorkman O. Hormones, exercise and regulation of splanchnic glucose output in normal man. In: Poortmans J, Nisset G, eds. Biochemistry of exercise IVa. Baltimore: University Park Press, 1981.

Young VR. Skeletal muscle and whole body protein metabolism in relation to exercise. In: Poortmans JR, Nisset G, eds. Biochemistry of exercise IVa. Baltimore: University Park Press, 1981.

HUMORAL REGULATION IN EXERCISE

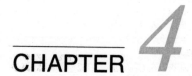

CHAPTER 4

GENERAL FEATURES

HYPOTHALAMIC AND PITUITARY HORMONES
  Hypothalamus and Posterior Pituitary Gland
  Growth Hormone
  Prolactin
  Endorphins
  Other Hormones

THYROID HORMONES

ADRENAL CORTEX
  Cortisol
  Aldosterone and Renal Hormones

CATECHOLAMINES
  Varieties of Catecholamine
  Varieties of Receptor
  Response to Exercise

PANCREATIC HORMONES
  Insulin
  Glucagon

ANDROGENS

FEMALE HORMONES
  Hormonal Changes During the Menstrual Cycle
  Performance and the Menstrual Cycle

OTHER HORMONES
  Prostaglandins
  Somatomedin

GENERAL FEATURES

While the central nervous system is well-adapted to the purpose of regulation against the acute problems of thermal and gaseous homeostasis associated with increased energy usage, the endocrine system plays a major role in adaptations to vigorous physical activity, ensuring delivery of appropriate amounts of fuel to the active muscles (Table 4-1). It is also implicated in many other aspects of long-term control during sustained activity. It is thus hardly surprising to find that exercise increases the blood levels of many hormones.

It should be stressed immediately that an increase in the blood concentration of a hormone does not neces- sarily imply an increased secretion of the substance in question. Other possibilities include hemoconcentra- tion, a decreased breakdown in the liver (because of reduced hepatic blood flow), a decreased excretion (caused by a reduced renal blood flow), or a decreased rate of uptake by target tissues (with no change in the rate of production). Moreover, the functional response depends not only on the blood concentration, but also on the proportion of the hormone that is bound to pro- teins, the blood flow to the target organ, and the num- ber of active receptor sites in the target organ. Finally, observed changes in the rate of hormone secretion may reflect a diurnal rhythm or an effect of emotion rather than a response to exercise.

TABLE 4-1   Hormones Possibly Involved in the Response to Physical Activity

Site of Production	Hormone	Main Functions
Hypothalamus	Somatoliberin	Stimulates release of somatotropin
	Somatostatin	Inhibits release of somatotropin
	Thyroliberin	Stimulates release of thyrotropin
	Corticoliberin	Stimulates release of corticotropin
	Luliberin	Stimulates release of lutotropin
	Prolactoliberin	Stimulates release of prolactin
	Prolactostatin	Inhibits release of prolactin
	Antidiuretic hormone	Released from posterior pituitary, increases renal water retention
Anterior pituitary	Somatotropin (growth hormone, GH)	Stimulates bone growth and fat mobilization
	Thyrotropin (thyroid stimulating hormone, TSH)	Stimulates production and release of thyroxine
	Corticotropin (adrenocorticotropic hormone, ACTH)	Stimulates production and release of adrenal cortical hormones
	Luteotropin (luteinizing hormone, LH)	Stimulates production of testosterone by testes, promotes development of corpus luteum in females
	Prolactin	Stimulates renal water retention, fat mobilization, and (in female) lactation
	Endorphins	Relieves fatigue, elevates mood
Thyroid gland	Thyroxine	Stimulates mitochondrial function, cell growth
	Calcitonin	Reduces blood calcium, phosphate levels
Adrenal cortex	Cortisol and others	Promotes fat utilization, conserves glucose, reduces inflammation
	Aldosterone and others	Promotes renal sodium and water retention
Adrenal medulla	Epinephrine, norepinephrine	Enhances cardiac output, vasoconstriction, glycogen breakdown, fat mobilization
Pancreas	Insulin	Promotes glucose uptake by cells, increases glycogen storage
	Glucagon	Promotes glucose release from liver, mobilizes fat, increases cardiac output
Parathyroid glands	Parathyroid hormone	Increases blood calcium, decreases blood phosphate
Testes	Testosterone	Increases muscle mass, decreases body fat, increases muscle glycogen and red cell production in male subjects (females produce androgens in adrenals)
Liver	Somatomedin	Activated by somatotropin, stimulates cartilage and bone growth
Kidneys	Angiotensin	Increases central blood volume
Various tissues	Prostaglandins	Function varies with specific chemistry of prostaglandin, e.g., vasodilation, bronchodilation or constriction, increase of cardiac output

Based in part on collected data of D. Lamb

Our knowledge of the mode of action of hormones is expanding rapidly; in general, they alter (1) the rate of synthesis of specific enzyme proteins, (2) the rate of synthesis of adenosine 3':5'-cyclic adenosine mono phosphate (cyclic AMP) and prostaglandins (thus exerting an indirect effect on enzyme activity or membrane permeability), or (3) the permeability of cell membranes.

HYPOTHALAMIC AND PITUITARY HORMONES

Hypothalamus and Posterior Pituitary Gland

The hypothalamus secretes various "tropins" and "statins" that augment or depress the function of other endocrine glands. Since the activity of many of the target glands is enhanced by exercise, an increased output of tropins seems probable, although there is as yet little direct experimental evidence of this. An increased output of antidiuretic hormone from the posterior pituitary gland probably contributes to the suppression of urine formation when exercising under warm conditions. Regulation of the hypothalmic-pituitary hormonal axis is shown in Figure 4–1.

Growth Hormone

The growth hormone of the anterior pituitary gland has many important functions. It stimulates anabolism, strengthening muscle ligaments and tendons, while increasing bone thickness. It also enhances the synthesis of an inactive form of adipolytic lipase (the enzyme responsible for mobilizing depot fat), and in muscle counteracts the effects of insulin, either by inhibiting the membrane transport of glucose, or, more probably, by inhibiting glycogen breakdown (glycolysis) secondary to the increased blood concentrations of glucose and free fatty acids which it induces (Fig. 4–2). In the liver, glycogen storage is increased, perhaps because of increased gluconeogenesis.

A substantial (20- to 40-fold) increase of growth hormone levels is seen after 20 minutes of exercise at 40 to 50 percent of maximum oxygen intake. Subsequent hepatic degradation of growth hormone occurs with a half-time of approximately 30 minutes. Among suggested triggers to release of the hormone, we may note the psychological stress of either competition or experiment, the rise of core temperature, changes in plasma amino acids or glucose, and some consequence of anaerobic effort (such as an accumulation of lactate or hydrogen ions). Amino acids are a potent stimulus to growth hormone secretion under resting conditions,

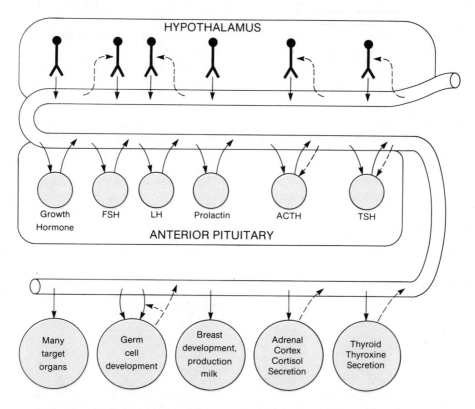

Figure 4–1 Regulation of hypothalamic/pituitary hormonal axis. Negative feedback is shown by interrupted lines. Heavy solid lines are neural connections, light solid lines are hormonal connections.

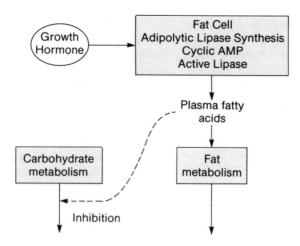

Figure 4–2 Diagram illustrating possible mode of action of growth hormone. Some authors believe growth hormone has two components—one (AcG) accelerates the formation of free fatty acids from depot fat. The other (InG) opposes this process and also inhibits key enzymes in carbohydrate breakdown (glyceraldehyde 3 phosphate and alpha glycerophosphate dehydrogenase).

and the release of triggering substances such as arginine seems a plausible hypothesis. Growth hormone also facilitates the entry of amino acids into active muscle cells, functioning as a linear amplifier of anabolism. There have been several recent reports of athletes who have been given injections of growth hormone in an illegal attempt to stimulate muscle hypertrophy (Chapter 14). Since the hormone is a natural body secretion, the detection and policing of this form of "doping" is extremely difficult.

Metabolic regulation by growth hormone is important in sustained exercise, when reserves of muscle and liver glycogen are becoming depleted. Muscle glucose uptake is decreased, because the phosphorylation of glucose by the enzyme hexokinase is inhibited (glucose must be converted to glucose-6-phosphate to cross the cell membrane). This action of the hormone serves to stabilize a falling blood sugar. Conversely, an increased output of growth hormone can be delayed or prevented by feeding a subject large doses of glucose or sucrose. Growth hormone also contributes to the late mobilization of fat during prolonged exercise, and by sustaining blood sugar it may enhance the output of insulin.

Prolactin

Prolactin mobilizes fat and has an antidiuretic effect upon the kidneys. Increased blood levels are seen following exercise. Occasional authors have attributed athletic amenorrhea (Chapter 10) to an increased secretion of prolactin, although this hypothesis is not now widely accepted.

Endorphins

Knowledge of the endorphins has grown rapidly over the 10 years since their discovery, although their precise functions remain a matter of controversy. They are produced in the intermediate lobe of the pituitary gland, and have some chemical similarity to the opiates. The nature and extent of endorphin responses can be tested by giving a blocking agent (naloxone). Release of endorphin is increased by both long-distance endurance exercise and heavy weight-lifting, but the response appears to be unchanged by training. It has thus been hypothesized that (1) such substances may contribute to the runner's "high," and (2) a chemical addiction to long-distance running is at least a technical possibility. An increase of beta-endorphins may depress respiration and the sensation of fatigue during prolonged exercise; it may also contribute to the increased output of growth hormones and prostaglandins and may be a factor in exercise-induced amenorrhea.

Other Hormones

The anterior pituitary secretes other trophic hormones (see Fig. 4–1), including follicle-stimulating hormone and luteinizing hormone (FSH, LH), adrenocorticotrophic hormone (ACTH), and thyroid-stimulating hormone (TSH). The secretion of each of these substances is apparently modified by vigorous and sustained exercise.

THYROID HORMONES

Thyroxine secretion is stimulated by pituitary thyrotropin. Blood concentrations of the latter are increased before, but not during, exercise. Since the blood stream half-life of the thyroid stimulating hormone (TSH) is approximately 1 hour, it may be that the anticipatory secretion of TSH accounts for the increased secretion of thyroxine during exercise. The free thyroxine level rises approximately 35 percent, but because degradation is also enhanced, physical activity may not increase the total of free and bound thyroxine in the blood.

One important function of thyroxine is to "uncouple" carbohydrate metabolism, so that the energy content of the foodstuff is liberated as heat rather than generating the anticipated number of high-energy adenosine triphosphate (ATP) molecules. Changes of thyroxine secretion may thus help acclimatization to very cold or very hot climates by modifying the rate of basal metabolism (Chapter 12). The thyroid hormone can also help in mobilizing fatty acids, and in promoting cardiac hypertrophy.

Training increases the plasma concentration of free thyroxine, but degradation is also accelerated, the half-life decreasing from 7 to 4 days. For some reason, basal metabolism remains unchanged by physical conditioning.

ADRENAL CORTEX

Cortisol

Cortisol is the most important of a group of glucocorticoids secreted by the adrenal cortex (Fig. 4–3). It mobilizes both fat and protein, thus conserving carbohydrates and at the same time elevating blood glucose. The primary mechanism of action of cortisol is probably to stimulate production of the hepatic enzymes involved in deaminating aminoacids, thus enhancing the rate of glucose production in the liver. Prolonged administration of cortisol leads to a wasting of muscle and a weakening of bone, (caused by both a loss of calcium and a reduction of the organic matrix). Within the muscle, glucose uptake is inhibited, and carbohydrate usage is decreased. Within adipose tissue, the synthesis of lipase is enhanced, and lipolysis is thus increased. Inactive forms of lipase are also activated by a chain reaction involving epinephrine, adenyl cyclase, and cyclic AMP. Excessive secretion of cortisol gives a general stress response with suppression of immune reactions, a reduction in the eosinophil count, and involution of the thymus. Lastly, water balance may be disturbed by sodium retention and potassium excretion.

Moderate levels of exercise have little effect on blood cortisol levels, but if exercise is heavy and prolonged, concentrations rise. If activity is very prolonged, there is ultimately a fall in blood cortisol levels that coincides with impending exhaustion of the adrenal cortex. Surgical removal of the adrenal glands has little impact on adjustment to moderate effort, but it does shorten the maximum working time. During brief exhausting effort (e.g., exercise at 140 percent of maximum oxygen intake), increased concentrations of cortisol are seen within 1 minute, and in such circumstances it is thought that the triggering intermediary is a locally secreted catecholamine (see section on Varieties of Catecholamine) rather than pituitary adrenocorticotropic hormone.

Training apparently increases the mass of the adrenal glands. The release of glucocorticoids at any given intensity of effort is diminished in a well-conditioned individual, but the time to exhaustion of the glands is increased.

Aldosterone and Renal Hormones

Aldosterone is the most important mineralocorticoid secreted by the adrenal cortex (Fig. 4–4). It encourages the retention of sodium ions and thus fluid, leading to an expansion of extracellular fluid volume and a rise in blood pressure. During exercise, there is a substantial increase in the secretion of this hormone, probably triggered by a fall of central venous pressure and/or a decrease of renal flow. The output of aldosterone is further boosted by heat acclimatization, with an associated decrease in the sodium content of sweat.

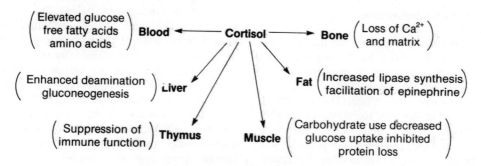

Figure 4–3 Sites of action of cortisol.

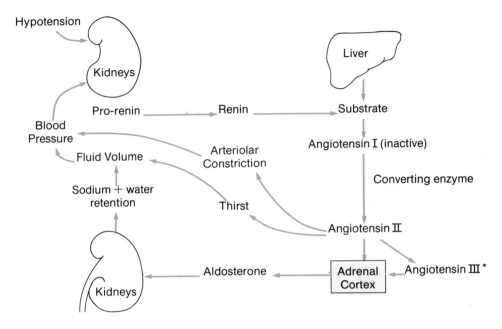

Figure 4–4   Schematic of aldosterone and angiotensin regulation of fluid volumes.

  * Note: Angiotensin III has 7 rather than 8 polypeptide links and is a more powerful stimulant of aldosterone output than Angiotensin II.

The decrease of renal flow stimulates the kidneys to release pro-renin, which is activated to renin; acting on a hepatic substrate, the latter forms the hormone angiotensin I. Converting enzyme in turn converts this substance to angiotensin II (an active form), and some is further modified to the yet more active compound angiotensin III. Angiotensin II and III in turn stimulate release of aldosterone from the adrenal cortex. At the same time, angiotensin II boosts arterial blood pressure by arteriolar constriction and a stimulation of thirst. In distance events such as a marathon race (where renal flow is severely curtailed), plasma renin may reach astronomic levels.

CATECHOLAMINES

Varieties of Catecholamine

Much of the older research on the naturally occurring catecholamines adrenaline (epinephrine) and noradrenaline (norepinephrine) is based on urinary assays. However, such figures give only a partial picture of the total output, since a large fraction of both norepinephrine and epinephrine secretions are metabolized before they are excreted. Brain catecholamines are excreted mainly as 3 methoxy-4 hydroxy-phenyl glycol (MHPG), while catecholamines from other sites appear as a mixture of MHPG and vanillylmandelic acid (Fig.

4–5). The sympathetic nerve endings secrete largely norepinephrine, and they are called into action by either an irradiation of impulses from the motor cortex or a fall of central blood pressure. The adrenal medulla yields 75 percent epinephrine and 25 percent norepinephrine; it is stimulated by either emotional stress or a drop of blood glucose to less than 60 mg per deciliter.

Varieties of Receptor

The functional role of the sympathetic nerves in increasing cardiac output, sustaining systemic blood pressure, and redistributing blood flow to the working muscles is well-recognized. The tissues have two main types of catecholamine receptors: alpha receptors (which yield an excitatory response) and beta receptors (where the response is inhibitory, except in the heart, where it remains excitatory). The beta receptors are further subdivided into type one (stimulated rather equally by epinephrine and norepinephrine, and yielding an increase of myocardial contractility, increased activity of lipolytic lipase, and an inhibition of gut motility) and type two (stimulated by epinephrine, and yielding bronchodilatation together with a stimulation of glycogen breakdown in skeletal muscle). Many post-coronary patients are treated by beta-blocking agents. They thus fail to show the normal increase of heart rate during exercise, and they may also complain of muscular weakness because of a smaller exercise-induced

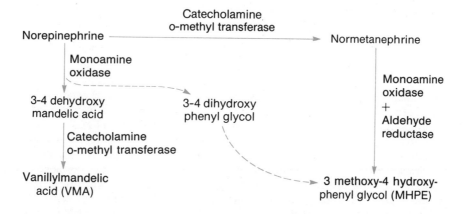

Figure 4–5 Pathways for metabolism of catecholamines.

mobilization of fat and glycogen. However, the body has alternative mechanisms which allow some glycogen breakdown to continue after beta-blockade, both in muscle (a calcium ion activation of the enzyme phosphorylase) and in liver (responses to hypoxia and secretion of the hormone glucagon). Likewise, the pituitary hormones and testosterone permit some continuing usage of fat.

Response to Exercise

During laboratory exercise, norepinephrine output is usually greater than that of epinephrine. However, significant amounts of epinephrine are produced under the stress of competition, or if oxygen consumption approaches maximal values. Exhausting activity may lead to an eventual decline of plasma epinephrine, suggesting that the adrenal medulla has become exhausted.

Training reduces plasma catecholamine levels at a given power output. It does not change the response at a given percentage of maximum oxygen intake, but there is an increase in the epinephrine content of the resting adrenal gland, presumably leaving it less vulnerable to exhaustion.

PANCREATIC HORMONES

Insulin

The feedback loops involved in the supply of glucose and free fatty acids to the exercising tissues are quite complex (Fig. 4–6). Insulin regulates the transfer

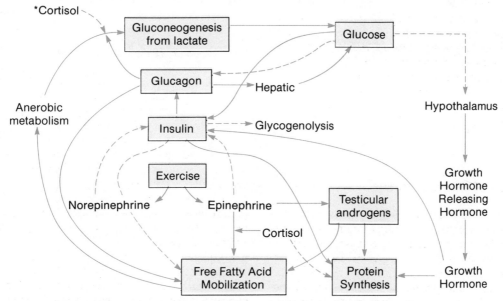

Figure 4–6 Interaction of hormones in glucose regulation during exercise. Negative feedback shown by interrupted lines.
* Cortisol blocks the entry of glycose into many types of cells. However, it facilitates conversion of amino acids into glucose in the liver.

of glucose from the blood stream into tissues, such as skeletal muscle. It promotes muscle glycogen storage and is essential to the process of glycogen "super-compensation" before a distance race. It also promotes the uptake of glucose by adipocytes (Figs. 4–7 and 4–8).

Plasma insulin levels drop by as much as 50 percent during and immediately after exercise. This reflects both a decrease of pancreatic secretion and an increased uptake of the hormone by the skeletal muscles. The insulin delivery to the working muscles is nevertheless increased, since local blood flow is increased 20- to 30-fold during physical activity. The combination of a reduced visceral flow and low plasma insulin concentrations favors the release of hepatic glycogen during vigorous exercise. Training typically curtails the depression of plasma insulin during exercise, possibly because of a lesser secretion of catecholamines.

Habitual physical activity helps to control blood glucose and reduces the need for insulin in diabetic patients, particularly in those with maturity onset diabetes. Several mechanisms are involved, including (1) the direct metabolic breakdown of sugars immediately following a carbohydrate meal, (2) an increased avidity of the muscles for glucose, and (3) the sparing of functionally weak insulin-secreting cells in the pancreatic islets following the ingestion of sugar. Provided that food intake is increased appropriately to match energy usage, most diabetics respond well to an exercise regimen. However, care must be taken that an increased local blood flow to a depot of injected insulin in an active limb does not lead to an excessively rapid absorption of the hormone, with a sudden fall of blood glucose (a hypoglycemic crisis).

Glucagon

Glucagon has the opposite type of action to insulin, raising blood glucose by activating enzymes that break down liver glycogen (Fig. 4–9). It also helps to increase myocardial contractility and releases fatty acids into the blood stream by an action upon the enzyme adenyl-cyclase within the adipocytes.

Short periods of exhausting exercise give rise to a 2-fold increase of blood glucagon, and some elevation of readings persists for 30 minutes after activity has ceased. While this hormone probably contributes to the mobilization of hepatic glycogen, animals are able to deplete their liver glycogen even after release of glucagon has been checked by surgical removal of the pancreas.

Highly trained subjects increase blood glucagon levels less than untrained individuals when exercising at any given fraction of maximum oxygen intake.

ANDROGENS

The unfortunate interest of many athletes in muscle-building by the illegal use of drugs has sparked a vigorous study of naturally occurring androgens such as testosterone (secretion 0.1 mg per day in women, 5 to 10 mg per day in men) and androstenedione (secretion 2 to 4 mg per day in women, 1 to 2 mg per day in men), along with synthetic analogues, such as danabol, which exaggerate the anabolic properties, while minimizing the virilizing effects of testosterone. Human research has been hampered by the reluctance of investigators

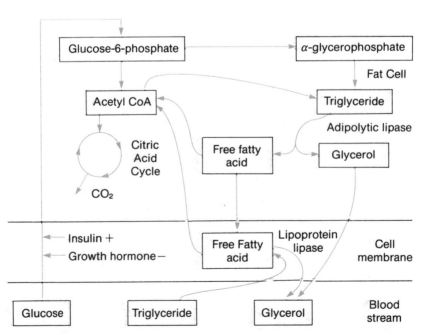

Figure 4–7   Regulation of glucose and fat usage at the membranes of the fat cell.

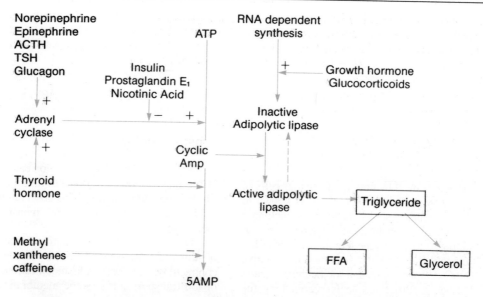

Figure 4–8 The various hormones involved in activation of adipolytic lipase (based in part on Harper, 1969).

to give the gross overdoses (100 mg per day or more) sometimes taken illegally by strength athletes, but it is now widely believed that massive doses of steroids do enhance muscle development (Chapter 14).

At the cellular level, androgens induce a stimulation of amino acid uptake, with synthesis of the fundamental cellular building blocks ribonucleic acid (RNA) and deoxyribonucleic acid (DNA), a growth of individual muscle fibers, and a facilitation of glycogen storage. Body fat content is decreased, red cell formation is stimulated, bone thickness is increased, and aggressive behavior is stimulated.

Adolescent boys show a rapid development of strength coincident with puberty, and this has been attributed to an increased secretion of testosterone by the interstitial cells of the testes. Androgens are sometimes given to older men to encourage the rebuilding of muscles following immobilization or injury, although it is less clearly established that such therapy is necessary or effective.

It is now generally agreed that testosterone levels are low in distance runners. This is possibly due to an inadequate intake of food energy, since a drop of serum testosterone has also been described in wrestlers who engage in severe dieting. In untrained subjects, exercise has little acute effect upon androgen levels, but in Olympic-caliber contestants the acute response is an increase of blood concentrations. There is no evidence

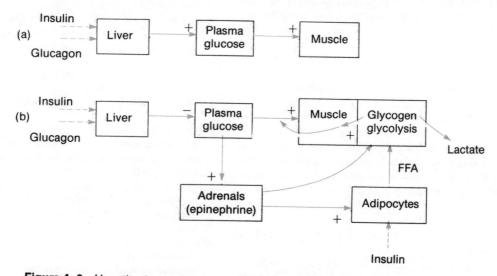

Figure 4–9 Hypothesized role of glucagon (a) during exercise, and (b) effect of glucagon suppression. Based in part on concepts of Wasserman and Vranic.

of an increased output of the pituitary regulator luteo-tropin, and the most likely explanation seems to be a checking of hepatic breakdown of androgens during vigorous exercise.

FEMALE HORMONES

Hormonal Changes During the Menstrual Cycle

Estrone is produced by both the follicular cells of the ovaries and by the adrenal glands. It is known to induce female secondary sex characteristics, including the feminine pattern of subcutaneous fat deposition, and it is also supposed to encourage female patterns of be-havior (although it is hard to disentangle the relative importance of hormone output and sociocultural factors to such behavior). Progesterone is secreted by the corpus luteum during the second half of each menstrual cycle. Changes in the relative proportions of proges-terone and estrone towards the end of the cycle disturb fluid balance, giving rise to water retention and the premenstrual tension syndrome.

Performance and the Menstrual Cycle

There have been numerous attempts to document changes of performance during the menstrual cycle, but the reported effects have been small, and sometimes it has been difficult to distinguish hormonal responses from associated problems of personal hygiene. In gen-eral, skilled performance deteriorates during the phase of premenstrual tension, but certain skills may actually be performed better during the phase of menstrual flow. Some athletes now use hormone preparations to mani-pulate the timing of their menstrual cycles, in the hope of facilitating their participation in major competitions.

Female reactions to intensive exercise have been studied particularly in the context of primary amenor-rhea (a failure to initiate menstrual cycles at the normal age of puberty) and secondary amenorrhea (the cessa-tion of menstruation during a period of hard training). One postulated explanation of the menstrual distur-bances is a negative energy balance; Rose Frisch has argued that a certain minimum of body fat is neces-sary to normal menstruation. This could be viewed as a method of protecting the body against pregnancy when food is in short supply. A second hypothesis (no longer widely accepted) has been an increase of blood prolac-tin concentrations. There may also be some decrease in blood levels both of estrone and progesterone (see further, Chapter 10); however, the primary cause of the menstrual disturbance is far from resolved.

Many athletes welcome amenorrhea as a means of avoiding the inconvenience of menstruation. The main drawback is a decrease of bone density. So far as is known there are no other harmful, long-term sequelae

to the exercise-induced disturbance of menstrual rhythm. Normal cycles return when training is modera-ted, and there is no evidence that subsequent fertility is impaired.

OTHER HORMONES

Prostaglandins

Ergometer cycling to exhaustion causes an increase in the plasma concentration of some prostaglandins. The practical importance of this observation for women is that it may lead to painful menstruation (dys-menorrhea).

Other effects of prostaglandins include an increase of skin and muscle blood flow, an increase of cardiac contractility, a decrease of fat mobilization, and changes of ion transport across some membranes.

Somatomedin

Somatomedin is secreted by the liver in response to a pituitary somatotropin. Since somatotropin levels are known to increase during exercise, an increased out-put of somatomedin might be inferred. The latter hor-mone encourages sulphation of chondroitin, and thus stimulates the growth of cartilage and bone.

FURTHER READING

Atria A. Endocrine function tests. Springfield, Ill: CC Tho-mas, 1970.

Galbo H. Catecholamines and muscular exercise. Assessment of sympathoadrenal activity. In: Poortmans J, Niset G, eds. Biochemistry IVb. Baltimore: University park Press, 1981:5.

Haymaker W, Anderson E, Nanta WJH. The hypothalamus. Springfield, Ill: CC Thomas, 1972.

Herber JV, Sutton J. Endorphins and exercise. Sports Med 1984; 1:154–174.

Kochakian CD. Anabolic—androgenic steroids. Berlin: Springer Verlag, 1976.

Lamb DR. Androgens and exercise. Med Sci Sport 1975; 7:1–5.

Lefkowitz RJ, Caron MG, Michel T, Stadel JM. Mechan-isms of hormone receptor-effector coupling: — the β adrenergic receptor and adenylate cyclase. Fed Proc 1982; 41:2664–2670.

Luyckx AS, Pirnay F, Krzentowski G, Lefebvre PJ. Insulin and glucagon during prolonged muscular exercise. In: Poortmans J, Niset G, eds. Biochemistry of exercise IVa. Baltimore: University Park Press, 1981:131.

Milledge JS, Bryson EI, Catley DM et al. Sodium balance fluid homeostasis and the renin-aldosterone system dur-ing the prolonged exercise of hill walking. Clin Sci 1982; 62:595–604.

Newsholme EA, Crabtree B. General principles of hormonal regulation of metabolism. In: Poortmans J, Niset G, eds.

Biochemistry of exercise IVa. Baltimore: University Park Press, 1981:46.

Robison GA, Butcher RW, Sutherland EW. Cyclic AMP. New York: Academic Press, 1971.

Shephard RJ, Sidney KH. Effects of physical exercise on plasma growth hormone and cortisol levels in human subjects. Exerc Sport Sci Rev 1975; 3:1–50.

Terjung RL, Winder WW. Exercise and thyroid function. Med Sci Sport 1975; 7:20–26.

Viru A. Exercise metabolism and endocrine function. In: Knuttgen HG, Vogel JA, Poortmans J, eds. Biochemistry of exercise, Volume 13. Champaign, Ill: Human Kinetics Publishers, 1983.

Von Euler VS. Sympatho-adrenal activity in physical exercise. Med Sci Sport 1974; 6:165–173.

Vranic M, Kawamori R, Wrenshall GA. The role of insulin and glucagon in regulating glucose turnover in dogs during exercise. Med Sci Sports; 1975; 7:27–33.

Wahren J, Bjorkman O. Hormones, exercise and regulation of splanchnic glucose output in normal man. In: Poortmans J, Niset G, eds. Biochemistry of exercise IVa. Baltimore: University Park Press, 1981:149.

Winder WW, Premachandra BN. Thyroid hormones and muscular exercise. In: Poortmans J, Niset G, eds. Biochemistry IVb. Baltimore: University Park Press, 1981:131.

APPLIED EXERCISE PHYSIOLOGY

NEUROMUSCULAR ASPECTS OF EXERCISE

CHAPTER *5*

Forms of Sensory Feedback
Balance and Steadiness
Conscious Proprioception
Response Time

TESTING MUSCLE FUNCTION

Muscle Dimensions
Explosive Force
Isometric Force
Isometric Endurance
Isotonic Force
Isokinetic Force
Power Output Tests
Quantitative Electromyography
Normal Standards

THE SKELETAL SUPPORT SYSTEM

Ligaments and Tendons
Joints
Articular Cartilage
Joint Capsule and Synovial Fluid
Bone
Static Flexibility
Dynamic Flexibility

GENERAL CONSIDERATIONS

The muscle fibers of the body are essentially the transducers, whereby the substantial chemical energy stored in food is released and translated into body movement. The total bulk of the musculature is such that it constitutes the largest organ group in the body (approximately 40 percent of body mass, or 24 kg in a 60 kg young woman). It has a highly variable blood supply (10 to 20 ml per kilogram at rest. 1ℓ per kilogram in vigorous exercise) and the resultant increase of flow (0.25ℓ per minute rising to as much as 25ℓ per minute) can present a substantial challenge to circulatory homeostasis.

Isotonic and Isometric Movements

In animal experiments, a clear distinction can be drawn between isotonic contractions (where a muscle shortens rapidly with a negligible increase of tension) and isometric contractions (where a muscle develops a large increase of tension, with little change of length). Human movements are often a complex mixture of isotonic and isometric contractions. Nevertheless, we still distinguish some muscles specializing in fast movements (where individual fibers are implanted end-on to the tendons), and other more slowly contracting muscles (where fibers are implanted at an angle to their tendons). These are known as fusiform and pennate or bipennate insertion arrangements, respectively (Fig. 5-1).

Agonists, Synergists, and Antagonists

Distinction is drawn between agonists (muscles that initiate a given movement), synergists (that assist in performing the movement, for example by stabilizing body posture), and antagonists (that control the speed and accuracy of the movement, checking displacement of body part once the desired action has been completed).

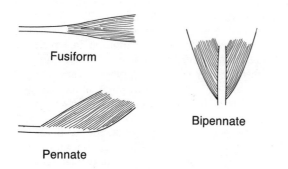

Figure 5–1 Fusiform and pennate types of fiber insertion. The fusiform pattern facilitates rapid movement; the pennate or bipennate form is designed for more powerful movements.

MUSCLE FIBER TYPES

Basis of Classification

Physiologists originally distinguished "red" and "white" muscles, on the basis of their color and thus their content of the red pigment myoglobin. More recently, individual fibers have been classified on the basis of their contractile properties (slow- or fast-twitch) and their metabolic characteristics (whether aerobic or anaerobic enzymes are predominant). In animals (and probably in man), one can separate Type I (slow-twitch, red, aerobic fibers), Type IIa (intermediate fibers, with a fast-twitch speed, but having both oxidative and glycolytic properties), Type IIb (fast-twitch, white glycolytic fibers) and Type IIc (undifferentiated fibers).

Inheritance of Fiber Types

In general, endurance athletes are selected because they have a high proportion of Type I fibers (at least in the muscles critical to their sport), while Type II fibers predominate in power athletes. Training may enable Type IIb fibers to assume Type IIa properties, but there is no sound evidence that Type II fibers can be converted to Type I, or vice-versa (except in experiments where the nerves supplying slow and fast twitch muscles have been transposed). This is one important reason why athletes are said to be "born" rather than "made" as a result of prolonged training.

Characteristics of Fiber Types

Some of the more important characteristics of the several fiber types are summarized in Table 5-1. Type I fibers have a good capillary supply, a large content of fat, myoglobin, and oxidative enzymes, but a limited content of glycolytic enzymes. Type II fibers have only limited fat stores, much less myoglobin, and (particularly in Type IIb) a smaller number of mitochondria with a low concentration of oxidative enzymes. The end result of these various differences is that Type I and Type II fibers have approximately the same maximum rate of adenosine triphosphate (ATP) regeneration. However, the metabolic characteristics of the Type I fibers give them a capacity for sustained, fatigue-resistant activity; Type II fibers are better fitted to brief bursts of anaerobic activity at a high-power output.

Typical Fiber Distribution

Opinions on an athlete's fiber distribution are often based on needle biopsy of the muscle, with staining of metabolic marker enzymes (for instance, the relative

TABLE 5-1 Some Characteristics of the Three Main Fiber Types

Variable	Muscle Fibre Type		
	Type I (Red) (Slow Twitch)	Type IIa (Intermediate) (Fast-Oxidative)	Type IIb (White) (Fast-Glycolytic)
Fiber size	Small	Large	Medium
Motor neuron size	Small	Medium	Large
Size of motor unit	540 fibers	440 fibers	750 fibers
Capillary	4 / fiber	4 / fiber	3 / fiber
Myoglobin content	High	Moderate	Low
Fat content	High	Moderate	Low
Enzyme content			
ATPase	Low	High	High
Glycolytic enzymes	Low	Moderate	High
Mitochondrial enzymes	Moderate	High	Very low
Time to peak tension	80 msec	40 msec	30 msec
Maximum Tension	Low	Moderate	High
Liability to Recruitment	High (mainly submaximal effort)	Medium	Low (mainly maximal effort)
Fatigue resistance	High	Moderate	Very low
Functions	Low tension, postural and endurance work.	Moderate tension, medium endurance	High tension, rapid powerful movements.

proportions of the oxidative enzyme succinic-dehydrogenase and the glycolytic enzyme phosphofructokinase) or enzymes that reflect twitch-speed (myosin ATPase, stained after acid and alkaline pre-incubation). Unfortunately, the specimen thus obtained is drawn from a very small part of a given muscle, and is not necessarily representative even of that muscle, much less the status of the body as a whole. In an average sedentary person, the most commonly sampled muscle (the vastus lateralis) contains approximately 50 percent Type I fibers, 35 percent Type IIa, and 15 percent Type IIb. A similar fiber distribution is reported for many other limb muscles, such as the gastrocnemius, rectus femoris, deltoid, and biceps; on the other hand, postural muscles such as the soleus contain 75 to 90 percent Type II fibers.

Signal for Fiber Differentiation

The signal for fiber differentiation in early development appears to be transmitted via the motor nerve; in animal experiments where nerves to a fast and a slow muscle have been transposed, a corresponding exchange of characteristics has developed with respect to not only enzyme patterns and twitch speed, but also the characteristics of the muscle proteins. It is not yet clear whether a chemical is transmitted down the motor nerve or whether a cue to appropriate differentiation is provided by the characteristic pattern of neural impulses in a given nerve. If the latter is the case, an unscrupulous endurance athlete might engage in "nerve doping," submitting to a pattern of electrical stimulation that would encourage the conversion of Type II to Type I fibers or vice-versa. Although there have been reports that

low-frequency neural stimulation (5 to 10 Hz, typical of a Type I motor unit) increases aerobic enzyme activity, myoglobin content, and fatigue resistance in the corresponding muscle, recent research suggests that the main source of benefit is an improved intramuscular capillary supply, without conversion of Type II into Type I fibers.

FINE STRUCTURE OF MUSCLE FIBER

Overall Pattern of Organization

The structure of a typical muscle fiber is shown schematically in Figure 5-2 and 5-3. The motor nerve terminates in the motor end plate, about halfway along the muscle fiber. Here, the nerve emerges from its myelin sheath to form a number of "terminal knobs" that are in intimate contact with the outer (sarcolemmic) membrane of the muscle fiber.

The sarcolemma, which bounds the entire muscle fiber, comprises a mass of cytoplasm in which are embedded longitudinally running thick and thin filaments that interdigitate with each other and are arranged in the format of a regular hexagonal lattice. Regular invaginations of the sarcolemma give rise to a system of transverse tubules (t-system) which, in effect, carry the membrane into the interior of the muscle fiber. The transverse tubules end in swellings (central sacs), each of which lies in close apposition with two lateral sacs. The latter run into sarcoplasmic recticulum, a longitudinally oriented system of membranous sacs that extend between successive systems of transverse tubules. Small ribosome granules give parts of the sarcoplas-

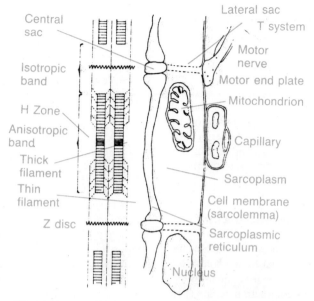

Figure 5-2 Schematic representation of muscle fiber.

mic reticulum a rough appearance. Here the muscle proteins are synthesized. Other parts of the sarcoplasmic reticulum provide binding sites for glycogen metabolizing enzymes.

The Oxygen Transport Pathway

Mitochondria are widely scattered through the sarcoplasm. Notice that the final steps of oxidative metabolism (for example, the breakdown of pyruvate to CO_2 and water) occur on the inner surface of the mitochondria. Oxygen must thus diffuse from capillaries in the immediate vicinity of the muscle fiber (4 to 6 capillaries per fiber, depending on fiber type), to within the mitochondria. An increase of muscle fiber size (e.g., with training) increases the length of the oxygen diffusion path *unless* there is also an increase in the number of mitochondria and/or capillaries per fiber; however, the metabolic impact of an increased oxygen

diffusion path length could be compensated by an increased activity of aerobic enzymes within a given mitochondrion. In general, the proportion of mitochondria found in unit volume of muscle tissue seems to increase in parallel with an individual's maximum oxygen transport. Energy is expended in transporting protons to the interior of the mitochondrion as part of the oxidation process (the so-called malate-aspartate shuttle, Chapter 3). The ATP yielded by glycogen breakdown is thus 37 moles per glucose equivalent, rather than the 39 moles calculated by looking at individual steps in the metabolic chain; 2 moles of ATP have been consumed during proton transfers.

Structure Under Light Microscopy

The contractile part of the fiber comprises a series of myofibrils, each approximately 1μ in diameter.

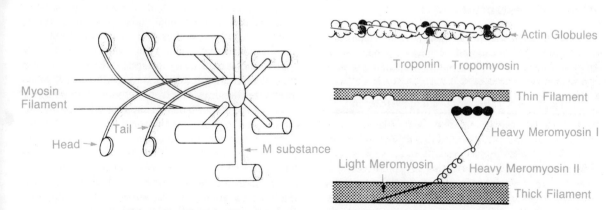

Figure 5-3 Schematic arrangement of thin and thick muscle filaments. The myosin molecules are wrapped around each other in the thick filaments, and are spaced as a regular hexagon by the M substance.

Many hundreds of myofibrils are found in a typical fiber. Light microscopy shows alternating dark and light bands that correspond to zones with differing ability to transmit polarized light; the normally transmitting isotropic (I band) and the anisotropic (A band). The reason for the special optical property of the A band is that rod-like structures are embedded in a medium of differing refractive index. Individual longitudinal segments of the fiber or sarcomeres are marked off by the Z discs or Zwischenscheiben, at the center of each I band. Toward the middle of the A band is a lighter H zone (Hellige = light), and at the center of the H zone is a narrow M line, or Mittelscheibe.

Structure Under Electron Microscopy

Electron microscopy confirms the filamentous nature of the muscle fiber. Interdigitating thick and thin filaments are arranged in a regular hexagonal lattice, sliding between each other as contraction occurs (Fig. 5-2). The main protein constituents of the two types of fiber are listed in Table 5-2. The thick filaments originate in the M structure (which contains M protein). Their main component is the long-chain protein myosin, but they also contain smaller amounts of C protein. The main constituent of the thin filaments is a long-chain (F) form of the protein actin. Polymerization from the globular (G) form of actin is facilitated by the presence of smaller amounts of β actinin within the filaments. The calcium-binding protein troponin is also found every eighth unit of the actin chain (a distance of 40 nm, or 40×10^{-9} m along the filament). A strand of tropomyosin is distributed longitudinally along the thin filaments, lying in a groove between two coils of F actin. Tropomyosin inhibits the interaction between actin and myosin by undergoing a slight lateral displacement within its central groove; this process is reversed as calcium ions react within troponin. Individual thin filaments originate in the Z discs that contain a further specific protein; alpha actinin.

Myosin Ultrastructure

The ultrastructure of the myosin molecule has now been studied in considerable detail. The long "tails" of its two protein chains are coiled around the thick

TABLE 5-2   Principal Muscle Proteins

Muscle Protein	% of Total Protein
Myosin	54 - 60
Actin	20 - 25
Tropomyosin	4.5 - 11
Troponin	2 - 5
α Actinin	2 - 10
β Actinin	
M protein	
C protein	

filament, while two shorter heads project towards the actin molecules. One part of each "head" has a strong ATPase activity (that is, an ability to convert ATP to ADP with release of energy), while a second part develops the reaction central to muscle contraction, a strong bonding (cross-bridge formation) with actin molecules (Fig. 5-3).

Growth and Hypertrophy

During the period of growth, the muscle can increase in length by adding sarcomeres; cross-section is increased by the splitting of myofibrils when they reach a critical size. There is no evidence that the number of independent muscle fibers can be increased by training (Chapter 9). Any increase of muscle cross-section thus reflects a combination of hypertrophy and fiber splitting.

CHEMICAL MECHANISM OF MUSCLE CONTRACTION

Neuromuscular Coupling

The cytoplasm in the terminal knobs of the motor nerve contains vesicles filled with acetylcholine. Periodically, a vesicle discharges into the neuromuscular cleft, inducing a local loss of negative change (depolarization) of the immediately adjacent sarcolemmal membrane; the electrical disturbance is quite small and is known as a miniature end-plate potential. However, when a nerve impulse reaches the motor end-plate there is a much more massive release of acetylcholine from the terminal knobs, and in the presence of calcium ions, the disturbance of membrane potential in the vicinity of the motor end-plate surpasses a threshold value. A wave of depolarization then passes along the entire length of the sarcolemma, with a corresponding disturbance of ionic balance across the membrane (an inward movement of sodium ions, and an outward movement of potassium ions). The electrical signal (a "propagated action potential") also penetrates inwards, via the transverse tubules. When the disturbance of membrane voltage reaches the triad of central and lateral sacs, it induces a substantial release of calcium. This diffuses longitudinally through the sarcoplasmic reticulum, bonding with troponin molecules along the length of the actin filaments, and thus allowing the formation of cross-bridges between actin and myosin.

The acetylcholine liberated at the neuromuscular junction is quickly hydrolyzed by the enzyme cholinesterase, forming choline and acetic acid. These compounds are readily reabsorbed by the terminal knobs of the motor nerves, allowing a resynthesis of acetylcholine. A "sodium pump" at the sarcolemmal membrane extrudes sodium ions and restores membrane potential. Relaxation of the muscle depends on the release of calcium from the contractile proteins and reabsorption of the calcium ions by storage sites in the sarcoplasmic reticulum. These various processes all consume ATP.

Cross-Bridge Formation

Muscle contraction depends on the formation of cross-bridges between actin and myosin. The bridges generate sufficient force to draw one set of filaments within the other. The maximum force is developed when the distance between two adjacent Z-discs is 2.0 to 2.5 μ (1 μ = 10^{-4} cm). Contraction is not possible if the sarcomere is elongated to a length (~3 μ) where the two types of filament no longer overlap (Inset to Fig. 5-4). Contraction is also impeded if there is too much overlap (sarcomere length <2.0 μ). When the thin filaments are activated by calcium ions, the heads of individual myosin molecules bind with receptor sites on the corresponding actin molecules, drawing the latter towards the equilibrium position for the head in question; once the equilibrium position has been passed, the actin-myosin bond ruptures and the myosin filament slides onwards toward the next actin receptor site. The minimum quantum of movement thus corresponds to the formation and rupture of a single actin-myosin bond—a longitudinal distance of approximately 1 nm, with a correspondingly slow speed of movement (10 nm per second, Fig. 5–5). However, each half sarcomere

has approximately 10 cross-bridges arranged in series, so that if all 10 cross-bridges are used, the total speed per half sarcomere is 2^9 times as rapid. Furthermore, individual sarcomeres are arranged in sequence with each other, so that the overall velocity of the fiber reaches $10^9 - 10^{10}$ nm per second (1 to 10 m per second!).

Energy Transfer

Energy stored within the terminal phosphate bond of ATP is needed for either the formation or the rupture or actin-myosin bonding (it is still debated which of the two processes is energy consuming). Release of the required energy is facilitated by a part of the myosin molecule, which functions as an ATPase. Under biological conditions of pH and ionic concentrations, the energy content of the ATP phosphate bond is approximately 46 kJ per mole. Given a 49 percent efficiency in the usage of this resource, the usable energy is 22.5 kJ per mole (Table 5–3). Since by Avogadro's hypothesis, each mole contains 6.02×10^{23} molecules, a single molecule of ATP yields 3.7×10^{-20} J. Further, a study of frog muscle estimated that a single actin-myosin bond yielded a force of 3×10^{-12} N. Since work = force × distance, a single ATP molecule should draw the muscle filament through 3.7×10^{-12}, or 1.23×10^{-6} cm. In practice, there is sometimes up to three times as much movement per molecule of ATP, partic-

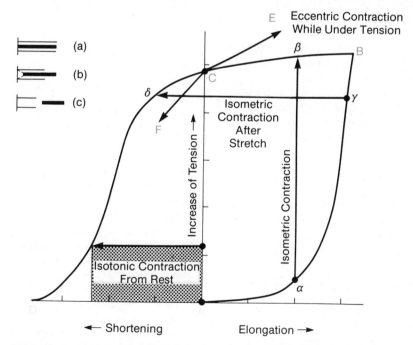

Figure 5–4 Length-tension diagram for muscle. Shaded area indicates isometric contraction followed by isotonic contraction when lifting a heavy load. In position *A*, cross-bridge formation is impeded; in position *B*, cross-bridge formation is optimal, while in position *C*, no cross-bridges can be formed. For comments on lettering, see text.

Displacement 10^{-6} mm in 100 msec (10^{-6} cm/sec)

10 bridges per half sarcomere.

Speed per fibril 2^9 (10^{-6} cm/sec) = $10^2 - 10^3$ cm/sec

Figure 5–5 Development of speed in a muscle fibril.

ularly under conditions of light loading, since not every possible cross-bridge is formed and broken down as the filaments slide over one another. In addition to this type of work, ATP is utilized in membrane pumping, extruding sodium ions from the interior of the muscle cells after depolarization and returning calcium ions to storage sites in the reticulum sarcoplasm. It costs approximately one molecule of ATP to pump five ions against a potential gradient of −80 mV. Further amounts of ATP are used in phosphorylating blood glucose prior to its transfer from the capillaries to the sarcoplasmic reticulum and in transporting protons to the interior of the mitochondrion for final oxidation (the malate–aspartate shuttle).

Muscle Heat Production

Muscle heat production has been studied under the somewhat artificial conditions of severe cooling in order to accommodate the recording characteristics of rather slowly reacting thermal probes. Four phases are identified:

1. *Activation Heat.* The heat of activation appears within 10 to 15 msec of stimulation and peaks within 20 to 30 msec. It reflects (a) the release of calcium ions and their interaction with the contractile proteins, and (b) internal shortening and thermoelastic effects within the muscle–tendon system even under nominally "isometric" conditions. This is supplemented by a phase of "labile" heat production (with a half-time of approximately 1.5 second), related to the speed of any movement which is allowed, and a "stable" heat production (which continues even during a sustained, tetanic contraction, reflecting inefficiencies in the transfer of ATP energy to actin–myosin bonding).
2. *Heat of Shortening.* Fenn first noticed that if a muscle is allowed to shorten, there is a second phase of heat production that is roughly proportional to the external work that is performed. A detailed explanation is awaited, but it can be envisaged as a form of internal viscous work, performed as one muscle filament slides a substantial distance over another.
3. *Relaxation Heat.* If the muscle has performed work against gravity (for example, in lifting a load), further eccentric work may be needed to assure a controlled descent of the load (in other words, the

muscle must continue to contract as it is being lengthened by the external load). This accounts for a phase of relaxation heat.
4. *Recovery Heat.* Finally, there is a phase of recovery heat. This reflects inefficiencies in the aerobic processes that use glycogen and fat to restore initial phosphagen reserves (ATP and creatine phosphate) within the active muscle fibers.

Warmup

Effects of Warmup. In theory, an increase of muscle and/or core temperature can improve physical performance in several ways. A rise of local temperature reduces the viscosity of the muscles, tendons, and joints, decreasing the internal work associated with a given movement (see the heat of shortening). The antagonists are also more completely relaxed after warmup, thereby not only reducing the resistance to movement, but also lessening the risk of physical injury (muscle and tendon tears).

An increase of muscle blood flow with warmup improves the local blood supply during submaximal work; a rightward shift of the oxyhemoglobin dissociation curve induced by the local increase of temperature allows a greater and more ready release of oxygen at any given partial pressure. Probably because of the muscle vasodilatation and the reduced cardiac workload, there is a reduced likelihood of cardiac dysrhythmias in the early stages of effort. The power of local chemical reactions is increased as predicted from the Law of Arrhenius (a doubling of the rate of reaction for a 10° C rise of local temperature). The mechanical efficiency of exercise is also improved, and this seems to be a specific response to the increase of intramuscular temperature, since passive stretching of the limbs does not have a similar effect. Finally, if the warmup involves a mild form of the intended exercise, performance may be improved by recent practice of the required skill.

Magnitude of Temperature Changes. The crucial factor during warmup is probably the rise of local muscle temperature. Typically, vigorous exercise gives a 2 to 3° C rise of intramuscular temperature within 5 to 10 minutes, but unless the conditions are particu-

TABLE 5-3   Calculation of Displacement
Produced by 1 Molecule of ATP

Energy content of ATP = 46 kJ/mol
49% transfer = 22.5 kJ/mol
1 g mol = 6.02×10^{23} molecules
1 molecule of ATP yields 3.7×10^{-23} kJ or 3.7×10^{-20} J
Force = 3×10^{-12} N per bond
Displacement = Work/Force
= $3.7 \times 10^{-20}/3 \times 10^{-12}$
= 1.23×10^{-8} m = 1.23×10^{-6} cm

larly adverse, the core temperature moves more slowly to its plateau, readings increasing by 0.5 to 1.0° C over 30 minutes of sustained activity. If the intensity of effort is expressed in absolute units, the rise of core temperature is greater in the unfit than in the fit. However, if the intensity of activity is expressed as a percentage of the individual's maximum oxygen intake, the increment of temperature is similar in fit and unfit.

Impact Upon Physical Performance. Performance times for speed events are improved by an appropriate warmup, although it is difficult to separate a true physiological response from the athlete's prior belief in the necessity for a warmup. Accuracy, movement time, range of motion, and strength are all improved, yielding an overall gain of up to 10 percent in performance. Some authors find a similar margin of benefit from light exercise, diathermy, or warm showers as from a vigorous, active warmup. Others believe that passive heating diverts blood flow to the skin, with an adverse effect upon subsequent physical performance. Obviously, if the preparatory exercise is too intense, the definitive performance may be adversely affected by an accumulation of lactate or a depletion of glycogen reserves.

The cooling of the muscles to pre-exercise temperatures may take as long as 60 minutes. An athlete can thus benefit from a warmup, even if it proves necessary to conduct this away from the competition site.

REGULATION OF MUSCLE CONTRACTION

Basic Pattern of Innervation

The muscle fiber has a characteristic dual pattern of innervation, a large (α) motor nerve passing to the fiber proper, and a smaller (γ) motor nerve supplying a variable sensitivity tension receptor (the spindle organ) arranged in parallel with it (Fig. 5–6). Sensory feedback is provided from the spindle receptors (generally a positive feedback to the central nervous system, encouraging initiation or continuation of muscle contraction) and from the Golgi organs (tension receptor fibers in the tendon which inhibit contraction).

The muscle fiber can thus be called into action in three ways:

1. *Voluntary Movement.* A novel "voluntary" movement may be initiated in the motor cortex, with nerve impulses travelling down the pyramidal tract to the anterior horn cells of the spinal cord. Here, there is activation of agonist and inhibition of antagonist neurons, with an appropriate modulation of impulses passing via the α motor fibers to the corresponding muscles.

2. *Automatic Movement.* A learnt, or familiar ("au-

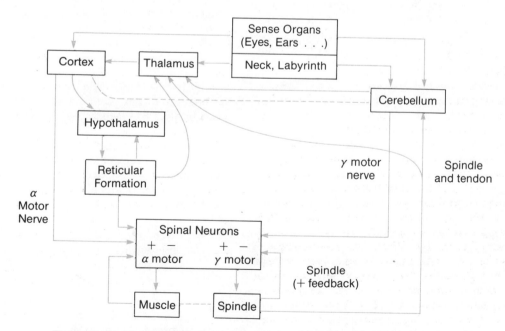

Figure 5–6 Simplified diagram showing control loops for muscle fibers. Note: Movement can be initiated in four ways: (1) discharge via α motor nerve ("voluntary movement"), (2) discharge via γ motor nerve ("learned" or "automatic" movement), (3) simultaneous α and γ motor nerve discharge ("co-activation"), (4) stretching of muscle spindle, with positive feedback via γ loop.

tomatic") movement may be initiated in the cerebellum. Impulses travelling via the extrapyramidal pathways and the γ motor fibers then cause a contraction and thus a shortening of the spindle organs within a specific muscle; this increases spindle tension, increasing the sensory feedback to the central nervous system. A complex pathway within the brain then activates the pyramidal tract and α motor fibers, causing the main muscle belly to contract (the γ-loop mechanism).

3. *Coactivation.* In practice, there is often simultaneous (coactivation) of α and γ motor fibers so that muscle fibers and spindles contract in parallel. If the external resistance remains at the anticipated level, the speed of spindle shortening then remains appropriate to muscle length throughout the movement, and the γ-loop feedback mechanism is not activated. However, if the force of the primary muscle movement is excessive (for instance, kicking against a football that is no longer in the expected position) the main muscle shortens more than the spindle. Tension drops in the latter, and a reduction of muscle force is made. The γ feedback loop ensures that errors of matching are reported to the cerebellum, and storage of this information allows a more precise movement to be made if a similar action is performed on a future occasion.

4. *Passive Stretching.* Passive stretching of the tendon (for example, the "patellar tap" used by the clinician when testing reflexes) also increases spindle tension. Sensory feedback from the spindle receptors to the spinal cord then initiates a contraction via the α motor fibers. However, if the tendon tension becomes excessive (for example, kicking a rock in mistake for a football), the golgi receptors inhibit the contraction to avoid muscle and tendon damage.

Stability of Control Loop

Bioengineers have speculated that the combination of long–lever arms (the limbs) and a long, relatively slowly conducting neural control loop (from the spindle receptors to the brain and back to the appropriate muscles) leaves the various joints of the body very vulnerable to unwanted tremor. The usual method of overcoming the problem of control oscillation in machines, which have been designed by human engineers is to introduce an "advance of phase" (that is to say, the machine is set to respond not to the signal, but rather to its differential; the rate of change in signal intensity).

A similar type of signal differentiation seems one function of the human γ loop. Because the sensitivity of the receptor is adjusted by a shortening of the spindle organ as soon as the main muscle contraction begins, the spindle organ receptors respond to the rate of change of tension, rather than to the absolute level of tension. A second control option adopted in some human-designed machines is a damping of the signal. This is accomplished in the γ-loop system by sending

inhibitory impulses to an appropriate level in the spinal cord; these impulses effectively check an oscillation before it becomes established. Damping originates in the midbrain and is vulnerable to a deterioration of this part of the brain due to aging or disease. Thus, in the clinical condition of Parkinson's disease, a degeneration of midbrain nuclei reduces the strength of inhibitory impulses. The muscles become unduly stiff, and there is also a tendency to a coarse tremor which becomes exacerbated whenever a movement is attempted ("intentional tremor"). Boxers sometimes develop a Parkinson-type syndrome because of cerebral injuries sustained during pursuit of their sport.

The Motor Unit

The motor unit comprises all of the muscle fibers supplied by a single anterior horn cell in the spinal cord. It is thus the smallest functional unit that can be activated within any given muscle. Depending on the size of the muscle under consideration, the number of fibers that are innervated by a single neuron ranges from 1 to 2,000. A given anterior horn cell innervates either fast- or slow-twitch fibers, but not both.

Nerves supplying fast–twitch fibers have a high electrical stimulation threshold, a rapid rate of discharge, and a rapid speed of conduction (>90 m per second; however, they show only transient bursts of activity. Nerves supplying slow–twitch fibers have a much lower stimulation threshold, a slow rate of firing, and a relatively slow rate of conduction (50 to 80 m per second).

If a sharp, powerful movement is made, the phasic (fast–twitch) motor units are recruited, but in submaximum effort the tonic (slow–twitch) motor units are selectively called into play, at least until the corresponding glycogen reserves are exhausted. The slow–twitch fibers are also recruited first during a mild isometric effort, but at discharge frequencies above 30 Hz, an increasing proportion of fast–twitch fibers are used. Patterns of muscle fiber recruitment are often inferred from glycogen depletion as seen in muscle biopsy specimens, although when interpreting such information account must also be taken of fat usage in aerobic work, and of interfiber differences in the efficiency of effort. The tension yielded per mole of ATP is greater for slow- than for fast-twitch fibers.

Modulating Muscle Force

A given motor unit responds to a single stimulus in an "all or none" fashion. However, there are various possible tactics for ensuring an appropriate gradation of muscle force:

(1) The number and type of motor units that are recruited may be varied.

(2) The frequency of activation of individual units may be increased so that force is augmented by a preexisting stretch of series elastic elements (a *summation* of contractions, leading on to a partial or complete *tetanus,* Fig. 5–7).

(3) The interstimulus interval may be reduced, so that the force of contraction is increased by what has been termed a *catch-effect* (this probably reflects an incomplete return of calcium ions to storage sites in the sarcoplasmic reticulum following the previous contraction, Fig. 5–2).

(4) Energy may be stored and later released from series elastic elements (particularly strong tendons, which are stretched if the muscle contracts against an external resistance).

The externally-measured force can be further increased by release of any central inhibition of motor neurons (for example, the athlete who develops a more powerful contraction in response to self-hypnosis), relaxation of antagonistic muscles, an improved choice of external loading and speed of contraction (the power output from a given muscle is usually greatest when it is operating at intermediate loads, Fig. 5–8), an improved synchronization of motor unit activity (for a peak effort, all units must contract in phase), an increase of muscle temperature (in a cold muscle, much effort is expended in overcoming internal viscosity), and an improvement of the local oxygen supply.

An alteration in the pattern of fiber recruitment is usually the most important modulating tactic. Because of differences in the number of fibers innervated, the total fiber cross-section and the force developed per unit of cross-section, there may be a tenfold difference of force between fast and slow motor units. The practical advantage of selective fiber recruitment (option 1) rather than rate-coding of the nerve impulses (options 2 and 3, above) is that the loading of individual fibers is kept quite low, and there is less likelihood that fatigue will develop due to an occlusion of the local blood supply. The fourth option of energy storage is evoked by the experienced sprinter; the extensor muscles start contracting before the foot hits the track, and forcible elongation of the contracting muscle stores energy in the elastic elements of the tendo Achilles, thereby providing additional power for the next stride. There have also been suggestions that forcible stretching of the muscle may in some way increase the efficiency of transfer of ATP energy to actin-myosin bonding, but this hypothesis has yet to be confirmed.

Role of the Antagonists

The action of the antagonist muscles is modified according to the precision of movement that is required. Complete relaxation of the antagonists allows a free, ballistic movement at a speed determined by the natural frequency of the part. For example, the extended lower limb has a natural frequency of 2 to 3 Hz, corresponding to the pace selected during relaxed distance running. In contrast, in a carefully controlled action such as movement of a typewriter carriage to a specif-

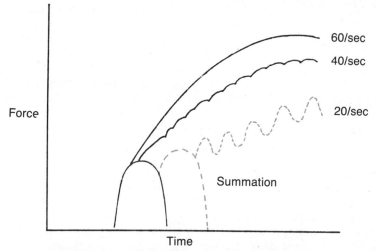

Figure 5–7 To illustrate summation and partial tetanus.
Note: The force of muscle contraction can be varied by changes in
    (a) type of fiber recruited
    (b) number of units recruited
    (c) rate of electrical discharge (as above)
    (d) synchronization of discharge
    (e) speed of shortening (see Fig. 5–8)
    (f) control of movement by antagonists
    (g) stored energy of stretched tendous
    (h) central inhibition
(After Shephard RJ. Physiology and biochemistry of exercise. New York: Praeger, 1982; Fig. 3.3. Courtesy of the publisher.)

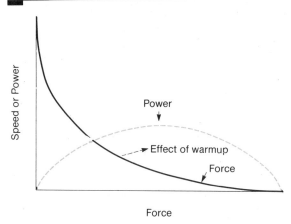

Figure 5–8 The relationship between speed of contraction, force, and power of skeletal muscle. If speed = 0, contraction is isometric (maximum force). If force = 0, contraction is isotonic (maximum velocity).

ic position, displacement of the limb is braked by periodic bursts of contraction from the antagonists. Ballistic movements are economical, since the agonists contract only when the movement is initiated. In contrast, during a speed event such as a 50- or 100-meter dash, the limbs are thrust forward at a pace which exceeds their natural frequency, and the necessary sustained contraction of the agonist muscles makes such exercise mechanically very inefficient.

Stride length is proportional to leg length, while the natural frequency of the leg and thus its speed of comfortable, ballistic movement, varies as $\sqrt{1/L}$ (where L = length of stride). A tall runner thus has some advantage when operating under ballistic conditions, taking longer if slightly less frequent strides.

Impact of Leverage

In real-life situations, leverage is an important variable, greatly modifying inferences that might be drawn from the relationship between muscle length and contractile force as seen in an isolated muscle (Fig. 5–4). Leverage is usually optimal around the midpoint of movement at a given joint. Thus, many subjects are unable to lift a heavy load from a crouching position because leverage in this situation is insufficient to allow the quadriceps muscle to lift the combined mass of the body plus an external load.

It is usually convenient to think of torque (turning moment, equal to force × leverage) about a given joint. Many lever systems in the body (such as the forearm) are designed for fast rather than for powerful movements (Fig. 5–9). The distance between the muscle insertion and the fulcrum is then kept short relative to the lever arm available to the moving part and any external load. One example of a more powerful arrangement is the ankle joint. Here, the calcaneum provides the gastronemius with a substantial lever, since this muscle must often lift the entire body mass plus some external load.

Electromechanical Coupling

The sequence of electrical and mechanical events occurring during a muscular contraction is illustrated in Figure 5–10. There is an initial *latent period* of some 4 msec following the propogation of an end-plate potential over the entire surface of the muscle sarcolemmal membrane. Muscle tone remains unchanged during this interval. It is suggested that 1 msec is required for the wave of electrical depolarization to penetrate the transverse tubules and initiate a release of calcium ions into the lateral sacs, and a further 2 to 3 msec is required for the calcium ions to diffuse through the sarcoplasmic reticulum to active sites on the troponin molecule. A slight "latency relaxation" may be seen at this stage. This is followed by a phase of increasing rigidity within the muscle filaments (the "active state"), as crossbridge formation occurs. However, the development of an external tension, which can be recorded by the usual type of dynamometer (see section on Isometric Force) lags behind the active state, since it is first necessary to stretch the elastic elements of the tendons, which are effectively arranged in series with the muscle fibers. Finally, membrane pumps restore the sodium–potassium distribution across the sarcolemma and return calcium ions to their storage sites in the sarcoplasmic reticulum. During the recovery phase, persistence of tension in the elements of the tendons again causes the dynamometer readings to lag behind the chemical processes of recovery.

The minimum disturbance needed to initiate a propogated action potential across the sarcolemma is a reduction of the normal 80 mV negative potential gradient beneath the motor end plate to a figure of −40 to −50 mV. If there is a larger electrical change, this accelerates calcium release into the sarcoplasmic reticulum, but the speed of the process initiating a contraction apparently "saturates" when the membrane potential drops to about −25 mV. The normal gradient of −80 mV is restored as sodium ions are pumped out of the muscle fiber, the recovery process taking about 50 msec.

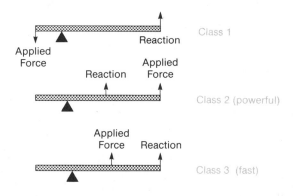

Figure 5–9 Three classes of lever. Note that class 2 levers give a powerful movement, and class 3 a fast movement.

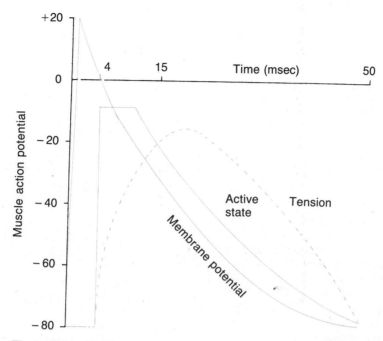

Figure 5-10   To illustrate time course of membrane potential, active state, and tension in muscle fiber.

Contracture and Fatigue

Repeated stimulation of an isolated nerve muscle preparation gives rise to a state of *"contracture"*, with an incomplete relaxation of the muscle fibers between individual contractions. This reflects a local lack of ATP, due in turn to an inhibition of glycolysis as the pH of the muscle falls; energy seems needed to restore the normal plasticity of the relaxed muscle fiber. Occasionally, a local depletion of ATP stores may also halt the calcium pumping that is needed during the recovery process. There is then a failure of electromechanical coupling, although a contraction can still be induced by local application of an appropriate concentration of mineral ions.

Humans show a superficially similar type of fatigue to that observed in the frog nerve-muscle preparation, with a progressive diminution in the magnitude of individual muscle contractions during a bout of repeated "isotonic" weight lifting. Chemical factors may contribute to the problem (oxygen lack, phosphagen depletion, inhibition of glycolysis, and ultimately glycogen depletion), but often there is a psychological overlay of "central inhibition" that can be overcome by hypnosis, strong encouragement, or fear (Chapter 3). If the effort is initially submaximal, the time to exhaustion can be extended by an alternation of activity between adjacent motor units. However, there is a progressive increase in the total electrical activity recorded from the muscle (the electromyographic root mean square voltage) as exhaustion is approached. Either less appropriate motor units are recruited in an attempt to continue the task or there is a decrease in the tension developed by individual muscle fibers.

During a maximal isometric contraction, fatigue may develop at the neuromuscular junction. Over the first minute of effort, activity ceases in the high-frequency (fast–twitch) motor units, and low frequency (slow–twitch) units are recruited in their place. If the contraction is sustained, the basis of fatigue changes to a local deficiency of ATP and other pH related problems. At this stage, additional fibers are recruited to make good the declining tension in those units that were first activated. Because of incomplete relaxation of the fatigued fibers, less energy is needed to sustain than to develop tension. Prior exercise often shortens the time to fatigue. Contributory factors include a depletion of local glycogen stores (first in slow, then in fast–twitch fibers), an increase of intracellular fluid, a loss of potassium ions, and a disturbance of intracellular buffering.

Recovery from fatiguing work generally follows the time course associated with its biochemical causes, reflecting phosphagen regeneration (completed in less than 2 min), lactate removal (half-time of 10 to 15 min) and glycogen replenishment (1 to 2 days). Because of the slow rate of glycogen replenishment and the need to allow for a repair of minor tissue injuries, there are advantages to alternating a day of heavy training with a lighter "work-out" (Chapter 3).

Length-Tension Diagram

Since work is the product of force and distance, the work that can be performed by a muscle fiber is shown by the relationship between its length and the tension that can be developed (the length–tension diagram, Fig. 5–4). The diagram may be considered as beginning with the muscle relaxed and at its resting length (point A). Passive stretching of the tissue will then progressively increase the resting tension, as conditions move to the right along the curve AB. An isometric contraction may be initiated at any point along the line AB, the corresponding maximum tensions β_1---β_n forming a line CB.

Notice that the peak isometric tension is developed when the system is under only a slight stretch, that is when the contraction is initiated at a little to the right of point A. This is one explanation for the "wind up" practised by many power athletes, although in some cases the competitors may also attempt to store elastic energy by stretching appropriate tendons. Note further that in the body the theoretical advantage of stretching the muscle suggested by an *in vitro* length-tension diagram is sometimes offset by poor leverage.

An isotonic contraction can also be initiated from point A, with a maximum shortening of A-D. Alternatively, if the muscle is first stretched passively, the isotonic contraction may be initiated from any point along the curve AB, the corresponding maximum shortening being indicated by the points δ_1---δ_n along the curve DC.

If the muscle is stretched while it is contracting (the process of eccentric contraction), the maximum force passes outside the boundary CB, as indicated by the line E. This situation is seen, for instance, when the shoulder muscles are used to lower the body gently to the ground. Repeated eccentric contractions (as in downhill treadmill running) can cause muscle damage, with release of intracellular constituents (myoglobin and creatine kinase), plus soreness postexercise (Chapter 3).

The final possibility is a forcible shortening of the muscle while it is contracting (a co-centric contraction). This reduces the maximum tension below the boundary CB, as indicated by the line F.

Lifting Work

In real-life activities such as the lifting of a heavy mass, a combination of isometric and isotonic contraction is likely. Consider a woman who is lifting a 30-kg suitcase. She first develops a force sufficient to counter the local gravitational acceleration (30×9.81 newtons), and then lifts the mass through a distance of 1.3 meters, using a combination of leverage and muscle shortening. The work performed is the product of force and distance ($30 \times 9.81 \times 1.3$ Nm, 383 Nm or 0.383 kJ).

Notice that a traditional weight-lifting session (3 sets of 10 repetitions using a load of 30 kg) would perform a fairly small total amount of work (30×0.383 kJ, or 11.5 kJ), and if spaced over 10 minutes, the power output (1.15 kJ per minute, 20 J per second or 20 W) would also be very low. Plainly, a standard weight-lifting session is not an effective method of training the cardiovascular system.

Design of Exercise Machines

When designing an exercise machine such as a bicycle, an appropriate choice of gear ratios is necessary. Sometimes gearing is chosen for subjective comfort, or to facilitate local blood flow. However, a further important consideration is to match the characteristics of the machine to the force–velocity curves of the active muscles, so that the rider delivers the maximum possible work per pedal revolution. If the required force is too high, little muscle shortening can occur before the limit CB of Figure 5–4 is reached, and if the external resistance is too low extensive shortening is possible but little work is performed. The optimum arrangement is usually to develop 25 to 35 percent of the maximum voluntary force (that is, 25 to 35 percent of the isometric force which can be developed when initiating a contraction from the resting point A).

Explanation of Length-Tension Diagram

The form of the length-tension diagram for a muscle can readily be understood in terms of cross-bridge theory (Fig. 5–4). If individual muscle fibers are stretched excessively, the thick and thin filaments no longer interdigitate to the same extent; cross-bonding is thus decreased, and finally is no longer possible. Conversely, if interdigitation is increased excessively by forcible shortening of a muscle, this also interferes with cross-bridge formation, possibly because the sarcoplasmic reticulum is distorted, hampering the movement of calcium ions to binding sites on the troponin molecule. The extent of interdigitation of the thick and thin filaments is optimal when the muscle is at or a little above its normal resting length.

Velocity of Contraction

The relationship between the speed of muscle shortening (V) and loading takes the form of a hyperbola (Fig. 5–8). The velocity of contraction is very high at low loads, but drops to near zero as maximum isometric force is approached. The corresponding mathematical expression is $V = (P_o - p) b / (p + a)$ where P_o is the maximum isometric tension, $(P_o - P)$ is the applied tension, and a and b are constants. Useful external work is proportional to PV, wasted internal work is proportional to (aV), and the constant b describes the relationship between the total work performed and external loading of the system.

The wasted internal work reflects in part the viscosity of the muscle sarcoplasm, which impedes sliding of the thick and thin filaments over one another. The force–velocity hyperbola is thus displaced upwards and to the right by an increase of local muscle temperature (greater force at a given speed, or greater speed at a given force). This is one reason why athletes find it beneficial to warmup prior to competition. Maximum benefit is obtained from a warmup which involves no more than 5 minutes of moderate activity.

Afferent Information

Afferent information involved in the coordination of muscular activity (proprioceptive input) is derived from local muscle and tendon tension receptors (the spindle organs and golgi receptors above), from tension receptors in the neck muscles, position receptors in the labyrinth, pressure receptors in the skin (particularly the soles of the feet), visual impulses from the eyes, and sounds detected by the ears (Fig. 5-6).

A portion of the afferent information is coordinated at the spinal level. For example, a gentle stimulation of the sole of the foot gives an extensor thrust, a part of the normal reflex of walking. More painful stimulation of the foot causes an involuntary withdrawal of the limb (the flexor withdrawal reflex). Reflexes such as the knee jerk caused by forcible stretching of the patellar tendon are also processed in this fashion.

Most of the more complicated movements are based upon a referral of afferent signals to the higher centers of the brain. Here, they can be interpreted against a background of cumulative experience (the process of "conditioning"). For example, the head is normally turned in reflex fashion towards a noise such as the slam of a door. If there are interesting sequelae such as the appearance of a well-built football player on each occasion that the sound is heard, the reflex persists, but if there are never any interesting sequelae (e.g., if the door is in an adjacent apartment that cannot be seen), after a time the sound is ignored (the process of "habituation" or negative conditioning).

Voluntary and Automatic Movement

Some authors have attempted to distinguish between "voluntary" and "automatic" movements. The famous neurologist, Hughlings Jackson, even described a hierarchy of movements ranging from the "most voluntary" (such as speech) to the most automatic (such as breathing). The extent of the voluntary control of movement is an interesting topic for philosophical discussion. In the case of breathing, it is possible to isolate regions of the brain which have intrinsic signals with a respiratory rhythm; in other words, irrespective of the environmental situation or the level of physical activity, we are constitutionally endowed with a drive to activate the respiratory muscles. Nevertheless, even with a process as automatic as breathing, the inherent drive is strongly modulated by various afferent signals, as is discussed in Chapter 7.

It is unclear how far other motor programs are inherited. Some studies of "identical" (monozygous) twins have suggested that they develop very similar movement patterns even when they are reared independently, but this could reflect similarities of body build

rather than the inheritance of specific motor programs. From the practical point of view, most physiologists would argue that even apparently voluntary movements do not arise *de novo* in the cerebral cortex. All are called into play by afferent stimuli, although the chain of events between the stimulus and the resultant action may be long and complicated.

Cerebral Processing of Movement Skills

Part of the information involved in the more immediate control of movement is passed to the thalamus, whence it is relayed to the sensory cortex (yielding a conscious appreciation of movement) and to the motor cortex (yielding an appropriate modulation of the pyramidal tract stimulation of the α motoneurons). A further part of the information is transmitted to the cerebellar cortex. Here it can (1) initiate extrapyramidal, γ motoneuron activity (co-activation, or a γ-loop drive to the limbs) (2) be compared with existing γ-loop programs, and (3) be used to improve, up-date, or add to the body's store of γ-loop motor programs.

When a task is first being learned (for example, the playing of a piano or the operation of a word-processor), the required movements must be monitored closely by the motor cortex. However, as skill is developed, the necessary actions shift closer to the popular concept of an automatic movement; attention turns from detailed control of motor output to an overall appreciation of the initiating signal, and muscle tone is modulated via the γ loop rather than the α motor pyramidal pathway.

Forms of Sensory Feedback

A continuous input of sensory data from the eyes, the labyrinth and other proprioceptors allows the prepackaged discharge of the γ efferent fibers to be modified in the light of the subject's immediate situation (Fig. 5-6). Let us suppose that an unanticipated resistance is encountered when a familiar movement is repeated. The α motor neuron discharge no longer causes the expected amount of muscle shortening, and the decrease of γ afferent fiber discharge is less than anticipated. Thus, an error signal is reported to the sensory cortex. A decision can then be taken, either to allow a corrective increase in the force of contraction (via the γ-loop), or to abort the movement. In either event, it is likely that some alteration will be made to the movement program as stored in the cerebellum, so that the same situation can be addressed more effectively on a future occasion.

The practical contribution of vision and pressure sensations to the control of movement can be illustrated by the difficulties that arise when these forms of feedback are withdrawn, as in the patient with the condition of tabes dorsalis, a syphilitic degeneration of the dorsal spino-cerebellar tracts. Individuals who develop this particular disorder are quite capable of balancing while they keep their eyes open, but if they close their eyes (for instance, to wash their hair) a lack of compensating secondary information from pressure receptors in the feet causes them to lose their balance, tumbling into the wash basin. Likewise, paraplegics who have been enabled to stand by electrical stimulation of the paralyzed muscles in the lower limbs find some difficulty in balancing unless a pressure feedback is provided from the soles of their feet.

Balance and Steadiness

The γ loop contributes substantially to balance in a normal person. As the body moves out of equilibrium, there is an increased input from γ afferent fibers on the side of the body where the spindle organs are stretched, and a diminished input from the contralateral afferents. A reflex adjustment of muscular tone thus pulls the body back to a more stable posture.

Typically, there is a slight sway about the equilibrium position while standing, because of the time required to initiate compensating changes of muscle tone around the long control loop. The extent of this sway can be assessed by a device known as an ataxiameter. If a given posture is to be maintained for some time, the energy cost of maintaining balance can be reduced by locking the knee joints.

The ability to maintain dynamic balance is tested by an apparatus known as a stabilometer, which is in essence a short board pivoted on a central roller. The task of the subject is to stand astride the board and prevent it from rotating. Scores are expressed as the period over which ground contact has been avoided, or the cumulative angular rotation in 60 seconds. Favorable scores generally reflect sensitive static and dynamic receptors in the inner ear and/or good γ loop responses. Certain categories of athlete such as water skiers, gymnasts, and sailors achieve above-average results on the stabilometer. This may be partly a question of selection by either neural sensitivity or body build (a low center of mass is plainly an advantage), but there is also evidence that the sensitivity of the inner ear and/or the central control mechanism can be modified by learning. For instance, a pronounced rocking sensation is experienced on returning to dry land after a week's yachting holiday.

Hand steadiness is important to many fine skills. It can be evaluated very simply by having a subject pass a brass probe down a tapered slot, noting the distance travelled before electrical contact is made with the side walls of the slot. The natural frequency of oscillation is 8 to 9 Hz for the elbows and fingers, 10 to 11 Hz for the wrist and 3 to 4 Hz for the forearm. Oscillations at these frequencies become apparent when impulse traffic around the gamma loop is excessive. The cause is sometimes overarousal, with a spread of impulses from the reticular formation of the brain to the anterior horn cells of the spinal cord. There have

been instances where nervous athletes have sought to steady their hands by drinking a depressant drug (alcohol) immediately prior to competition, and two pistol-shooters were reportedly disqualified on this basis at the Mexico City Olympic Games of 1968; more recently, anti-adrenergic drugs have also been taken with a view to decreasing arousal. A second possible explanation for excessive oscillation (tremor) in older people is the loss of normal inhibitory impulses from the midbrain, owing to trauma, specific degenerative conditions such as Parkinson's disease and Huntington's chorea, and general aging.

Conscious Proprioception

A portion of overall proprioceptive input (see section on Afferent Information) is passed via the thalamus to the sensory part of the cerebral cortex. These signals allow a subject to make judgments about limb position, the amplitude and direction of limb displacement, and the velocity of movement of both the limb and external objects.

Conscious proprioceptive sensitivity is increased by external loading (e.g., the mass of a bat or racquet) presumably because the added inertia increases stimulation of the spindle receptors, and thus the flow of afferent information. Conversely, kinesthetic skills are reduced and limb positions are poorly judged when underwater or on space missions, because stimulation of the spindle receptors and other proprioceptive endorgans is greatly reduced and the readings that are reported to the brain during any given body movement do not have the anticipated values.

Kinesthetic skills are very important to performance in rapidly moving ball games. In such situations, a main aim is to synthesize information from the retina, the neck, and the ocular muscles. If viewing time is short (less than 240 msec), reliance is placed upon the processing of retinal images alone. However, the level of skill shows a dramatic improvement if a longer viewing time allows the combination of the retinal images with information derived from the increased size and clarity of the approaching ball plus proprioceptive stimulation contributed by movement of the head and convergence of the eyes.

One limit to kinesthetic skill is the discriminating capacity of the retina. Two objects can be distinguished only if their image at the retina is separated by a distance of at least 4.5 μ. The equivalent angular resolution is about 1 minute. The more distant a target, the smaller the angle it subtends at the retina. Sports enthusiasts thus try to extend their performance by using a nearby reference point (e.g., the spot system in bowling).

Response Time

The time required for response to a signal is influenced by both the sensory and the motor sides of any reflex loop. For example, the braking of a car in response to a red traffic signal involves a light reaction time of 170 to 200 msec, and a movement time of 170 to 200 msec as the foot is lifted from the gas pedal and applied to the brake. Some tasks also require an initial movement of the eyes to feed the signal to the central nervous system. Sometimes a subject is offered several cues and must make a choice before responding (a multiple choice reaction time). This usually lengthens reaction time. Alternatively, there may be a single cue, but a choice between responses. This lengthens movement time.

The simplest reactions depend solely on the length of the reflex arc, the speed of nerve conduction, and the number of intervening synapses; each synapse adds a finite delay of some 20 msec. In the athlete, times are generally lengthened by a need to choose between several stimuli and to effect skilled movements. Responses are speeded by training and by an appropriate level of arousal or expectancy. Athletes generally have faster reactions than nonathletes. This advantage is particularly marked among sprint contestants, and is limb specific (e.g., the runner responds relatively more rapidly with the legs than with the arms, while the reverse is true of a tennis player). Reaction and movement times reach a minimum between 20 and 30 years of age and, perhaps for sociocultural reasons, are slower in women than in men.

Most competitors adopt a "sensory set" rather than a "motor set," concentrating upon the initiating signal (the starter's pistol) rather than the task to be performed. If a sensory set is adopted, the starting signal is probably calling forth a preprogrammed cerebellar motor program without substantial involvement of the cerebral cortex. There is some evidence that this speeds the response relative to a "voluntary" movement.

TESTING MUSCLE FUNCTION

Muscle Dimensions

Since there is a general relationship between the cross-section of a muscle and the force that it can develop, one simple method of assessing muscle strength is to determine muscle dimensions.

When recruiting mineworkers from poorly nourished African tribes, Wyndham found that a simple determination of body mass provided a useful indication of strength and thus productivity. Likewise, a recent survey of recruits to the Canadian Armed Forces found that body mass gave almost as useful an indication of the ability to undertake heavy work as did the performance of more complicated isotonic lifting tasks. The measurement of body mass has the important advantage that little cooperation of the subject is required. Moreover, the test result is uninfluenced by learning or motivation. The main disadvantage is that in overnourished subjects, excess mass is likely to be fat rather than muscle. In such circumstances, it may be preferable to calculate lean body mass, using either a direct measurement of this variable or one of the fat estimation techniques discussed in Chapter 3 (lean mass = total body mass × [(100-Fat percent)] × 1/100). Total body potassium as measured by whole body counter shows a fair correlation with explosive force, but the correlation with the summed isometric force of selected large muscle groups is only r = 0.50. One problem is that body fat screens out radiation from the underlying ^{40}K, reducing the apparent amount of muscle in the obese individual. Training may reduce the fat screen, and it also increases the ^{40}K content of lean tissue, both of which changes exaggerate the apparent muscle content of the well-conditioned individual.

Local muscle mass can be estimated by measuring circumferences relative to well-standardized bony landmarks. Thus clinicians commonly evaluate quadriceps wasting by measuring the circumference of the thigh 12.5 cm above the condyles of the knee. Such scores show only a limited relationship to tests of running, throwing, jumping ability, and muscle force, although precision is improved if allowance is made for the size of the underlying bones and the thickness of overlying fat by measuring inter-condylar diameters and skinfold thicknesses respectively. Other possibilities include obtaining soft-tissue radiographs or ultrasound pictures of the limbs showing the relative dimensions of muscle, fat, and bone. Interestingly, during the period of recovery from a limb injury, force returns to wasted muscles faster than bulk. Presumably, a part of the recovery is attributable to a greater activation (or a lesser inhibition) of the motor neuron pool rather than to a hypertrophy of the wasted muscles.

Explosive Force

Two popular field tests of explosive strength are a "vertical jump and reach" and the standing broad jump. Scores for both of these tests are greatly influenced by height, body mass, motivation, practice, and immediate environmental conditions. More precise measurements of explosive force can be obtained from a force plate. Typically, this type of instrument has a stack of 3 piezo electric crystals mounted at each corner of a rigid plate. Deformation of the crystals during jumping develops a voltage which indicates the direction and magnitude of the applied force.

The forces developed during a vertical jump average about 1.3 kN in a young woman and about 1.7 kN in a young man. C.T.M. Davies estimated the power developed by the jumper at 2.4 kW for a woman and 3.9 kW for a man. Of course, this intensity of effort is sustained for only 0.2 seconds. During a staircase sprint, he noted a power output of 0.7 kW in women and 1.0 kW in men; during exhausting exercise on a cycle ergometer, the output of useful power dropped to only 0.2 to 0.4 kW.

Isometric Force

Because elastic structures are arranged in series with a muscle, it takes a finite time to develop a true isometric contraction (see section on Electromechanical Coupling). Chaffin has defined isometric force as a force that can be sustained for 3 seconds. The recording device may be a simple mechanical dynamometer (where the force is exerted against a strong, spring-loaded plate), or a cable tensiometer (where a mechanical or an electrical gauge determines the tension developed in a steel cable). With the latter type of device, it is important to consider the angulation of the cable relative to the limb and the length of the lever arm allowed by the position of the cable harness relative to the axis of rotation of the joint (Fig. 5–9). Results are best expressed as a turning moment, or torque (Nm), about the axis of rotation.

The maximum scores recorded are further influenced by such variables as the joint examined, the degree of immobilization of other adjacent body segments, any jerking or inertial artefacts, and the intrinsic motivation of the subject relative to the urging of the observer. In general, the maximum force that can be developed by the adult is proportional to the cross-section of muscle, although there is substantial interindividual variation within the range 30 to 70 N/cm². Longer muscles also have more cross-bridges, and thus can develop a greater force, although this may be masked by a longer lever arm for the cable tensiometer attachment. The ratio of observed force to cross-sectional area in fact seems largely independent of gender, training, or fiber type, although lower values are found in older individuals, probably because the contractile tissue of the muscle has become diluted by inactive constituents such as fat and connective tissue.

The commonest isometric measurement is of hand grip force. Scores vary somewhat with the design of the dynamometer that is used and the separation of the grip plates that is chosen, but typical readings are approximately 350 N in a young woman and 500 N in a young man. Clarke found a correlation coefficient of 0.69 between handgrip force and the averaged strength of a number of other large muscle groups as assessed by cable tensiometer. In other words, the handgrip test described approximately half of the interindividual variation in large muscle strength; however, much of this seemingly useful correlation was due to a mutual dependence upon body mass. Reliance upon the handgrip test places women at a substantial disadvantage, since the ratio of leg to arm strength is greater in women than in men. If the dominant hand is used, grip force may also be biassed upwards by local training responses to sport or to daily work.

If efforts are repeated over a short period of time, the maximum force that can be developed decreases progressively. When 6 contractions are made per minute, the readings drop to a plateau that is approximately 85 percent of the initial value over the course of 4 minutes, while at a rate of 29 contractions per minute, scores settle down progressively to 60 percent of their initial level.

Isometric Endurance

The scores in field tests of isometric endurance such as a flexed arm hang from parallel bars are strongly influenced by both body mass and motivation. In the laboratory, one can note the time for which a dynamometer or a tensiometer is held to within 20 N of a predetermined value (usually a fixed percentage of the individual's maximum isometric force).

A curve of roughly exponential form relates force to endurance time (Fig. 5–11). An effort of less than 10 to 15 percent of maximum voluntary force can be held almost indefinitely. With stronger contractions, endurance decreases rapidly, reaching a minimum of 20 seconds endurance at 100 percent of maximum force. Effort is halted by local weakness and pain as an intramuscular accumulation of lactate inhibits the glycolytic enzymes. Limitation of blood flow to the active muscles begins when effort reaches some 15 to 25 percent of maximum isometric force, and vascular occlusion becomes complete when 60 to 70 percent of maximum isometric force is exerted. The endurance time thus depends on (1) the extent of residual blood flow to the muscle, (2) local stores of oxygen and phosphagen at the onset of the contraction, (3) the rate of usage of energy, and (4) any diffusion of lactate and other metabolites away from the active muscle fibers. If a muscle is strengthened by training, a given tension can be developed at a smaller fraction of its maximum voluntary force, and blood flow is thus impeded to a lesser extent. This is one reason why the anaerobic

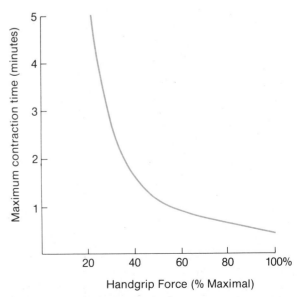

Figure 5–11 Relationship between maximum contraction time (minutes) and intensity of continuous isometric contraction (% of maximal force).

threshold of well-trained individuals is set at a higher fraction of maximum oxygen intake than in sedentary subjects.

Since local intramuscular stores of oxygen are very small, there is little possibility of sustaining fat metabolism during isometric contraction. Glycolysis also has only one-thirteenth to one-eighteenth of the efficiency calculated for a complete combusion of carbohydrate to carbon dioxide and water (Chapter 3). Nevertheless, it seems unlikely that muscle glycogen reserves would be exhausted by less than 4 to 5 minutes of maximal isometric effort (a sequence of 10 to 12 maximal contractions, each sustained to exhaustion). Effort is halted rather by the local accumulation of acid metabolites, with a resultant inhibition of key enzymes in the glycolytic sequence. Recovery occurs at about the same speed as would be anticipated following rhythmic work, being 87 percent complete 40 minutes after an exhausting isometric effort.

Isotonic Force

Many practical problems arise when measuring maximum isotonic force, including a need to control body posture and to allow for a loss of energy in the acceleration and deceleration of body parts; some authors are thus content to infer the isotonic value from its correlation with isometric force (r = 0.8).

Common field tests of performance such as speed sit-ups and push-ups combine elements of both isotonic muscle force and isotonic endurance. Laboratory measurements include the maximum load that can be lifted through a specified distance and the maximum load that can be lifted ten times through the same range. Such values are usually determined by incremental loading of a pulley system or heavy weights mounted in a rigid lifting frame. Because of the incremental protocol, there is some danger that subjects will be exhausted before the true maximum isotonic force has been attained. Moreover, the reported result is inevitably influenced by the speed of muscle contraction adopted by the subject and the consequent inertia of the load.

Isokinetic Force

Torque generators allow force measurements while a joint is being rotated at a predetermined speed. If a high speed of rotation is selected, recruitment of Type II fibers predominates, while at lower speeds there is a proportionately greater recruitment of Type I fibers. Attempts to determine the peak force generated during an isokinetic movement are often unsatisfactory due to overshoot of the recorder. The alternative of using a heavily over-damped recording is not much more satisfactory, and the current approach is thus to integrate the forces developed over a specified range of joint movement (in essence, making a measure of isokinet-

ic power output). A fair proportion of the total work is often performed against the mass of the limbs, and many authors thus apply a "gravity correction" to the dynamometer read-out.

Power Output Tests

A further potential approach to the assessment of isotonic performance is to measure the work that can be performed over a brief interval. Bar Or has proposed recording the power output developed on a cycle ergometer over 5 seconds and 30 seconds of all-out exercise. The 5–second score corresponds approximately with anaerobic power (depletion of local reserves of oxygen and phosphagen), while the 30 second score is related to anaerobic capacity (the halting of glycogen powered effort by the local accumulation of acid metabolites). A similar type of test can be carried out by running up a flight of stairs at maximum speed. If the rate of ascent is timed with photocells, the power output can be deduced as the product of body mass, the height climbed per second, and an assumed efficiency of climbing. A third possibility is a timed uphill treadmill run. With this approach, the speed and slope are set so that a person with a normal aerobic capacity is able to continue running for approximately 45 seconds; the muscle endurance can then be assessed in arbitrary units per kilogram of body mass from the individual's total running time.

Quantitative Electromyography

Electromyograms display the action potentials recorded over (plate electrodes) or within (needle electrodes) a given muscle belly. Plate electrodes give a good idea of total muscular activity about a given joint, although results can be distorted by a change in the relative contributions of superficial and deep muscles. Needle electrodes are helpful in determining which particular fibers are active in a given movement. When quantifying the extent of muscle activity, data are commonly presented as the root mean square (RMS) of electromyographic potential.

There is a fairly close relationship between this RMS voltage and the force that any given individual can develop in the muscle group under investigation (Fig. 5–12). However, if a person is strong, there is less electrical activity per unit of force than if she or he is weak. A plot of electrical activity against tension thus provides a submaximal test of muscular strength. This approach is particularly useful in workmen's compensation investigations, since scores are relatively independent of the subject's cooperation. Electrical activity increases as a person becomes fatigued, and the RMS–force relationship becomes alinear above 90 percent of maximum voluntary contraction. Action potentials are also larger for concentric than for eccentric exercise.

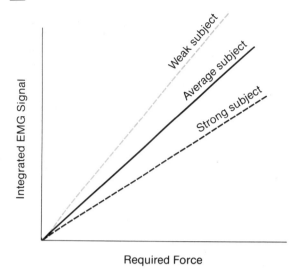

Figure 5–12   Use of the integrated EMG in assessing muscle weakness. A weak subject develops a greater EMG signal for any required force.

Normal Standards

Since the muscle force developed by an adult is proportional to the cross-section of the active fibers, we might anticipate that body size would influence muscle strength as the square of stature. However, if a person is followed over the period of growth, the exponent is often as high as 2.9 to 3.0, rather than 2.0. One possible explanation is the addition of more cross-bridges as a muscle becomes longer. A standard exponent of 3.0 cannot necessarily be used when making interindividual comparisons; one further complication is that tall individuals tend to have thin, poorly-muscled ectomorphic body builds; shorter people are often more muscular and mesomorphic. Debate continues as to how far these inherited characteristics can be modified by power or endurance training.

The maximum isometric force that the average woman can develop is 50 to 60 percent of the male value for the upper limbs, 40 to 45 percent of the male value in the trunk, and about 65 percent of the male value in the lower limbs. Since the typical man is 10 percent taller than a woman, a strength advantage of 20 percent (the H^2 hypothesis) or 30 percent (the H^3 hypothesis) can be attributed to size alone. Boys show a sudden spurt of strength at puberty, and it could be that much of their residual advantage over adolescent girls is hormonal. However, it remains difficult to disentangle any biochemical handicaps of the female from those sociocultural factors that have traditionally discouraged women from developing and manifesting muscle strength.

The dominant arm is usually 5 to 10 percent stronger than its counterpart, but in some sedentary individuals there is surprisingly little difference of performance between the two limbs. Men increase their strength to about 25 years of age, subsequently maintain a plateau to about 45 years, and show a progressive loss of muscle force with further aging. Women often reach their peak strength at 13 to 14 years of age, but again it is unclear whether the cause of this early peaking is biological or sociocultural.

Grip strength shows a diurnal rhythm, being larger in the afternoon and evening than in the morning. This reflects not only an increase of body temperature (and thus a decrease of muscle viscosity), but also an increase of cortical arousal. Hand grip readings can be increased 5 to 25 percent if central inhibition is released by such techniques as verbal encouragement or hypnotic suggestion.

THE SKELETAL SUPPORT SYSTEM

The effectiveness of the muscles as energy transducers depends ultimately upon the transmission of substantial forces through tendons and joints to the rigid lever arms of a bony or cartilaginous skeleton.

Ligaments and Tendons

Ligaments and tendons are formed of white fibrous tissue, particularly long parallel fibers of collagen. Their stiffness varies from perhaps 2 N per millimeter at low forces to 20 N per millimeter when large forces are applied. The maximal strength of a tendon is typically about four times the strength of the corresponding muscle. Nevertheless, it is protected from tearing by the inhibitory Golgi organ reflex (see section on Basic Pattern of Innervation 5–1). If stretched forcibly by external forces, a tendon can be lengthened by approximately 4 percent, without significant injury.

Further stretching does cause tears, usually at the point of insertion, where the collagen merges with the fibro-cartilage of bone. Disuse leads to a weakening of both the body of the tendon and its insertion; conversely, training strengthens a tendon, increasing its content of mucopolysaccharides and hydroxyproline, thickening collagen fibers and decreasing the number of unwanted cross-linkages between adjacent fibers.

Joints

There are three types of joint: fibrous, cartilaginous, and synovial. The fibrous joint is exemplified by the bones of the skull, the cartilaginous joint by the articulations of the vertebral column, and the synovial joint by the elbow articulation. In a cartilaginous joint, limited movement is possible through deformation of a plate of white fibrocartilage which separates the adjacent bones. Examination of an intervertebral disc reveals a mixture of fibrous tissue and cartilage, with the fibers arranged at right angles to the imposed stress; this design gives a tension resistance of 2 N per square millimeter, but a compression resistance that is ten times as great. Normally, the fibrocartilage is protected by the support of surrounding muscles, but a combination of factors such as fatigue, poor coordination, excessive stress, and previous injury may cause the elastic limit of the cartilage to be exceeded. When this happens to the fibro-cartilages of the knee joint, the result is a "torn cartilage." In the vertebral column, rupture of an intervertebral disc allows the softer center of the disc (the nucleus pulposus) to project backwards, pressing on the spinal cord and causing pain or loss of nerve function (a "slipped disc").

Articular Cartilage

The articular surfaces of bones are covered by a thin layer of hyaline cartilage. This consists of fine fibrils embedded in a ground substance of mucoproteins; it ensures relatively friction-free movement about the axes of rotation of a joint and can also be deformed, thus absorbing a proportion of external forces. Vigorous physical activity causes a seepage of fluid into the cartilage from the underlying bone, increasing its thickness by 13 to 14 percent within 10 minutes, a useful by-product of a preliminary warmup. More permanent increases in the thickness of articular cartilage are induced by training, but if the underlying bone is exposed through trauma, it undergoes proliferation; the resulting bony protruberances (exostoses) cause stiff and painful joints (osteoarthritis). Most elderly people show some radiographic evidence of osteoarthritis, but the resultant degree of incapacitation varies markedly from one individual to another.

Joint Capsule and Synovial Fluid

The synovial fluid normally forms a very thin viscous lubricating film over the joint surfaces. However, if the joint is injured or inflamed, fluid may accumulate in excessive amounts, with reflex inhibition of contraction in surrounding muscles. Four types of nerve endings have been described in and around joints. Types I and II, in the joint capsule, register position and speed of movement respectively. Type III, in the ligaments, also records position; Type IV consists of freely-branching pain endings.

Bone

Bone contains organic matter (collagen fibers embedded in a specific group of mucopolysaccharides, the glycosaminolysans), and an inorganic phase (apatite, crystals of $Ca_{10}(PO_4)_6(OH)_2$). An internal architecture of reinforcing bars and braces gives a typical bone great strength with minimal mass. Resistance to tension, compression, and shearing forces has been estimated at 12.2, 16.6, and 4.9 kN per square centimeter,

respectively. Unlike most engineering structures, bone shows little deterioration with age, since remodelling proceeds on a continuous basis. This remodelling allows specific adaptation of bones to athletic or occupational challenges.

The ratio of organic to inorganic matter drops from 1:1 in a child to 1:4 in a young adult and 1:7 in an elderly individual. During the period of growth, moderate activity apparently encourages the development of longer and heavier bones; intense activity leads to a shorter and lighter pattern of architecture—presumably, moderate compression stimulates growth at the epiphyses, but excessive pressure has an inhibitory effect.

Maintenance of a normal bone composition as an adult depends on continued weight bearing. Bed rest, space travel, and even prolonged swimming lead to a loss of both calcium and collagen from bone, and it is suggested that normal breakdown and resynthesis of bone is regulated by the piezo-electric potentials that are developed through weightbearing. Physical disuse is associated with an increased number of osteoclasts in the bone, with a two- to threefold increase over the normal rate of breakdown. The impact of athletic amenorrhea has already been noted (Chapter 4). Aging also leads to bone atrophy, although there is evidence that this process can be arrested, if not reversed, by regular load-bearing physical activity.

Static Flexibility

Static flexibility is a measure of the possible range of movement at any given articulation. In some instances (such as the elbow) a limitation is imposed by contact between opposing soft or bony tissues, but at other joints the limitation arises from the elastic resistance of the muscle sheath, tendon, joint capsule, or supporting ligaments, together with the overlying skin. A typical measure of static flexibility is the familiar "sit and reach" test, in which the forward reach is measured relative to a board contacted by the feet.

Women generally have better flexibility than men, and both sexes show a deterioration of about 20 percent over the normal span of working life. An unusual range of movement does not confer any great advantage in normal adult life, but may be very important to the performance of some athletic feats. In extreme old age, loss of flexibility may be the critical factor which leads to loss of independence; the older individual may no longer be able to bend the back sufficiently to put on shoes and stockings, and may lack the hip flexibility needed to climb into a bath.

Dynamic Flexibility

Dynamic flexibility is an inverse function of the resistance encountered when moving the body part at a normal operating speed for the joint in question. It depends largely upon the elasticity and resistance to deformation of the joint tissues, with negligible contributions from inertia, viscosity, and frictional resistance. Dynamic flexibility is increased acutely by a warmup, and is also improved by habitual activity, but like static flexibility, it deteriorates with aging.

FURTHER READING

Baldwin KM. Muscle development: neonatal to adult. Exerc Sport Sci Rev 1984; 12: 1–20.

Bigland-Ritchie B. EMG/force relations and fatigue of human voluntary contractions. Exerc Sport Sci Rev 1982; 9: 75–118.

Bonnet M, Requin J, Semjen A. Human reflexology and motor preparation. Exerc Sport Sci Rev 1982; 9: 119–158.

Booth FW, Nicholson WF, Watson PA. Influence of muscle use on protein synthesis and degradation. Exerc Sport Sci Rev 1982; 10: 27–48.

Bourne GH. The structure and function of muscle. New York: Academic Press, 1973.

Carlson FD, Wilkie DR. Muscle physiology. Englewood Cliffs, NJ: Prentice-Hall, 1974.

Cavagna G. Storage and utilization of elastic energy in skeletal muscle. Exerc Sport Sci Rev 1977; 5: 89–130.

Clarke HH. Muscular strength and endurance in man. Englewood Cliffs, NJ: Prentice Hall, 1966.

Ernst E, Straub FB. Symposium on muscle. Budapest: Akademiai Kiado, 1968.

Gans C. Fiber architecture and muscle function. Exerc Sport Sci Rev 1982; 10: 160–207.

Gentile AM, Nacson J. Organizational processes in motor control. Exerc Sport Sci Rev 1976; 4: 1–34.

Goldspink DF. Development and Specialization of skeletal muscle. London: Cambridge University Press, 1980.

Goodman MN, Ruderman NB. Influence of muscle use on amino acid metabolism. Exerc Sport Sci Rev 1982; 10: 1–26.

Goodwin GM. The sense of limb position and movement. Exerc Sport Sci Rev 1977; 4: 87–124.

Grinnel AD, Brazier MAB. The regulation of muscle contraction excitation - contraction coupling. New York: Academic Press, 1981.

Hayes KC. Biomechanics of postural control. Exerc Sport Sci Rev 1982; 10: 363–391.

Hettinger T. Physiology of strength. Springfield, Ill: CC Thomas, 1961.

Hill AV. First and last experiments in muscle mechanisms. London: Cambridge University Press, 1970.

Knuttgen HG. Neuromuscular mechanisms for therapeutic and conditioning exercise. Baltimore: University Park Press, 1976.

Komi PV. Physiological and biomechanical correlates of muscle function: effects of muscle structure and stretch-shortening cycle on force and speed. Exerc Sport Sci Rev 1984; 12: 81–122.

Kulig K, Andrews JG, Hay JG. Human strength curves. Exerc Sport Sci Rev 1984; 12: 417–466.

Matthews PBC. Mammalian muscle receptors and their central actions. London: Arnold, 1972.

Petrofsky JS. Isometric exercise and its clinical implications. Springfield, Ill: CC Thomas, 1982.

Phillips CG. Corticospinal neurones: Their role in movement. London: Academic Press, 1977.

Pollack GH, Sugi H. Contractile mechanisms in muscle. New York: Plenum Press, 1984.

Porter R, Whelan J. Human muscle fatigue: physiological mchanisms. London: Pitman, 1981.

Rohmert W. Muskelarbeit and muskeltraining. Stuttgart: Gentner Verlag, 1968.

Schmidt RA. Control processes in motor skills. Exerc Sport Sci Rev 1977; 4: 229–261.

Stein RB, Pearson KG, Smith RS, Redford JB. Control of posture and locomotion. New York: Plenum, 1973.

Sugi H, Pollack GH. Cross bridge mechanism in muscle contraction. Baltimore: University Park Press, 1979.

Tonomura Y. Muscle proteins, muscle contraction and cation transport. Baltimore: University Park Press, 1972.

Varga E, Kover A, Kovacs T, Kovacs L. Molecular and cellular aspects of muscle function. Budapest: Akademiai Kiado, Budapest, 1981.

Vrbova G. Influence of activity on some characteristic properties of slow and fast mammalian muscles. Exerc Sport Sci Rev 1980; 7: 181–213.

Zachar J. Electrogenesis and contractility in skeletal muscle cells. Baltimore: University Park Press, 1971.

EXERCISE AND THE CARDIOVASCULAR SYSTEM

CHAPTER 6

The transport of oxygen from the atmosphere to the working tissues and thus the maximum rate of aerobic metabolism is restricted by the conductance of a closely linked system of pathways in the cardiorespiratory system (Fig. 6-1). Firstly, there is the maximum external ventilation, governed by the bellows function of the chest. Part of the effort expended by the chest muscles is "wasted" in ventilating the dead space of the airways and unperfused alveoli; a part of the delivered oxygen is consumed by the respiratory muscles themselves. The next link in the transport chain is the exchange of gas between the lungs and the pulmonary capillaries. Then there is the pumping ability of the heart, and the manner in which the maximum cardiac output is distributed between the working muscles and other parts of the body. Finally, there is the passage of oxygen from the muscle capillaries to the inner surface of the intramuscular mitochondria (where the protons liberated by metabolic processes are finally oxidized to water).

In disease states, any one of these various factors can become the critical variable limiting maximum oxygen intake. In a normal, healthy, young person the main limitation to large muscle aerobic activity is imposed by blood transport. This point is readily appreciated from an examination of oxygen partial pressure gradients (Fig. 6-2). In respired air, the partial pressure of oxygen is normally 20 kPa (150 Torr in the older units); in the pulmonary capillaries the figure has dropped to approximately 13 kPa, but the main pressure gradient is from here to the venous end of the muscle capillaries, where a typical reading during maximal exercise is only 0.6 to 0.7 kPa. As in an analogous electrical circuit, the main limitation of transport occurs over that part of the system where there is a large pressure drop. This chapter will discuss reactions of the cardiovascular system to exercise; respiratory factors are considered in Chapter 7.

The blood transport of oxygen depends upon (1) maximum heart rate, (2) maximum cardiac stroke volume, (3) blood hemoglobin level, (4) distribution of cardiac output, and (5) the completeness of oxygen extraction in the active muscles.

CARDIAC PERFORMANCE

Heart Rate

The resting heart rate is increased by such factors as anxiety, a warm room, recent exercise, or eating a heavy meal. However, if readings are obtained in the early morning while the subject is still sleeping or has just wakened, there is a fair relationship between heart rate and physical condition; such values range from 65 to 70 beats per minute in an untrained subject to less than 30 beats per minute in occasional exceptionally well-trained endurance athletes.

Physical activity leads to a rapid-onset increase of heart rate. In a large muscle activity such as treadmill running, cycling, or stepping there is an approximately linear relationship between the "steady state" heart rate and the intensity of effort (expressed as a percentage of maximal oxygen intake) from 50 to at least 90 percent of maximum effort. This finding provides one of the cornerstones of several techniques for the "prediction" of maximum oxygen intake from submaximum test data. Among limitations of such predictions, we may note that the heart rate corresponding to any given level of oxygen consumption (Fig. 6-3) is increased by (1) small muscle exercise, (2) anxiety, and (3) high room temperatures (Chapter 2); there are also substantial inter- and intra-individual variations of response.

The maximum heart rate varies with the duration of exercise and with age (Fig. 6-4). In a brief effort, such as turning a tight corner in down hill skiing, readings of 250 to 260 beats per minute may be sustained for a few seconds. The maximum rate that is more usually discussed is that observed during performance of a treadmill maximum oxygen intake test of several minutes duration. Under such conditions, 200 to 210 beats per minute are possible in a child, but in a young woman the average expectation is a maximum of some 198 beats per minute; by the age of 65 years, there is a further decrease to a maximum of about 170 beats per minute (note that the effects of aging upon maximum heart rate is somewhat less than the popularly described equation of 220 − age in years). Factors that set a ceiling of cardiac rhythm remain uncertain; one factor may be the rate of relaxation of the heart, and thus diastolic refilling of the ventricles.

The maximum heart rate is sometimes decreased a little (5 to 10 beats per minute) by athletic training, and it is also less when exercising at high altitudes. Low values are further seen when there is a peripheral muscular limitation of effort (for instance, in arm ergometry). In certain cases of ischemic heart disease, the maximum may be reduced by a poor oxygen supply to the cardiac pacemaker (the "sick sinus" syndrome). More commonly, the post coronary patient faces a suppression of normal mechanisms for an increase of heart rate because of administration of drugs such as propranolol; chemicals of this type block the beta-adrenergic sympathetic drive to the cardiac pacemaker (Chapter 4). Propranolol treatment thus invalidates the use of heart rate when prescribing exercise for cardiac patients (Chapter 13).

Stroke Volume

The stroke volume may be calculated quite simply if the cardiac output is divided by the corresponding heart rate. The fraction of the ventricular contents ejected at each beat may also be estimated more directly by echocardiography or radionuclide angiography.

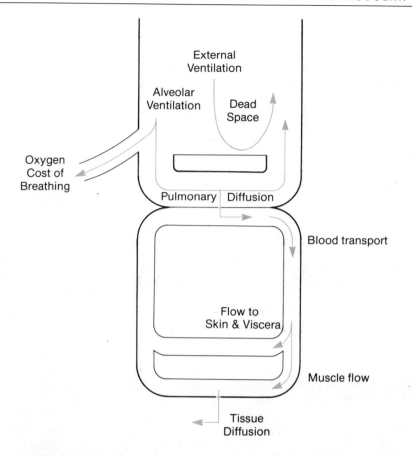

Figure 6–1 Bottlenecks to oxygen and carbon dioxide transport in the cardiorespiratory system.

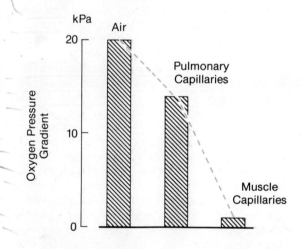

Figure 6–2 Oxygen partial pressure gradient from air to the muscle capillaries.

volume while lying supine, but an upright posture causes a progressive increase of stroke output from the resting figure of 80 mℓ to a plateau of about 110 mℓ at 40 to 50 percent of maximum oxygen intake (Fig. 6-5). During uphill treadmill running, the stroke output is well maintained from 50 percent through to 100 percent of maximum oxygen intake. However, in cycle ergometry (probably because a large proportion of the total work is performed by a single muscle group, the quadriceps), there is a tendency for stroke volume to diminish between 70 and 100 percent of maximum effort; this trend is particularly obvious in older individuals, possibly because ischemia of the myocardium limits the maximum force that can be developed by the ventricles.

The magnitude of the stroke volume plateau is reduced by hot conditions and by arm work. In both of these circumstances, the venous filling ("preloading") of the ventricle is diminished by a pooling of blood in the leg veins. Echocardiography has confirmed impressions formed earlier from radiography. Ejection of the cardiac contents is always incomplete; at the end of the diastole the ventricle may contain 160 mℓ of blood, and if the heart is functioning normally, 50 to 55 percent of the blood is expelled by the end of systole. One of the characteristics of a heart that is severely

The resting stroke volume is approximately 80 mℓ per beat if the subject is sitting or standing, but rises to about 110 mℓ per beat if the supine position is adopted. Exercise has little effect on the magnitude of stroke

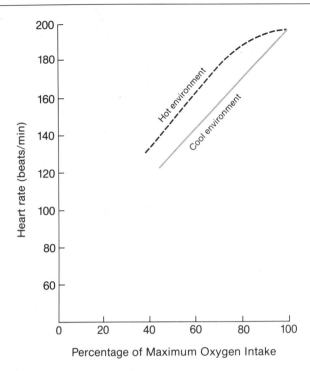

Figure 6-3   Likely effect of adverse environment upon relationship between heart rate and oxygen intake.

affected by coronary vascular disease is a reduction in this ejection fraction.

The increase of stroke volume with exercise is accommodated by both an increase of end-diastolic volume and an increase of ejection fraction. Early studies of isolated heart preparations by the English physiologist, Starling, led to the description of a standard curve relating stroke volume and diastolic filling (the so-called Starling's Law of the Heart, Fig. 6-6). It was envisaged that if the heart began to fail in its pumping function for any reason such as a poor oxygen supply, the resultant increase of diastolic filling induced a compensating increase of stroke volume ("compensated heart failure"). However, if there was

a further increase of diastolic filling, a point of diminishing returns was reached (the stage of "decompensated heart failure"), where stroke volume began to decrease rather than to increase. Starling's hypothesis can be explained in modern terms if we think of an extension of the muscle fibers to the point that the individual actin and myosin filaments no longer overlap and are thus unable to interact effectively with each other (Chapter 5). The increase of systolic emptying during physical activity reflects a leftward shift from the resting to the exercise stroke volume–diastolic filling relationship. This is mediated by catecholamines and/or sympathetic nerve stimulation, and is one expression of an increase of myocardial contractility.

Simple indices of myocardial contractility were once derived by relating the waveform of precordial or carotid vessel pulsation to heart sounds, on the basis that an increase of myocardial contractility at any given heart rate shortened the time required to open the aortic valves or to complete cardiac ejection. More precise data such as the speed of circumferential shortening in the ventricular wall are now obtained from the echocardiogram.

Cardiac Output

The cardiac output is plainly the product of heart rate and stroke volume. The "gold standard" of cardiac output measurement is based on an application of the Fick principle, which relates the steady state oxygen

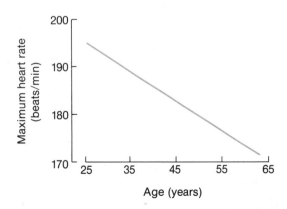

Figure 6-4   Influence of age upon maximum heart rate.

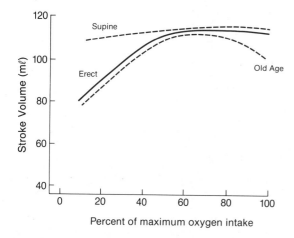

Figure 6–5 Influence of posture and age upon cardiac stroke volume.

consumption ($\dot{V}O_2$) to the oxygen content of both arterial and mixed venous blood (Ca, O_2 and $C\bar{v},O_2$). The venous sample must be well mixed, and is best obtained by catheterization of the pulmonary artery:

$$\text{Cardiac Output} = \dot{V}O_2/(Ca, O_2 - C\bar{v}, O_2)$$

Exercise testing laboratories are naturally reluctant to carry out cardiac catheterization on all of their volunteers. One useful alternative is to carry out analogous calculations, based on the rebreathing of carbon dioxide or of acetylene:

$$\text{Cardiac Output} = \dot{V}CO_2/(C\bar{v}, CO_2 - Ca, CO_2)$$

Under resting conditions, the cardiac output is typically 3.0 to 3.5 ℓ per minute per m² of body surface area (a figure of 4.8 to 5.0 ℓ per minute in a woman with a surface area of 1.5 m²). The maximum cardiac output is about 19 ℓ per minute in a young woman and 25 ℓ per minute in a young man. Some male endurance athletes have maxima as large as 35 ℓ per minute, while in the elderly of both sexes, the maximum value is 20 to 25 percent smaller than in a typical young adult.

Before echocardiography became widely available, heart size was deduced from cardiac radiographs (Fig. 6-7). The cardiac volume was approximated from linear measurements made in the postero-anterior and lateral planes. A typical finding was a volume of 10 to 11 mℓ per kilogram of body mass in a young woman or man, but values as high as 14 mℓ per kilogram were noted in some endurance athletes. Much of the large size of the cardiac shadow in athletes reflects a large stroke volume, but there is also some increase in the thickness of the heart wall, whether due to selection or training. This has given rise to an extended discussion of the supposed dangers of an athlete's heart. Certainly, dilatation of the heart due to cardiac failure is an adverse sign, and in some clinical conditions such as pulmonary or aortic stenosis, hypertrophy of the heart wall can develop to the point that the coronary blood flow is inadequate and local oxygen lack is occurring. There have also been reports that hypertrophy of the interventricular septum is associated with sudden death during vigorous sports, but there is little evidence that the more uniform ventricular hypertrophy seen in a typical endurance athlete is unhealthy.

Hemoglobin Level

Approximately 1 percent of blood oxygen is normally carried in physical solution; the remaining 99 percent is combined reversibly with red cell hemo-

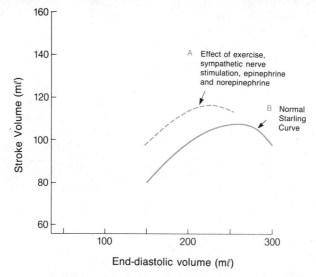

Figure 6–6 The relationship between end-diastolic volume and cardiac stroke volume. *A*, normal Starling curve; *B*, after exercise, sympathetic nerve stimulation, or administration of catecholamines.

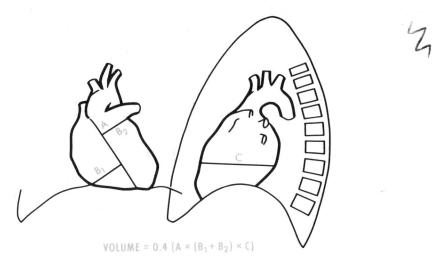

VOLUME = 0.4 (A × (B₁ + B₂) × C)

Figure 6–7   To illustrate radiographic method of calculating heart volume. (From Shephard RJ. Physiology and biochemistry of exercise. New York: Praeger, 1982. By courtesy of the publisher.)

globin. The oxygen pumped around the circulation with each liter of blood thus depends on the hemoglobin level and the affinity of the hemoglobin for oxygen (the latter being modified somewhat by blood temperature, pH, and the 2:3 diphosphoglycerate concentration).

When fully saturated with oxygen, each gram of hemoglobin carries 1.34 mℓ of oxygen. Thus a young woman with a hemoglobin level of 13.8 g per deciliter of blood could carry 18.5 mℓ of oxygen attached to her hemoglobin, and a further 0.2 mℓ of oxygen in physical solution in the plasma. Normally, the blood leaving the woman's lungs is 97 percent saturated with oxygen, and thus carries 18.1 mℓ of oxygen per deciliter. Under resting conditions, the arteriovenous oxygen difference is only 4 to 5 mℓ per deciliter, but in vigorous effort a figure of 13 to 14 mℓ per deciliter is observed. A cardiac output of 19 ℓ per minute allows the transport of 2.5 to 2.6 ℓ per minute of oxygen.

A young man typically has a hemoglobin level as high as 15.6 g per deciliter. This gives him a 13 percent advantage over a woman in terms of blood oxygen transport. The hemoglobin differential is probably due in part to the fact that the man loses no blood in menstruation, and in part to a greater secretion of androgens in male subjects. An increase of hemoglobin concentration is sometimes seen in athletes who take anabolic steroids (Chapter 4). In contrast, some endurance competitors are anemic, or have incipient anemia (as indicated by a reduced iron saturation of carrier proteins in the plasma). Athletic anemia has been blamed upon several factors, including (1) an expansion of plasma volume, (2) fads of diet (including a suppression of iron absorption by a high fat intake), (3) a reduced production of red cells in the bone marrow, (4) loss of iron in sweat (probably not a major factor), (5) increased breakdown of red cells due to mechanical trauma, and (6) loss of hemoglobin in the urine.

Some endurance competitors have attempted to boost their performance by "blood doping" (retransfusion of their own blood after allowing a few weeks for natural regeneration of a normal red cell count). Early efforts were not always successful in augmenting performance, because the blood deteriorated while in storage, but with modern methods of preservation, this procedure can give the dishonest competitor a substantial advantage in endurance events. A similar type of advantage has been sought in experiments where hemoglobin has been boosted by training at high altitudes, or by breathing low oxygen mixtures. A practical limitation to the augmentation of hemoglobin concentration is set by the viscosity of the blood which rises steeply, thus reducing maximum cardiac output if the red cell count is pushed to more than 30 percent above its normal figure.

BLOOD PRESSURE

Resting Blood Pressure

If blood pressure is measured by a mercury sphygmomanometer, it remains permissible to report readings in mm Hg rather than in the usual SI units (7.5 mm Hg = 1 kPa). In the adult, a typical resting pressure is 120/80 mm Hg. Figures are lower in the child (for instance, 105/70 mm Hg at age 10) rising slowly through maturation and adulthood to old age. A diagnosis of hypertension implies an increased resting pressure. A diastolic reading of more than 90 mm Hg is suggestive of hypertension, and if the diastolic figure is more than 100 mm Hg the condition is well established. However, in reaching such a diagnosis it is important to ensure that measurements are made under standard conditions, with the patient lying both rested and relaxed. Approximately 20 percent of adults claim to have been told by doctors that their blood pressure is too high, which may be true if a hasty reading is taken in the anxious surroundings of a medical consulting room; nevertheless, in four out of five individuals a normal pressure can be recorded under relaxed conditions.

A high resting blood pressure increases the risk of various forms of cardiovascular disease, including cerebrovascular catastrophes and myocardial infarctions. Regular exercise leads to a small, but statistically significant and therapeutically useful, decrease of blood pressure (5 to 10 mm Hg). A reduction of obesity (through a combination of exercise and dieting) also decreases the resting blood pressure.

Pulse Pressure

The pulse pressure reflects (1) the size of the cardiac stroke volume, (2) the elasticity of the vessels into which the blood is expelled, (3) the speed of cardiac ejection, and (4) any special features such as a narrowing of the aortic valve (a low pulse pressure) or of the aorta (a high pulse pressure). A fit individual usually has a substantial pulse pressure because of (1) and (3).

Hypotension

The adaptability of the circulation is sometimes tested by a tilt table test, in which a person is suddenly moved from a horizontal to a vertical posture. In a fit person, there is a reflex increase of tone in the leg veins, so that blood pressure is well maintained. However, venous tone deteriorates with lack of exercise, and an unfit person may show a substantial drop of blood pressure when the same procedure is carried out.

Prolonged standing gives rise to a drop of blood pressure through a combination of pooling of blood in the leg veins and exudation of fluid into the working muscles. On occasion, the drop in pressure may be sufficient to cause a loss of consciousness (a "faint"). The situation is readily corrected by lying down. The blood pressure is then sufficient to restore blood flow to the brain. Pressures can be boosted further, if necessary, by elevating the legs. There may be pallor and shivering for a few minutes, but the subject should not be swathed in an excess of blankets—overheating of the body merely encourages venous pooling.

On occasion, psychological factors contribute to the sudden drop of blood pressure (a "vasovagal attack"). In one recent example in the author's laboratory, a capillary prick of the finger reminded a young man of driving a nail into his finger, and there was a rapid loss of consciousness. The heart rate was very slow, owing to a profound vagal discharge, and wide vasodilatation of the muscle vessels contributed to the fall of pressure.

Hot and humid shower areas leave the subject particularly vulnerable to a fall of blood pressure immediately following exercise. In postcoronary patients, this environment may cause not only a loss of consciousness, but also depression of the ST segment of the electrocardiogram and ventricular arrhythmias. Two of four cardiac emergencies in the Toronto Rehabilitation Centre cardiac program have occurred during recovery from exercise sessions.

Exercise Blood Pressure

Because the blood pressure rises sharply during isometric activity, many people exclude older individuals from isometric training programs. The rise of blood pressure is largely an attempt to reestablish perfusion of a muscle when the local blood flow has been impeded by the muscle contraction. Obstruction of blood flow begins when the muscle develops 10 to 15 percent of its maximum voluntary force, and vascular occlusion has become virtually complete when exertion is 70 percent of maximum force. A second factor sometimes restricting the circulation is the performance of a Valsalva maneuver (forcible expiration against a closed glottis as part of isometric straining). Although the blood pressure can reach an alarmingly high level during a sustained isometric effort, it is not valid to argue against isometric exercise simply on the supposed danger of hypertension, since some muscle training response can be induced by very brief (6 to 10 second) contractions that cause little increase of blood pressure.

The blood pressure also rises during sustained rhythmic exercise (Table 6-1), in part because exhausting effort causes an increased secretion of catecholamines (Chapter 4), and in part because some muscles are contracting at a substantial fraction of their maximum voluntary force even during an apparently isotonic effort. The ability to sustain cardiac output against a rising peripheral pressure (after-load) depends on the condition of the myocardium and the adequacy of coronary blood flow. In healthy young subjects, stroke volume is often maintained to 100 percent of maximum effort, but in older individuals with an impaired coronary blood flow, the stroke volume diminishes when the intensity of exercise exceeds 70 to 80 percent of maximum aerobic effort. One of the interesting features of cardiac rehabilitation in postcoronary patients is that an improvement of pump function allows them to develop a higher peak exercise systolic pressure.

It is usual to monitor the blood pressure regularly during exercise. If a sphygmomanometer cuff is used while the subject is active, it is often difficult to detect the diastolic reading, whether muffling (Phase IV) or disappearance (Phase V) of the Korotkov sounds be accepted as the appropriate end-point. However, fairly accurate estimates of systolic pressure remain possible. A sudden drop of systolic pressure during heavy effort indicates that the heart muscle no longer has an adequate oxygen supply to meet its work-rate. It is an ominous sign and an urgent indication to halt an exercise test. Patients with aortic stenosis (and thus a heavy after-loading of the myocardium) are particularly vul-

TABLE 6-1   Systolic Blood Pressure in Relation to Age and Work Rate

Age (y)	Rest (1MET) (kPa)	Work Rate and Systolic Pressure			
		4 METs* (kPa)	6 METs* (kPa)	8 METs* (kPa)	10 METs* (kPa)
25	16.0	19.3	20.8	22.3	23.8
35	16.3	19.6	21.6	23.5	25.2
45	16.7	20.2	22.4	23.5	24.8
55	17.0	20.9	23.4	25.5	27.5

* MET is the ratio of the observed oxygen consumption to basal metabolic rate
Based on data of S.M. Fox, personal communication to the author

nerable to this type of response. However, when a brief bout of exercise (5 to 10 minutes) is carried to centrally-limited exhaustion, there is often a rather similar type of situation just before the test is concluded. Reduced blood flow to the brain accounts for confusion and at least a part of the observed incoordination; an eventual loss of consciousness follows.

Cardiac Work Rate

Cardiac muscle, like skeletal muscle, requires a renewal of its adenosine triphosphate (ATP) reserves if the actin–myosin bonding that is the basis of its pumping action is to continue. The total energy needs of the heart include small costs associated with its basal metabolism, the pumping of mineral ions such as sodium and calcium during activation and repolarization of the myocardium, and internal work associated with fiber shortening. However, the main sources of energy consumption are pumping and tension maintenance.

The pumping work can be calculated as the product of systolic pressure and the volume of blood that is expelled from the ventricle. Since pressure is not constant over the cardiac cycle, the information is most conveniently presented as a pressure–volume diagram. If Standard International (SI) units are used, pressure (Pa) has the dimensions N per square meter and volume is m^3, so that the area within the diagram is the work performed in joules (N • m). The power output (watts, or Joules per second) depends greatly upon the contractility of the heart, and thus the speed of fiber shortening.

Tension work is examined using the law of LaPlace (which was originally intended for thin-walled structures such as bubbles); this law states the relationship between intraventricular pressure Pv and wall-tension T as a function of the principal radii of the heart r_1 and r_2:

$$Pv = T (1/r_1 + 1/r_1)$$

From the equation, we might infer that tension work would be augmented by an increase of heart size, whether due to cardiac dilatation or hypertrophy.

However, hypertrophy also increases wall thickness and thus the stress carried per unit cross-section of cardiac muscle is reduced. The situation is further complicated if exercise or training induces an increase of myocardial contractility, since there is then an increased rate of energy expenditure associated with any given heart size. Within the relatively thick ventricular wall, the tensions associated with any given intraventricular pressure are greatest towards the inner, endocardial surface. This sector of the heart muscle is at a further disadvantage from the viewpoint of oxygenation, since the arterial supply must penetrate the contracting muscle from the superficially-placed main coronary arteries. It is thus hardly surprising that the subendocardial tissues are particularly vulnerable to ischemia and myocardial infarction.

The power output of the heart (w) can be calculated as:

$$W = \left[\int_{V_d}^{V_s} P_V \delta V + \alpha_o' \int T \delta t \right] f_h/60$$

The first term in this equation corresponds to the area of the pressure–volume diagram, integrated between end-diastolic and end-systolic dimensions. It can be approximated as the product of the mean ejection pressure and the cardiac stroke volume. The second term is the average wall tension, integrated over the contraction phase of the cardiac cycle, and multiplied by an arbitrary constant α to convert it to SI units. Notice also that since the dimensions of a power measurement are J per second, the heart rate f_h (beats per minute) must be divided by 60 when making this calculation.

Since the main purpose of the heart is to pump blood rather than to sustain intraventricular pressure, the first term represents the useful component of cardiac work, while the efficiency is given by the ratio of this first term to the total power output. At rest, the efficiency may be as low as 3 percent, but it rises to 10 to 15 percent during vigorous exercise. Because of the increase in efficiency during physical activity, a substantial exercise-induced increase of cardiac output can be accommodated with only a small increase in the total power output of the heart. On the other hand, an anxiety-generated rise of blood pressure leads to a drop in efficiency and a large increase of cardiac work. It is thus logical to encourage the postcoronary patient to engage in moderate exercise, rather than to remain sitting at home in a state of anxiety.

When carrying out exercise tests on a person with an impaired oxygen supply to the myocardium, it is useful to relate ECG changes to the cardiac work rate. If there were no changes of stroke volume, blood pressure, or ejection time, the heart rate would provide an index of cardiac power output. Some animal experiments have used this measure, but it is unlikely that all of the other variables concerned with cardiac work-rate will remain constant during vigorous exercise. In humans, it is thus more usual to use the "double product" or the "tension–time index" (the product of systolic pressure times heart rate) to approximate the cardiac work-rate.

The resting oxygen consumption of the heart (30 to 35 mℓ per minute) accounts for a substantial fraction of basal metabolism. In vigorous exercise, a cardiac oxygen consumption of 150 to 200 mℓ per minute is likely. Again, this represents a significant change upon the total process of oxygen delivery, although if 150 mℓ of oxygen are consumed in pumping 20 ℓ of blood, the cost of 7.5 mℓ per liter is still much less than the oxygen that is delivered (the latter being at least 120 mℓ per liter). There is little danger of reaching the point where the cost of pumping blood exceeds the extra oxygen introduced into the body by a further increase of cardiac activity.

Effect of Increasing Cardiac Output

There are three basic tactics that can be used to increase cardiac output: (1) an increase of heart rate, (2) an increase of stroke volume via an increase of end-diastolic volume, and (3) an increase of myocardial contractility (and thus a more complete emptying of the heart).

An increase of heart rate inevitably increases the nonproductive, isovolumic component of cardiac work, and it also leads to an increase of myocardial contractility. It is thus the least economical method of increasing cardiac output. An increase of end-diastolic volume is also costly, since the tension term in the cardiac work calculation is increased through the LaPlace relationship. At a first glance, an increase of myocardial contractility might be thought an expensive tactic; however, the direct effect of increasing oxygen consumption in the cardiac muscle fibers is often offset in practice by a decrease in mean ventricular volume.

As in skeletal muscle, a slow velocity of contraction improves efficiency at heavy work-rates, perhaps because the rate of hydrolysis of the actin–myosin cross-bridges is slower during the phase of the cardiac cycle when tension must be sustained. A reduction of contractility may thus be helpful in meeting the double challenge of old age—an increased energy demand from a chronic rise in after-loading and an impaired energy supply.

ELECTROCARDIOGRAM

General Considerations

The electrocardiogram is frequently recorded during exercise, both as a means of accurately determining the heart rate and as a safety precaution. However, if the observer lacks medical qualification, it is important not to express an opinion on the normality of the ECG. In one recent court case, a person who had a heart attack while exercising successfully sued a physical educator who had told him a few weeks earlier that the exercise ECG was normal; unfortunately, a cardiologist retained for the trial was able to point to a minor abnormality that had not been observed at the time of testing. Despite this medicolegal problem, those conducting exercise tests should become as familiar as possible with normal and abnormal ECG tracings, so that they know when to refuse and when to halt an exercise test.

Lead Systems

There has been much discussion concerning the optimum lead system for exercising subjects. At rest, the cardiologist records up to 12 lead combinations, either in sequence or simultaneously. During and immediately following exercise, most of the electrical anomalies in left ventricular function can be detected using a bipolar lead system (CM-5). One electrode is placed over the manubrio-sternal juction (Fig. 6-8), and the second is located over the apex beat (fifth interspace, 9 to 10 cm to the left of the sternum); the grounding electrode is attached to the nape of the neck. Some authors prefer to use three bipolar electrode positions (C2, C4, and C6), while others read from the full range of 12 positions. In general, an increase in the number of recording electrodes increases the probability of detecting small abnormalities of ventricular repolarization, but it also greatly increases the proportion of false-positive tests (where an apparent abnormality such as ST segmental depression is reported for an individual with a normal heart and coronary circulation).

Those who are inexperienced in exercise testing encounter much difficulty from an electrical baseline that wanders with respiration. The variations of baseline voltage reflect a varying electrical impedance at the skin surface. Respiratory artefacts can be largely overcome by a preliminary light abrasion of the dermis with a device such as a dental burr; this removes much of the dry, electrically-insulating keratin. Residual difficulties can be resolved by means of an electronic averaging device. Typically, this superimposes 16 or 32 similar ECG waveforms to give a clear averaged trace.

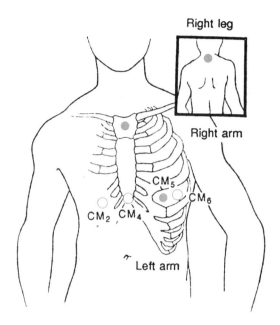

Right leg

Right arm

CM₅

CM₆

CM₂   CM₄

Left arm

Figure 6–8   To illustrate the recommended placement of electrodes for exercise tests (lead CM_5). The lead labeled "right arm" is attached over the upper part of the sternum (manubrium sterni). The lead labeled "left arm" is attached over the apex beat (in the space between the fifth and sixth ribs, 3 to 4 inches to the left of the midline). The lead marked "right leg" is attached at the back of the neck. Alternative placements for leads CM_2, CM_4, and CM_6 are also indicated. (From Shephard RJ. Endurance fitness. Toronto: University of Toronto Press, 1977. By courtesy of the publisher.)

The ECG recorder should meet the minimum specifications of the American Heart Association with respect to its responsiveness at high and low frequencies. A poor low frequency response may give the appearance of ST depression to a perfectly normal tracing. Tape recorders and telemeters are particularly likely to lack the required frequency response characteristics.

Resting Electrocardiogram

The resting ECG of an athletic individual has several characteristic features, including large P and T waves and left axis deviation (a prominent R wave in Lead I and a large S wave in Lead III). These findings generally reflect left ventricular hypertrophy and a large stroke volume. A substantial proportion of athletes also show a prolonged P-Q interval and some notching of the R wave (right bundle branch block).

A careful inspection of the resting tracing can pick out some pathologies where exercise is unwise (Fig. 6-9). A prominent Q wave and ST elevation may indicate an acute myocarditis or a recent anterior infarction (although both changes are also possible in a normal heart). A recent posterior infarction may give rise to ST depression; whether it is initially elevated or depressed, the displacement of the ST segment is corrected as the individual recovers from the infarction. Recent pulmonary embolism may be shown by a rapid heart rate and such signs of right heart strain as inverted T waves over the right ventricle. Bursts of rapid ventricular rhythm (ventricular tachycardia) with independent P waves and broadened QRS complexes can progress to ventricular fibrillation, particularly if the premature beats occur in the vulnerable early phase of ventricular repolarization (immediately following the peak of the T wave). The Wolff-Parkinson-White syndrome also increases the risk of ventricular fibrillation. In this condition, an electrical short circuit in the a-v node gives rise to premature and abnormal excitation of the ventricle. The P waves are normal, but the P-R interval is less than 120 msec and the QRS complex shows a very abnormal waveform.

In atrial flutter, there is a rapid succession of P waves, with one in three or four beats being transmitted to the ventricle. In atrial fibrillation, the P waves are replaced by small and irregular f waves, while the ventricular complexes have a slow, irregular timing. Exercise should proceed with care in both of these conditions. Other conduction disturbances that require a cautious approach to exercise include sinuatrial block, marked atrioventricular block, and left bundle-branch block. With sinuatrial block, some of the impulses arising in the sinus fail to depolarize the atria. In older subjects, this may be an indication of ischemia in the sinus pacemaker, and the sick sinus syndrome can develop where the heart rate fails to increase as expected during vigorous exercise. However, excessive vagal tone can also give rise to a sinuatrial block in endurance athletes. Atrioventricular block can arise from excessive vagal activity. Usually, the P-R interval gets progressively longer (Type I block), until only a proportion of impulses are transmitted to the ventricles (Type II block); some ventricular complexes are missing, and an occasional QRS complex may appear without a preceeding P wave (ventricular escape). Ultimately, the atria and ventricles develop a completely independent rhythm (Type III block); progression to this stage usually signals some abnormality of the myocardium, and it may herald a Stokes-Adams attack (where there is complete ventricular standstill, or asystole). An increase of serum potassium (as in freshwater drowning) lengthens the P-R interval, while an increase of sodium ions (as in saltwater drowning) shortens it. Left bundle branch block is seen as a broadening and/or a notching of the QRS complex, with a leftward shift in the electrical axis of the heart; it is usually associated with myocardial disease.

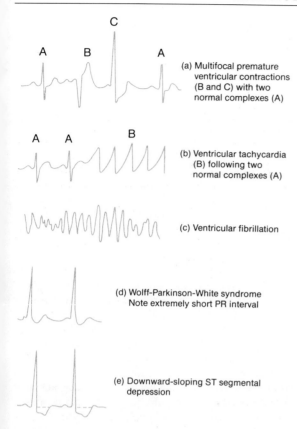

(a) Multifocal premature ventricular contractions (B and C) with two normal complexes (A)

(b) Ventricular tachycardia (B) following two normal complexes (A)

(c) Ventricular fibrillation

(d) Wolff-Parkinson-White syndrome Note extremely short PR interval

(e) Downward-sloping ST segmental depression

Figure 6-9   Some common ECG abnormalities.

Clinicians diagnose a sinus bradycardia if the resting heart rate is less than 60 beats per minute. However, such findings are common in endurance athletes. The mechanism seems to be a vagally-induced increase of potassium ion permeability in the sinuatrial node. Sinus arrhythmia is another "innocent" source of irregular heart rhythm that is seen more often in athletes than in sedentary subjects. The phenomenon is characterized by a quickening of heart rate during inspiration and a slowing during expiration; however, a more steady pace develops as exercise is begun. It is not clear whether sinus arrhythmia is caused by cyclic variations of venous return or whether there are cyclic changes in vagal and sympathetic nerve tone.

Premature contractions may arise in the sinus, atrium, a-v node, or ventricle. Ventricular beats are usually ectopic (arising other than in the normal pathway for the conduction of electrical impulses); in consequence, the QRS complex is broadened and shows an abnormal waveform. Contributory factors include nicotine accumulation in a heavy smoker and an excessive sympathetic discharge in an anxious individual. Added beats of this sort usually become less frequent as exercise is begun, and although fears have been expressed that they may presage sudden death, in fact the effect upon prognosis is small if any, once

allowance has been made for coexistent ST segmental abnormalities (as will be discussed).

Exercise Electrocardiogram

The main features of interest in an exercise electrocardiogram are the onset of ST segmental depression, and the appearance of premature ventricular contractions (see Fig. 6-9).

The behavior of the ST segment is often analyzed by computer—after a series of closely matched ECG waveforms have been superimposed and averaged, the extent of ST segmental depression is measured electronically at a fixed interval of 60 to 80 msec following the QRS complex. Depression of the ST segment arises in essence because of a slowing in repolarization of the left ventricle. A very small phase difference between the repolarization process in right and left ventricles suffices to cause a substantial ST segmental displacement. The usual cause of the delay in repolarization is a slowing of the sodium pump, secondary to myocardial ischemia. However, a similar appearance is possible with any factor that modifies the rate of repolarization. For example, the plasma electrolyte balance may be disturbed by hyperventilation or the use of diuretics; other drugs such as digitalis act more directly to inhibit the membrane pump.

There has been much discussion of an appropriate criterion that will distinguish a true- from a false-positive ECG test result. If activity is monitored during both exercise (to at least 85 percent of maximum oxygen intake, Table 6-2) and recovery, the best discrimination of normal from abnormal is obtained when the criterion of a positive test is an ST depression of 0.1 mV at the junction between the ST segment and the T wave (Fig. 6-10). Acceptance of a lesser criterion (e.g., 0.05 mV of horizontal ST segmental depression) improves sensitivity (the percentage of ischemic hearts detected), but worsens specificity (the proportion of abnormal test results attributable to myocardial disease). The finding of a 0.1 mV ST depression approximately doubles the risk of a cardiovascular emergency over the next 5 to 10 years. Nevertheless, the findings from mass screening of the general public are sufficiently inconsistent that care must be taken in

TABLE 6-2   Relationship of Sensitivity and Specificity to Intensity of Exercise ECG Tests

Type of Test	Sensitivity* (%)	Specificity† (%)
Submaximal step test (double master)	35 - 60	69 - 100
Symptom-limited maximum	71 - 80	88 - 97

* Proportion of patients with myocardial ischemia detected by test
† Proportion of patients with abnormal test having myocardial ischemia

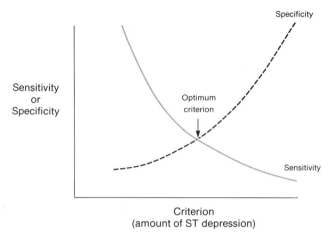

Figure 6–10   The relationship between criterion of ischemia, sensitivity and specificity of test.

presenting supposedly abnormal test results to an individual. As many as two-thirds of those with exercise-induced ST depressions are in fact free of ischemic heart disease, and unwise comments from the test administrator can create an unnecessary cardiac neurosis. When testing the general population, inherent probabilities are such that a negative result is much more likely to be correct than a positive response (Table 6–3).

The best approach is probably to reserve formal interpretation of an exercise ECG for those with high risk of cardiac disease. This tactic automatically increases the proportion of positive tests that are correct. It is also possible to look at the form of the ST segmental change; a horizontal or downward sloping segment is more frequently associated with ischemia than is an upward sloping segment. Finally, possible artefactual causes of ST depression, such as hyperventilation and the use of diuretics, should be considered before reaching a diagnosis (Table 6-4).

The proportion of exercise-induced ST abnormalities that are observed in the general population rises with age. By 65 years, at least 20 percent of people show an "abnormal" response. Apparently the proportion of false positive records is much higher in women than in men.

Occasionally, authors have continued with exhausting exercise until very deep ST depression (0.5 to 1.0 mV) has been produced. In the specific instances reported, there were no adverse consequences, but it is more usual to halt exercise if the depression exceeds 0.2 mV. The corresponding oxygen consumption is described as a "symptom-limited" maximum oxygen intake, and since the ischemic limitation has arisen from the work-rate of the heart, it is usual practice to note the corresponding pulse pressure product. Sometimes the appearance of ST depression is clearly linked to the onset of cardiac (anginal) pain (Chapter 13). In other subjects, the myocardial ischemia at first inspection seems "silent." Nevertheless, many such individuals can be taught to recognize a mild chest, arm, or throat discomfort that is associated with the ECG change, and this knowledge is helpful to them in regulating the intensity of subsequent daily exercise bouts.

The premature ventricular contractions of the anxious patient generally become less frequent with exercise. However, an abnormality of rhythm that appears for the first time during exercise—whether a heart block or a series of extrasystoles—should be regarded seriously, as it may progress to ventricular fibrillation. It is usual to halt exercise if more than three premature ventricular contractions are seen in any 10-second interval. Particularly adverse signs are a run of extrasystoles, a multifocal origin (as shown by a

TABLE 6-3   The Influence of Disease Prevalence on the Proportion of False-Positive and False-Negative Exercise ECG Test Results

Test Result	Ischemia Absent	Ischemia Present	Test Errors (%)
50 per 1,000 with myocardial ischemia			
Positive	95	40	70.4
Negative	855	10	1.2
425 per 1,000 with myocardial ischemia			
Positive	58	340	14.6
Negative	517	85	14.1

TABLE 6–4   Some Factors Causing False-Positive
and False-Negative Exercise ECG Test Results

False-Positive Results	False-Negative Results
Hyperventilation	Insufficient exercise intensity
Cigarette smoking	ST elevation at rest
Glucose and carbohydrate loads	Abnormalities of ventricular conduction
Diuretics, potassium loss	Nitroglycerine and other vasodilators
Abnormal stress on left	
ventricle	
ST depression at rest	
Abnormal ventricular conduction	
(e.g., left ventricular bundle	
branch block)	
Antidysrhythmic drugs	
(e.g., procainamide,	
quinidine)	
Digitalis therapy	

varying QRS waveform) and occurrence early during repolarization ("R on T" phenomenon). Causal factors are local hypoxia and the secretion of catecholamines. Oxygen lack causes a local and temporary unidirectional blockage of electrical transmission, facilitating re-entry of the ECG signal into the ventricular muscle, while the catecholamines lower the threshold for abnormal pace-making stimuli.

There is some relationship between the development of exercise-induced extrasystoles and the risk of sudden cardiovascular death, particularly in patients who have sustained a myocardial infarction. However, in the normal adult it is less clear that the appearance of premature ventricular contractions adds to the information on risk yielded by an analysis of exercise-induced ST segmental depression.

CARDIAC EMERGENCIES

Nature and Risk of Cardiac Emergencies

Exercise may provoke ventricular fibrillation, asystole, or myocardial infarction, the first of these emergencies being the most frequent. After surveying 74 North American stress-testing laboratories, Rochmis and Blackburn concluded that the risk of an emergency within 1 hour of testing was less than one in 10,000. Moreover, the 13 victims reported in their study were all individuals with known cardiac disease. This suggests that the risk to normal individuals is extremely low. Studies of joggers and of exercise programs at YMCAs indicate that the risk in the community is approximately one incident in 400,000 person-hours, about 7 times the resting hazard to a middle-aged individual. However, this disadvantage is probably offset by a beneficial effect on prognosis between exercise bouts (Chapter 13).

Ventricular Fibrillation

Ventricular fibrillation is an irregular writhing contraction of the ventricles (see Fig. 6-9) that is totally ineffective in expelling blood from the heart. Unless a normal cardiac rhythm is restored within 4 minutes, the brain sustains irreversible ischemic damage. Each minute reduces the likelihood of successful resuscitation, and it is thus important that health professionals be prepared to undertake cardiac resuscitation immediately it becomes necessary. Factors predisposing to ventricular fibrillation include an ectopic focus in the left ventricle, a rapid burst of extrasystoles, and a local environment that favors reentry of the electrical impulse. Electrical shock, freshwater drowning, myocardial ischemia, and an accumulation of catecholamines are all possible triggers.

The diagnosis is based on the absence of a pulse and the observation of irregular f waves on the electrocardiogram. The standard treatment is to apply one or more electrical "shocks" to the chest wall. A complete depolarization of the myocardium results, and the hope is that after ventricular repolarization has occurred, a normal cardiac rhythm will return. Defibrillators originally used alternating current, but a direct current condensor discharge has proved safer to both patient and operator. The machine is usually set to deliver a shock of 100 watt • second, but if this proves ineffective, the intensity can be increased progressively to 300 watt • second. The success rate of defibrillation depends greatly on the duration of myocardial hypoxia. If fibrillation has lasted for only a fraction of a minute, it is usually quite easy to restore a normal heart rhythm, but if the heart has become profoundly hypoxic, there may be little response unless its oxygenation is first improved by a preliminary period of cardiac massage.

Ventricular Arrest

Ventricular arrest may be a sequel to heart block, ventricular defibrillation, or saltwater drowning. The ECG shows no electrical activity. Sometimes the heart rhythm can be restored by a vigorous blow on the chest, but if this fails, cardiac massage must be begun immediately. It is important to place the patient on a rigid surface, since much of the effort expended by a rescuer can be dissipated in the springs of a mattress. A clenched fist is used to apply very vigorous pressure over the sternum some 60 times per minute. The free hand is used to protect the ribs and underlying viscera. If respiration has ceased, an assistant provides mouth-to-mouth resuscitation at a rate of approximately 20 breaths per minute. In small mammals such as the dog, quite substantial mean arterial pressures can be generated by external compression of the chest wall. In humans, the thorax is more rigid, and the blood pressure during resuscitation is quite marginal for survival; indeed, some observers believe that in older individuals massage is unlikely to be successful unless the thoracic cage is first ruptured by fracturing several ribs.

If the patient's condition does not improve quickly with external massage, a doctor may open the chest between the fourth and fifth ribs and begin internal massage. Intravenous sodium bicarbonate is commonly given to counter metabolic acidosis, and pressor amines can be administered to increase myocardial contractility.

Calcium chloride may also be helpful if contractions remain inadequate. The heart must be monitored carefully for a recurrence of the arrhythmia over the next 48 hours, and procainamide or lidocaine may be a useful means to reduce irritability at this stage. There is a danger of late swelling of the brain (cerebral edema); this is best countered by a deliberate reduction of the circulating blood volume and by hypothermia (to reduce metabolic demand).

DISTRIBUTION OF BLOOD FLOW

We have noted that the maximum arteriovenous oxygen difference depends in part on the distribution of blood flow between the muscles (where oxygen extraction is fairly complete) and tissues such as the skin and the kidneys (where flow is regulated to dispose of heat and waste products, rather than to deliver oxygen). We will now look at the blood flow to specific regions of the body during exercise.

Muscle Blood Flow

Variations of Flow. The blood flow to the skeletal muscles varies widely. Under resting conditions, they receive perhaps 2 to 3 ml of flow per 100 ml of tissue per minute, but in vigorous exercise, this is increased to as much as 100 ml per minute per 100 ml of tissue (more in red than in white muscle). The local flow is impeded as the force of muscle contraction rises and with some types of activity such as cycle ergometry, the perfusion of the most active muscles (the quadriceps) apparently peaks when the subject is developing approximatley 70 percent of maximum oxygen intake. During cycling, contractions are rhythmic, with a high proportion of the total blood flow occur-

ring during the relaxation phase; moreover, much of the oxygen needed for the 0.4 to 0.6 seconds of the contraction phase can be drawn from intramuscular myoglobin stores. The pumping action of the muscles plays an important role in assuring venous return, and can supply as much as 30 percent of the total energy needs of the circulation. For this reason, a cardiovascular problem arises during arm ergometry. A substantial amount of blood pools in the veins of the relaxed lower limbs, where the muscle pump is not functioning, and the resultant reduction of central blood volume limits both maximum cardiac output and maximum oxygen intake.

Regulation of Flow. Sympathetic stimulation reduces the perfusion of white muscle fibers by 80 percent, and red muscle fibers by 50 percent. It is assumed that during exercise a general sympathetic activation minimizes perfusion of the inactive muscles, and a local accumulation of metabolites counteracts this signal, assuring vasodilatation in the active regions. The increase of flow to the working muscles begins within 0.5 to 1.0 seconds of the onset of exercise, building to a steady-state level within 30 to 60 seconds. The precise metabolic signal for vasodilatation is still debated. Possible candidates include a decrease of local intravascular oxygen pressure, a decrease of intravascular pH, an extracellular accumulation of potassium ions, local changes of osmotic pressure, and an accumulation of phosphagen breakdown products. One suggestion has been that potassium ions interfere with the release of norepinephrine at the sympathetic nerve terminals.

Intermittent Contractions. If intermittent muscle contractions are held repeatedly for periods of 0.5 to 2.0 second, there is little cumulative fatigue, ischemic pain, or postcontraction hyperemia, but with a 4-second contraction per 8-second recovery cycle fatigue does develop and the postexercise blood flow becomes proportional to the number of contractions that have been made. Presumably, with the 4-second per 8 second rhythm of contraction and relaxation, it is no longer possible to make good the depletion of oxygen and phosphagen stores during the recovery interval. Attempts at compensation by an increase of systemic blood pressure serve mainly to increase blood flow to the skin and inactive muscles.

Capillary Supply. The muscle capillaries generally run parallel to the muscle fibers, being arranged with an average of 3 to 6 vessels per fiber. Under resting conditions, a cross-section of muscle shows a count of some 200 vessels per square millimeter, and during exercise this rises to perhaps 600 per square millimeter, with slightly higher figures in endurance athletes than in sedentary individuals. Given a total muscle mass of 30 kg, a capillary surface area of 300 to 600 m² may be anticipated. It is thus hardly surprising that in normal circumstances there is a fairly complete equilibration of gas pressures between the muscle capillaries and the surrounding tissues. Capillary transit times range widely from 90 msec to 43 sec, with a mean of 4.3

sec and a median of 8 sec; the dispersion among these values is sufficient that problems of equilibration are still possible in capillaries with a short transit time.

Oxygen Pressure Gradients. The local oxygen pressure needed to sustain aerobic metabolism within the interior of the muscle mitochondrion is very small (as low as 6 to 7 Pa or about 0.05 Torr for the NADH/NAD+ enzyme system, and approximately 24 Pa or 0.18 Torr for cytochrome c). To this must be added a gradient of approximately 13 Pa (1 Torr) facilitating diffusion from the surface of the mitochondrion to its interior, 90 to 100 Pa (0.7 Torr) for diffusion from the outer surface of the muscle fiber to the surface of the mitochondrion, 1.6 to 2.8 kPa (12 to 21 Torr) for diffusion from the intramuscular capillary to the outer surface of the most distant muscle fiber and a final pressure drop of 13 to 163 Pa (0.1 to 4.6 Torr) associated with delays in the dissociation of oxyhemoglobin in the tissues. The total of these several pressure gradients (1.8 to 3.1 kPa, 13 to 27 Torr, Table 6-5) agrees quite well with the partial pressure of oxygen which is found in venous blood leaving the active muscles. In other words, the driving pressure beyond the tissue capillaries is small; the system of oxidative enzymes and cofactors within the mitochondrion offers little impedance to the metabolic utilization of oxygen.

Role of Myoglobin. The pigment myoglobin plays an important role in transferring oxygen from the muscle capillaries to the mitochondrion. Because the myoglobin molecule contains only one heme group compared to the four of the hemoglobin molecule, it has a hyperbolic rather than a sigmoid-shaped oxygen dissociation curve (Fig. 6-11), and at the partial pressures of oxygen that are likely within the muscle capillaries (1 to 2 kPa), there is thus a transfer of oxygen from hemoglobin to myoglobin. Moreover, the myglobin molecules can themselves rotate within the muscle fibers, boosting the simple diffusional transport of oxygen by as much as 50 percent. Finally, the myoglobin provides a small store of oxygen (approximately 0.16 mℓ per 100 mℓ of muscle) that can be used during a brief contraction. For instance, if 10 kg of muscle are activated during cycling, 16 mℓ of oxygen are available per pedal revolution, or at 100 rpm a total of 1.6 ℓ per minute (typically, as much as one half of the total oxygen consumption).

Fluid Balance. Fluid tends to "leak" into the tissues at the arterial end of the capillaries; the intravascular hydrostatic pressure here is perhaps 4 kPa, compared with 1 kPa in the tissues (Table 6-6). This outward force is opposed by an osmotic pressure gradient of some 3 kPa drawing extracellular fluid back into the plasma. Thus, there is a net gradient of about 1 kPa in favor of fluid loss from the arterial end of the capillary loop. At the venous end of the capillaries, the hydrostatic pressure has dropped by approximately 3 kPa, but the osmotic pressure gradient remains largely unchanged. There is thus a 1 kPa gradient favoring reabsorption of fluid at the venous end of the circuit. Under resting conditions the two processes are essentially in equilibrium, with little tendency for the tissues to become waterlogged. However, the delicate balance of hydrostatic and osmotic pressures is easily upset by many factors, including an exercise- or a posture-induced increase of hydrostatic pressure within the capillaries of the leg muscles. During warm weather, a 2 to 10 percent increase in the fluid content of the leg muscles occurs over the first few minutes of vigorous exercise (a fluid loss of perhaps 0.4 mℓ per minute per 100 mℓ of active muscle). However, the process is self-limiting, since exudation not only increases the hydrostatic pressure within the extracellular spaces, but also boosts the osmotic pressure of the plasma.

Skin Blood Flow

The skin blood flow is capable of wide variation, increasing from 1 to 150 mℓ per minute per 100 mℓ of tissue as vasodilation occurs. In extreme heat, the total flow to the skin may be as large as 10 ℓ per minute. The increase of flow occurs by (1) a release of local vasoconstrictor tone, (2) a direct effect of warmth on the skin blood vessels, and (3) a local

TABLE 6-5   Oxygen Pressure Gradient from Muscle Capillaries to Enzymes on Interior Surface of Mitochondrial Membrane

Location	Local Gradient (Pa)	Total (cumulative) Gradient (Pa)
At NADH/NAD+ enzyme system	6 - 7	6 - 7
From Mitochondrial surface to NADH/NAD+	13	19 - 20
From Muscle fiber surface to mitochondrial surface	90 - 100	109 - 120
From Muscle capillary to muscle fiber surface	1680 - 2800	1789 - 2920
From Oxyhemoglobin dissociation to muscle capillary wall	13 - 163	1802 - 3083

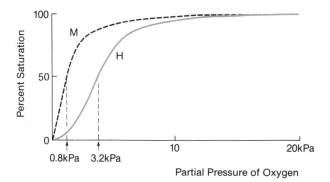

Figure 6–11   Comparison of the oxygen dissociation curves for myoglobin (M) and hemoglobin (H).

response to bradykinin (which is released whenever there is a significant secretion of sweat).

Much of the heat-induced increase of flow bypasses the normal capillary circulation, blood being returned directly to the venules through thick-walled and muscular arteriovenous anastomoses. Oxygen extraction is minimal when blood passes by this route, but substantial quantities of heat are lost through the superficial veins. Training increases the proportion of heat lost by sweating. Skin flow can then be decreased, and the maximum arteriovenous oxygen difference during vigorous exercise becomes correspondingly widened.

At rest, the skin flow is regulated largely in response to changes of core temperature, but during exercise both local and general skin temperatures play an important role. The vasoconstrictor pathway is responsive to temperature, while vasodilatation is influenced more by core temperature. There is thus a phase lag of up to 10 minutes in the vasodilator response to moderate exercise that corresponds to the time course of the rise in core temperature. The progressive increase of skin flow makes a major contribution to the upward drift of heart rate and downward drift of stroke volume that is observed when a subject performs prolonged work in a warm environment.

During brief periods of maximum effort, cutaneous vasodilatation may bring about a small increase of maximum cardiac output relative to that observed with maximum exercise in the cold, but even if vasodilatation is deliberately stimulated by wearing a heated water-filled suit, the skin flow of a vigorously exercising subject does not exceed 2.0 to 2.5 ℓ per minute. Under normal, warm conditions, the skin color of a person who is undertaking a maximum oxygen intake test changes from red to a bluish hue as arterial flow is reduced, and from blue to grey as tone is increased in the superficial venous capacity vessels. Because of the ultimate vasoconstriction, neither maximum cardiac output nor maximum oxygen intake are influenced greatly by brief heat exposure.

Under cold conditions, the blood flow to the extremities is greatly reduced by a closure of the arteriovenous anastomoses. The pathway of venous return is shifted thereby from superficial to deep veins; this arrangement allows heat exchange to occur between the arteries perfusing the limbs and the immediately adjacent veins.

TABLE 6-6   Balance of Hydrostatic and Osmotic Pressures at Arterial and Venous Ends of Muscle Capillaries

Site and Source of Pressure		Pressure		
		Intravascular (kPa)	Extracellular (kPa)	Gradient* (kPa)
Arterial				
Hydrostatic		4.0	1.0	+3
Osmotic		3.3	1.3	−2
Net Force				+1
Venous				
Hydrostatic		2.0	1.0	+1
Osmotic		3.3	1.3	−2
Net Force				−1

* Positive sign implies pressure gradient favoring leakage of intravascular fluids.

Visceral Blood Flow

A number of visceral organs receive more than their fair share of the total cardiac output at rest. The kidneys, for example, take more than 20 percent of the resting output. When endurance exercise is performed, the flow to all of the viscera is reduced. If physical activity is combined with exposure to a hot environment, visceral flow drops to only 25 to 30 percent of the resting value. Regulating factors include (1) an altered balance of sympathetic and parasympathetic discharge, and (2) an effect of any exercise-induced increase of serum catecholamines (Chapter 4) on the blood vessels.

The maximum possible redistribution of blood flow from the viscera to the working muscles is 2 to 3 ℓ per minute, approximately 10 percent of the total exercise cardiac output. The contribution that this makes to the blood flow demands of the active muscles is thus much smaller than the potential contribution from a reduction of skin blood flow. Nevertheless, visceral ischemia when exercising in the heat is sufficient to induce various functional changes, including a reduction in hepatic function (shown by a slower clearance of the dye indocyanine green), and a slower excretion of a renal test substance (para-aminohippuric acid). Constriction of the efferent arterioles in the renal tubules also increases the filtration pressure, stretching "pores" in the walls of the renal capillaries, and perhaps in consequence vigorous exercise usually gives rise to a substantial proteinuria.

Pulmonary Blood Flow

Pressure Range. Pressures in the pulmonary circuit are quite low. Even in the pulmonary artery, resting figures of 2.4/1.0 kPa are likely, and a threefold increase of blood flow can be accommodated without a significant rise of pulmonary arterial pressures. During maximum exercise, the pulmonary arterial pressures of a young person are unlikely to exceed 3.3/1.3 kPa.

Capacity Effects. The capacity of the pulmonary circuit is such that it serves a significant reservoir function. At rest, the lungs contain about 500 mℓ of blood; this increases to 1,500 mℓ during vigorous exercise. At the same time, the pulmonary capillary blood volume increases from 100 mℓ at rest to 200 mℓ during vigorous effort. The cross-section of the pulmonary capillary bed shows a threefold expansion, but since the cardiac output can increase to six times its resting value during maximum exercise, the speed of flow through the pulmonary capillaries is also augmented. In consequence, the average capillary transit time drops from 0.75 seconds at rest to approximately 0.3 seconds during maximum effort. In some of the shorter capillaries, the available time may then be insufficient to allow a full equilibration between alveolar gas

and blood. However, oxygen exchange occurs more rapidly than might otherwise be anticipated owing to (1) rotation of the red cells, (2) displacement of the red cells from their axial stream, and (3) a possible movement of hemoglobin and cytochrome molecules within the red cells.

Influence of Alveolar Pressures. The pulmonary arterial pressure is quite small relative to the vertical height of the lungs (Fig. 6-12), so that under resting conditions the alveolar gas pressure usually exceeds pulmonary arterial pressure in the upper part of the lungs (zone 1); with the exception of a few vessels in the angles between alveoli, there is thus a collapse of all blood vessels smaller than 30 μ in this part of the lungs. In the middle zone (zone 2), the paracapillary pressure is intermediate between pulmonary, arterial, and venous pressures, so that flow becomes possible whenever alveolar pressure falls (during inspiration), but it is interrupted as alveolar pressure rises (during expiration). In the lower part of the lungs (zone 3), even pulmonary venous pressure exceeds alveolar pressure, so that there is no longer any tendency for blood flow to vary with respiration. Finally, some authors distinguish a small zone 4, at the base of the lungs; here, flow is restricted by the increase of interstitial pressure as alveoli collapse.

The boundaries between the four zones are shifted by fluctuations of pulmonary capillary pressure over the cardiac cycle, by changes of alveolar pressure (for instance, with hyperventilation), and by any increase of pulmonary arterial pressure (with exercise, aging or exposure to low pressures of inspired oxygen). Because vigorous exercise raises the pulmonary arterial pressure, it tends to improve perfusion of the upper part of the lungs. The deeper ventilation associated with heavy effort also leads to an increase of the mean alveolar volume with less alveolar collapse. Together, these various changes improve the vertical matching of ventilation with perfusion and reduce the restriction of blood flow in zone 4. However, some horizontal mismatching of ventilation and perfusion persists at any given level within the lungs, even during all-out effort.

Pulmonary Edema. Normally, there is little tendency for fluid to escape from the pulmonary capillaries into the alveolar spaces. However, the delicate balance of osmotic and hydrostatic forces within the lungs can be upset if capillary permeability is increased by infection or oxygen lack or if pulmonary intravascular pressures are increased by hypoxia and exercise. Several of these factors provide the seeds for the acute pulmonary edema which has been observed at altitudes of more than 3,500 m (Chapter 11).

Blood Flow to Other Organs

Brain. During exercise, the cerebral blood flow remains relatively constant at its normal figure of 0.5 to 0.6 ℓ per minute, provided that an adequate systemic

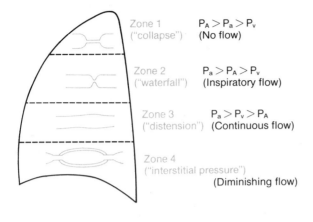

Zone 1 $P_A > P_a > P_v$
("collapse")   (No flow)

Zone 2 $P_a > P_A > P_v$
("waterfall")   (Inspiratory flow)

Zone 3 $P_a > P_v > P_A$
("distension")   (Continuous flow)

Zone 4
("interstitial pressure")
    (Diminishing flow)

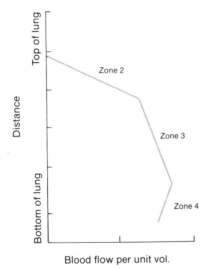

Figure 6–12 Relation of pulmonary alveolar interstitial pressure (P_A) to pressure at the arterial and venous ends of the pulmonary capillaries (Pa and Pv respectively).

blood pressure is maintained. Little measurable change occurs with either physical or mental activity, despite substantial alterations in cerebral activity; conceivably, flow is redirected from one part of the brain to another within the cranium, while maintaining a constant total cerebral flow. Any gains of mental performance during or following vigorous physical activity probably reflect an increase of arousal rather than an improvement of local blood flow to the brain.

Bone. The resting blood flow to bone is of a similar order to that for the brain, although it can be increased up to 40 percent in response to mechanical loading. If the nutrient arteries to a bone are damaged by mechanical trauma, degeneration may occur, with subsequent osteoarthritis. The scaphoid bone of the wrist joint (injured by falls on the outstretched hand) has only a single nutrient artery and is particularly vulnerable in this regard.

CIRCULATORY REGULATION

The primary function of the circulation is to maintain blood flow to the brain. The control system thus includes a typical cybernetic "feedback" loop from pressor sensors in the aorta and at the bifurcation of the common carotid arteries. If the blood pressure starts to fall, impulses are sent to controlling centers in the medulla oblongata, initiating corrective action (vasoconstriction and/or an increase of cardiac output). The vast blood flow demands of vigorous exercise present a major challenge to this regulatory system.

Neural Centers

Cardiac, vasoconstrictor, and vasodepressor centers have been described, based on responses to electrical stimulation of the medulla. The vasoconstrictor area has its own spontaneous electrical activity, but the discharge pattern is modulated by impulses that come from the cerebral cortex, the hypothalamus, and the medullary vasodepressor center. Comparing the circulatory control system with a regulator of human design, the vasodepressor center may be regarded as the comparator, matching reported systemic blood pressures to an arbitrary set point that will assure perfusion of the brain.

Anger, anxiety, and other emotional reactions initiate an increase of heart rate and blood pressure as part of a hypothalamic "fight or flight" response. Conditioned reflexes from the cortex may also induce a high heart rate (180 to 200 beats per minute) immediately prior to competition. This speeds the time needed to reach a steady exercise heart rate (the circulatory "on-transient"), reducing the size of the deficit in oxygen supply to the muscles at the beginning of exercise. However, anxiety-related increases of heart rate during submaximum exercise increase the cardiac work rate and lead to errors in the prediction of maximum oxygen intake from responses to submaximal effort.

Irradiation of impulses from the large pyramidal cells of the motor cortex to the cardiovascular centers also contribute to the increase of heart rate at the beginning of exercise.

The centers controlling body temperature are located in the hypothalamus. If body temperature is increased (e.g., by exercise), impulses are directed to the medullary cardiovascular control centers, inducing tachycardia, with an increase of blood flow to the skin and a decrease of flow to the viscera. On the other hand, cold exposure induces vasoconstriction in the skin and peripheral muscles, with tachycardia and a rise of blood pressure (although such vasoconstriction may later be reversed by a local accumulation of metabolites, or a cold-induced paralysis of the regulatory nerves).

In extreme environments, there may finally be an irradiation of impulses from the respiratory centers;

for example, severe hypoxia stimulates the carotid bodies, and an irradiation of impulses from the respiratory to the vasomotor centers causes an associated rise of systemic blood pressure.

Peripheral Receptors

The carotid and aortic pressure sensors respond to the rate of pressure change and the frequency of distension, rather than to the absolute level of systemic blood pressure. Although systemic pressures rise during vigorous rhythmic or isometric exercise, there does not seem to be any alteration in either the sensitivity of the peripheral pressure receptors or the set point of the medullary centers. However, exercise (particularly isometric contractions) reduces the slowing of the heart rate which is normally seen when suction is applied to the neck immediately over the carotid sinus.

Other pressure sensitive mechanoreceptors have been described in the great veins, atria, ventricles, and pulmonary arteries. Deliberate distension of the atria induces tachycardia (the ''Bainbridge reflex''), although it is unlikely that this is involved in normal responses to exercise, since physical activity causes little increase of the venous filling pressure. Possibly, information on venous filling relative to thoracic or total blood volume initiates mechanisms to regulate blood volume (such as an increased secretion of antidiuretic hormone and a decreased excretion of sodium ions).

Chemoreceptors have been postulated (but not as yet demonstrated) in the active muscles. Suggested stimuli include local increases of osmotic pressure and increases of intravascular potassium ion concentrations. Probably the main function of such receptors is to counter the general signal to muscle vasoconstriction at the onset of exercise.

Temperature receptors in the skin, particularly those around the nose, are probably responsible for the dramatic slowing of heart rate that occurs during diving and local cold exposure of the face (the ''diving reflex''). This reflex is said to be augmented by prolonged exercise, a fact which could account for the occasional hypotensive syncope in a marathon runner who is sprayed with cold water.

Patterns of Regulation

The heart is slowed by impulses passing down the vagus nerve to the sinuatrial pacemaker; it is speeded by a reduction of vagal discharge and a simultaneous increase in the activity of nerves liberating norepinephrine in the region of the sympathetic beta receptors. As shown by administration of cholinergic and beta-blocking agents, endurance training increases vagal drive while reducing sympathetic activity.

During exercise, an increase of sympathetic activity and a decrease of vagal discharge lead to aug-

mentation of heart rate, stroke volume, and myocardial contractility. Cardiac patients are often given beta-blocking drugs such as propranolol. There is then little or no increase in exercise heart rate, and despite an increase of stroke volume, the cardiac output response to a given submaximal exercise is reduced. However, there is surprisingly little decrease of maximum cardiac output or maximum oxygen intake after beta-blockade. In such patients, as in individuals where a slow heart rate is maintained by an artificial pacemaker, increases of end-diastolic volume and thus stroke volume often allow a surprisingly normal cardiac output response to exercise.

Blood vessels to the viscera have both sympathetic and parasympathetic innervation. The intramuscular vessels have adrenergic fibers (that release norepinephrine) and cholinergic sympathetic fibers (that liberate acetylcholine). The adrenergic receptors are of two main types. Alpha receptors give a constrictor response to either locally-secreted norepinephrine, or epinephrine reaching the muscles from the adrenal medulla. The beta receptors, in contrast, are without innervation and respond only to circulating epinephrine. Their stimulation causes vasodilatation. Currently, pharmacologists and sports physicians who wish to treat exercise-induced asthma without complaints of ''doping'' are interested in subdividing the beta-receptors to allow selective medication. For example, it is possible for a patient with exercise-induced bronchospasm to take salbutamol, a beta-2 blocker that relieves bronchospasm while having a minimal influence on beta-1 function in the heart. The cholinergic fibers are strongly activated in exercise; originating in the motor cortex, with relay stations in the hypothalamus and mesencephalon, they then bypass the medullary vasomotor centers. They cause vasodilatation in muscle, but constriction in the skin and visceral vessels. They also stimulate the sweat glands, which in turn secrete the vasodilator substance bradykinin.

Under resting conditions, the sum total of sympathetic activity leads to partial constriction in a substantial proportion of both arterioles and veins. This is important in maintaining both preloading of the heart and the systemic blood pressure, since either the viscera or the skin plus the muscles could easily sequester the entire blood volume. Local vasodilatation thus reflects (1) a release of vasomotor tone (either centrally mediated or in response to local changes of temperature and metabolism), (2) active cholinergic vasodilatation, and (3) during severe stress, the stimulation of beta-receptors.

The total reponse to exercise comprises an increase of cardiac output, vasodilatation in the active muscles, vasoconstriction in the viscera, inactive muscles, and (depending on temperature) the skin, with a reflex increase in the tone of the venous capacity vessels. An initial command from the cerebral cortex to the vasomotor center decreases the parasympathetic drive and increases sympathetic activity. There seems to be short-

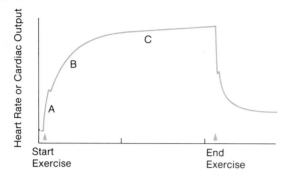

Figure 6–13 Typical pattern of adjustment of heart rate or cardiac output to exercise. After a very brief lag, there is an almost immediate adjustment amounting to 40 to 50 percent of the steady-state value (phase A). There is then a slower increase to a near plateau over 1 to 2 minutes (phase B). Thereafter, there is a slow upward drift (phase C). On stopping exercise, the return to resting values tends to follow the same triphasic curve.

lived vasodilatation in all of the body musculature, but after approximately 10 seconds, a marked vasoconstriction develops in the inactive muscles, presumably through stimulation of adrenergic alpha-receptors. In the active muscles, this signal is overridden by local metabolic factors. Meanwhile, cholinergic impulses constrict visceral and cutaneous vessels. The baroreceptors may check an excessive response to sympathetic activation, and in animals, denervation of the carotid sinus region increases the heart rate response to exercise. Similar ''braking'' of the cardiac response to exercise may occur in humans, since the maximum output of the heart is generally larger if the cutaneous vessels are dilated.

Speed of Adaptation

The speed of increase in cardiac activity with exercise (the ''on-transient'') has been examined most carefully with respect to heart rate. Tachycardia is initiated within 0.5 seconds of beginning a bout of exercise (Fig. 6-13), and if the intensity of effort is moderate, a steady-state heart rate plateau is reached within 1 to 2 minutes. The initial rapid increase of heart rate seems either a conditioned reflex or a response to the irradiation of cortical impulses (as discussed). The second, slower phase of adjustment reflects vasodilatation in the active muscles and an increased input to the vasomotor centers from muscle and joint proprioceptors. With more severe exercise, the heart rate continues to drift upward until the subject is exhausted. This final trend reflects (1) a rising core temperature, (2) a peripheral sequestration of blood, (3) the secretion of catecholamines, (4) recruitment of less efficient muscles as fatigue sets in, and (5) possible psychological reactions to exhaustion.

Recovery from exercise follows an analogous two- or three-phase curve with a rapid drop of heart rate

as the cortical drive to the muscles is halted, slower clearance of metabolites, and delayed elimination of body heat and catecholamines.

Adjustments of heart rate usually occur more quickly than changes in either stroke volume or ventilation.

FURTHER READING

Amsterdam EA, Wilmore JH, de Maria AN. Exercise in cardiovascular health and disease. New York: Yorke Medical Books, 1977.

Bajusz E, Rona G. Recent advances in studies on cardiac structure and metabolism. Baltimore: University Park Press, 1972

Barnard RJ. Long term effects of exercise on cardiac function. Exerc Sport Sci Rev 1975; 3:113–134.

Berne RM. The cardiovascular system. Section 2. In: Handbook of physiology. Bethesda, Md: American Physiological Society, 1979.

Bloomfield DA. Dye curves. The theory and practice of indicator dilution. Baltimore: University Park Press, 1974.

Carlsten A, Grimby G. The circulatory response to muscular exercise in man. Springfield, Ill: CC Thomas, 1966.

Caro CG, Pedley IJ, Schroter RC, Seed WA. The mechanics of the circulation. Oxford: Oxford University Press, 1978.

Dintenfass L, Julian DG, Searman GVF. Heart perfusion, energetics and ischemia. New York: Plenum Press, 1983.

Dowell RT. Cardiac adaptations to exercise. Exerc Sport Sci Rev 1983; 11:99–117.

Feigenbaum H. Echocardiography. Philadelphia: Lea & Febiger, 1973.

Fung YC. Biodynamics. Circulation. New York: Springer Verlag, 1984.

Guyton AC, Young DB. Cardiovascular Physiology III. International review of physiology. Baltimore: University Park Press, 1979.

Halhuber MJ, Gunther MJ, Ciresa M. ECG. An introductory course. Berlin: Springer Verlag, 1979.

Hudlicka O. Effect of training on macro- and microcirculatory changes in exercise. Exerc Sport Sci Rev, 1977; 5: 181–230.

Hwang NHC. Cardiovascular flow dynamics and measurements. Baltimore: University Park Press, 1977.

Jones N, Campbell EJM, Edwards RHT, Robertson DG. Clinical exercise testing. Philadelphia: WB Saunders, 1975.

Katz AM. Physiology of the heart. New York: Raven Press, 1977.

Keul J. Limiting factors of physical performance. Stuttgart: Thieme, 1973.

Kenner T, Busse R, Hinghofer-Szalkay H. Cardiovascular system dynamics. Models and measurements. New York: Plenum, 1982.

Larsen OA, Malmborg RO. Coronary heart disease and physical fitness. Baltimore: University Park Press, 1971.

Lubich T, Venerando A. Sports cardiology. Bologna: Aulo Gaggi, 1980.

Mirsky I, Ghista DN, Sandler H. Cardiac mechanics. Physiological, clinical and mathematical considerations. New York: Wiley, 1974.

Rushmer R. Cardiovascular Dynamics. 4th Edition. Philadelphia: WB Saunders, 1976.

Shepherd JT, Vanhoute P. The human cardiovascular system. Facts and concepts. New York: Raven Press, 1979.

Slutsky R, Froelicher V. The electrocardiographic response to dynamic exercise. Exerc Sport Sci Rev, 1978; 6: 105–124.

Thompson PD. Cardiovascular hazards of physical activity. Exerc Sport Sci Rev 1982; 10: 208–235.

Wade OL, Bishop JM. Cardiac output and regional blood flow. Oxford : Blackwell, 1962.

Wenger NK. Exercise and the heart. In: Brest AN, ed. Cardiovascular clinics. 2nd Edition. Philadelphia: FA Davis, 1985.

Wolf S, Werthesses NT. Dynamics of arterial flow. New York: Plenum Press, 1979.

EXERCISE AND THE RESPIRATORY SYSTEM

CHAPTER 7

The prime physiological limitation of oxygen transport in a healthy person occurs in the cardiovascular rather than the respiratory system. Nevertheless, respiratory function can limit performance severely in diseases such as emphysema, and even in the absence of disease, the unpleasant sensation of breathlessness may be the primary factor that causes a sedentary person to abandon an exhausting bout of exercise before the circulation is fully taxed.

EXTERNAL AND ALVEOLAR VENTILATION

Respiratory Minute Volume

The respiratory minute volume at rest is 3.0 to 3.5 ℓ per minute per m^2 of body surface area (5 to 6 ℓ per minute and 6 to 7 ℓ per minute BTPS[1] in a woman and in a man respectively). During maximum effort, figures of 70 to 90 ℓ per minute are likely in a sedentary young woman, and values reach 90 to 120 ℓ per minute in an average young man. In endurance athletes, peak exercise readings are as high as 120 ℓ per minute in women and 160 ℓ per minute in men.

These various figures all fall short of the corresponding maximum voluntary ventilations (MVV, see section on Maximum Voluntary Ventilation) as measured over 15 to 30 sec of all-out ventilatory activity. It has thus been argued that the power of the respiratory muscles does not limit performance. However, the maximum voluntary ventilation becomes smaller if it is tested over 15 minutes rather than over 15 seconds of activity, and presumably decreases even more over a 3-hour event such as a marathon run. It is less clear how far the decrease of MVV can be attributed to respiratory muscle fatigue and how far it is motivational. Strong urging after 15 minutes of flagging ventilation temporarily restores the 15 sec MVV, but this type of response is seen also with other types of muscle fatigue (Chapter 5); some authors have suggested that lactate levels in the respiratory muscles can rise as high as in the limb muscles during prolonged exercise.

It is also debatable how much benefit subjects could derive from making a greater respiratory effort, at least at sea level. Most authors find a fairly complete oxygen saturation of hemoglobin in the lungs, and in such circumstances an increase of alveolar gas pressures by

---

[1] Body temperature and pressure, saturated with water vapour—about 1.1 times the volume measured under ambient conditions and 1.2 times that measured under standard-pressure dry-gas conditions (STPD): respired volumes are traditionally expressed in BTPS units, although from the viewpoint of oxygen and CO_2 transport, the critical factor is the STPD volume.

further hyperventilation would be largely wasted effort, defeating its purpose by an increase in oxygen consumption of the chest muscles. There is some recent evidence indicating that endurance athletes with a large maximum oxygen intake economize on respiratory effort when exercising, allowing their alveolar oxygen pressures to drift down to a lower level than would occur in sedentary subjects. Dempsey has suggested that this is linked to a very rapid flow of blood through the pulmonary capillaries, incomplete equilibration and some unsaturation of arterial blood; however, even in such subjects it is unclear whether the unsaturation could be corrected by a larger respiratory minute volume.

At any given intensity of effort, the peak respiratory flow rate is approximately 2½ times the corresponding steady respiratory minute volume. If it is to function without inboard leakage at a facemask or mouthpiece, a respiratory demand system such as that used by fire-fighters and mine rescue workers must thus be capable of delivering respired gas at 3 times the anticipated maximum respiratory minute volume (Fig. 7-1).

In submaximum effort, there is a close linear relationship between ventilation and oxygen consumption to 50 to 60 percent of the maximum oxygen intake. At higher intensities of effort, a disproportionate increase of ventilation occurs. This corresponds approximately with the onset of anaerobic metabolism. Some authors have described two breakpoints in the curve (the aerobic and anaerobic thresholds, corresponding to average blood lactate concentrations of about 2 and 4 mmol per liter. Others point out that both intramuscular lactate concentrations and the appearance of lactate in the blood stream depend on the rate at which exercise is increased during testing (many tests of anaerobic threshold increase the work-rate at one minute intervals). Commonly, ventilatory variables show a gentle but continuous curvilinear relationship to the percentage of maximum oxygen intake that the subject is developing, and if objective "curve-stripping" techniques are applied, it becomes difficult to demonstrate one consistent breakpoint in the curve, let alone two. The detection of thresholds thus becomes an art rather than a science, with inspired interpretation of the course of ventilation, the ratio of ventilation to oxygen consumption (ventilatory equivalent), and the ratio of oxygen intake to CO_2 output (gas exchange ratio).

During light exercise, ventilation usually occurs via the nose. This routing serves to warm and humidify inspired air, filtering out both soluble vapors and major particles. The mouth begins to open at a ventilation between 30 and 40 ℓ per minute, and at large respiratory minute volumes the major fraction of the inspired air is taken in via the mouth. Respiratory experiments where light exercise is combined with the use of a mouthpiece are essentially artificial.

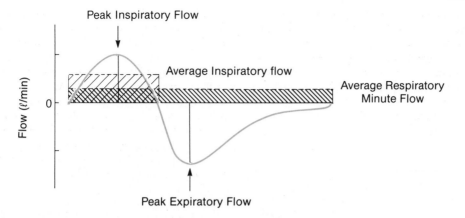

Figure 7–1 The relationship between peak inspiratory flow, average inspiratory flow, and average respiratory minute flow.

Respiratory Rate

The resting respiratory rate is commonly about 14 breaths per minute, although lower values are observed in some classes of athlete, particularly if their sport calls for a careful control of breathing (e.g., in rowing or swimming).

During exercise, the respiratory rhythm increases progressively, usually to a maximum of about 40 breaths per minute. This rate has been said to minimize the energy cost of breathing through an appropriate balancing of elastic against the resistive component of respiratory work (Fig. 7-2), although some recent research has queried this concept. The chosen value of 40 breaths per minute also increases the respiratory minute volume, while allowing a reasonable time for alveolar gas mixing. Much higher respiratory rates are sometimes observed during the performance of maximum voluntary ventilation tests (100 to 150 breaths per minute), but such a ventilatory pattern is very ineffective from the viewpoint of gas exchange.

In certain sports such as swimming and rowing, the breathing rate is inevitably tied to the pace of the primary task. In activities such as cycling, some people still link their breathing rate to the exercise rhythm (particularly if the required rate of limb movement is close to an appropriate respiratory rate); but in the majority of subjects, no such relationship is seen; there seems no fundamental linkage between the drive to the chest and the limb muscles.

Tidal Volume

The resting tidal volume is approximately 400 mℓ in a woman and 500 mℓ in a man. As the intensity of exercise rises, the tidal volume is also augmented, expanding at the expense of the inspiratory rather than the expiratory reserve. During maximum effort, the tidal volume is typically 60 percent of vital capacity (see section on Vital Capacity), with respiration extending from 30 to 90 percent of the potential inspired volume.

Under resting conditions, much of the tidal volume is directed to the upper lobes of the lungs, and the lower lobes tend to be collapsed. During exercise, there is an inspiratory shift of the mean chest position. This often opens up collapsed alveoli, giving a distribution of ventilation that is more uniform and better matched to perfusion. An increase of the mean alveolar gas

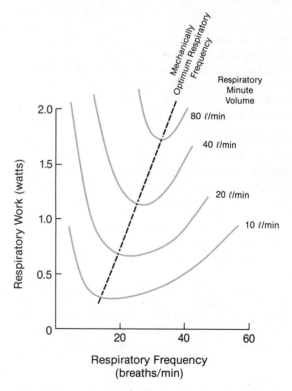

Figure 7–2 The relationship between respiratory work rate and breathing frequency at selected rates of ventilation. Note that as the respiratory minute volume increases, there is a progressive narrowing of the mechanically optimal range of respiratory frequencies. (Based in part on Milic-Emili and Petit).

volume also occurs, protecting the body somewhat against fluctuations of alveolar gas composition over the course of the respiratory cycle. A limit to the extent of inspiration is set by the fact that the muscles function less rapidly and less efficiently at the extremes of this range of movement (Chapter 5).

Ventilatory Equivalent

The ventilatory equivalent is in essence a measure of the efficiency of ventilation; it relates the respiratory minute volume (ℓ per minute BTPS) at any given intensity of effort to the corresponding oxygen delivery (ℓ per minute STPD [Standard temperature and pressure, dry gas]). Under resting conditions, 6 ℓ of ventilation deliver about 0.2 ℓ of oxygen (30 ℓ of ventilation per liter of oxygen delivered). During moderate exercise, the ventilatory equivalent drops to about 25 ℓ per liter. However, the efficiency of ventilation diminishes once the anaerobic threshold is passed; for example, if 90 ℓ of ventilation deliver 2.5 ℓ of oxygen, during maximum aerobic effort, the ventilatory equivalent is 36 ℓ per liter.

Partly because the anaerobic threshold is set at a higher fraction of maximum oxygen intake than in sedentary individuals, and partly because they have a lesser ventilatory response to accumulations of blood lactate, endurance athletes show a low ventilatory equivalent. Values are high in children, and are increased by small muscle exercise (since lactate production is then proportionately greater). In anxiety provoking situations, the respiratory minute volume for a given work-rate is also increased. The ventilatory equivalent can thus be reduced by habituation.

Respiratory Sensations

The factor limiting vigorous exercise in many older, sedentary individuals is an unpleasant shortness of breath, or dyspnea. Subjects generally become conscious of their breathing with the disproportionate increase of ventilation which occurs at the anaerobic threshold. One simple method of regulating the intensity of an endurance training prescription for an older person is thus to recommend exercise that causes slight breathlessness while still allowing the subject to engage in conversation.

Breathlessness becomes unpleasant when the tidal volume equals 50 to 60 percent of vital capacity. The sensation is aggravated by an increase in the resistance to breathing, whether internal (such as an exercise-induced bronchospasm) or external (for instance, the use of self-contained underwater breathing equipment.) The inspiratory muscles are weaker than those responsible for expiration, and perhaps for this reason an inspiratory resistance is generally regarded as more unpleasant than an expiratory loading. Moran Campbell has suggested that an important cause of breath-lessness is "length–tension inappropriateness"—in the terms of Chapter 5 there is a discrepancy between the signal sent to the respiratory muscles via the alpha-motor nerves and the resultant tension reported by the spindle organs.

Many athletes are conscious of some relief of breathlessness after they have been exercising for a few minutes (a phenomenon sometimes described as "second wind"). However, the timing of relief is so variable (2 to 18 minutes after the beginning of exercise in one series of experiments) that a single physiological explanation seems unlikely to cover all cases. Possible contributory factors include a "warmup" of the chest muscles, a catecholamine-induced bronchodilation, a decline of blood lactate (reflecting both an increase of muscle blood flow and some slowing of running pace), and a relief of anxiety once a contest is under way.

With prolonged, vigorous effort, a sharp and rather severe pain is commonly felt in the chest wall (the sensation of a "stitch"). Some authors have attributed this symptom to a spasm of the diaphragm, but a local ischemia of the respiratory muscles seems a more likely explanation. Particularly in conditions such as emphysema, where the work of breathing is increased, fatigue of the respiratory muscles can be sufficient to limit endurance performance. There has thus been some interest in specific isometric training regimens for patients with chronic obstructive lung disease. These have been designed mainly to strengthen the chest muscles.

Alveolar Ventilation

The proportion of the total respiratory effort "wasted" in ventilating the dead space is about 30 percent of a resting tidal volume of 500 mℓ. During exercise the absolute dead space increases owing to (1) physical expansion of the conducting airways, and (2) a shortening of the time available for equilibration of inspired and alveolar gas. However, the percentage of "wasted" ventilation decreases to 20 to 25 percent of the respiratory minute volume during exercise; the least wastage usually occurs at or near the breathing frequency adopted in vigorous work (30 to 40 breaths per minute, [Table 7-1]).

TABLE 7-1   Relationship of Breathing Frequency of Dead Space/Tidal Volume Ratio[*]

Respiratory Frequency (breaths/min)	Dead Space/Tidal Volume Ratio (arterialized capillary blood)
25[†]	0.23
32[**]	0.22[**]
35[†]	0.24
45[†]	0.29
55[†]	0.27

* Based on data of Shephard and Bar Or, for subjects performing near-manual exercise.
** Spontaneously selected frequency. Notice that this is optimal from the viewpoint of minimizing dead-space ventilation.
† Experimentally imposed frequency.

In some situations (such as snorkel diving) the normal respiratory dead space is increased by the external dead space of valves and equipment. There is then a compensatory increase of tidal volume; this is usually almost equal to the added dead space, although a small rise of alveolar carbon dioxide (CO_2) concentration provides a necessary increase of drive to the respiratory control centers.

There is normally a fairly complete equilibration of CO_2 between alveolar gas and arterial blood. Mean alveolar values rise slightly (0.13 to 0.26 kPa, 1 to 2 mm Hg) from the resting figure of 5.2 kPa (40 mm Hg) during light exercise, but drop progressively once the anaerobic threshold has been surpassed and lactate is escaping into the blood stream. Alveolar CO_2 concentrations show some oscillation over the breathing cycle even at rest, but this tendency is exaggerated by the larger CO_2 flux and the deeper breathing of vigorous exercise. In consequence, the end-tidal CO_2 pressure (often used as an estimate of arterial pressure) tends to exceed the true arterial pressure by 0.13 to 0.26 kPa (1 to 2 mm Hg).

The relatively large alveolar gas volume serves to damp out some of the potential respiratory fluctuations of alveolar gas composition. Nevertheless, a small oscillation of pH and P_{CO_2} readings can be detected in arterial blood, and Cunningham has argued that changes in this pattern of oscillation make an important contribution to the regulation of breathing during exercise.

PULMONARY DIFFUSION

The pulmonary diffusing capacity, or transfer factor, indicates the volume of gas that is exchanged between the alveoli and the pulmonary capillary blood per unit of time and per unit of pressure gradient. Unfortunately, most of the published literature is expressed in ml per minute per mm Hg rather than in SI units (mol/sec/Pa). The relevant pressure gradient is from alveolar gas (averaged over the breathing cycle and across spatial nonuniformities within the lung) to the mean pulmonary capillary pressure (Fig. 7-3) (averaged along the capillary, over the breathing cycle and across spatial non-uniformities within the lung).

Because of practical difficulties in integrating oxygen pressures along the pulmonary capillary, carbon monoxide (CO) is commonly used as a tracer gas to measure the rate of pulmonary diffusion. Given the high affinity of carbon monoxide for hemoglobin, the assumption can be made that the mean capillary pressure for this gas is approximately zero. In practice, the available hemoglobin takes a finite time to "mop up" intravascular carbon monoxide, and it is thus necessary to calculate the diffusing capacity $\dot{D}_L$ as the sum of two impedances arranged in series—the membrane diffusing capacity for carbon monoxide $\dot{D}_M$ and the rate of reaction of this gas θ with the pulmonary capillary blood volume V_C:

$$\frac{1}{\dot{D}_L} = \frac{1}{\dot{D}_M} + \frac{1}{\theta V_C}$$

Normally, $\dot{D}_M$ and θV_C each impose a rather similar barrier to CO transport. $\dot{D}_M$ is increased during exercise, because a larger proportion of the alveolar surface is covered by functional capillaries, and there is an associated increase of V_C as blood is transferred from peripheral to pulmonary reservoirs. The effective diffusing surface is further enlarged during exercise because of an increase in the uniformity of both ventilation and perfusion (and thus the matching of ventilation with perfusion) from the top to the bottom of the lungs. In consequence, the carbon monoxide diffusing capacity increases from perhaps 20 ml per minute per mm Hg in a young woman at rest to a maximum of some 60 ml per minute per mm Hg in maximum effort. Because of differences in water solubility and rates of reaction of the two gases with hemoglobin, the oxygen diffusing capacity is 1.23 times larger than the carbon monoxide diffusing capacity. Most authors further believe that except at high altitudes, the diffusing capacity is sufficiently large to allow a relatively complete equilibration of alveolar and arterial gas pressures. Any residual oxygen pressure gradients (1 to 3 kPa) reflect

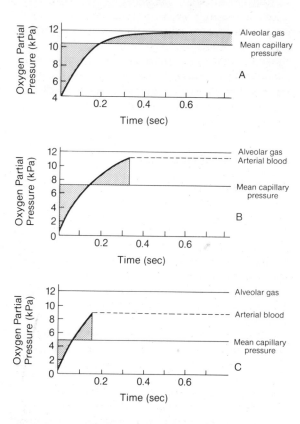

Figure 7–3 The concept of mean capillary pressure, illustrated for *A*, a typical capillary under resting conditions, *B*, a typical capillary during vigorous exercise, and *C*, a capillary with a short transit time during vigorous exercise.

not a problem of diffusion, but rather the direction of some of the venous blood (perhaps 1 to 2 percent) to zones of the lung with little ventilation, or to "shunts" that by-pass the lung completely. While equilibration across the pulmonary membrane is probably characteristic of the lungs as a whole, Dempsey has argued that particularly in endurance athletes there are occasional "short" capillaries where the rate of passage of the red cells is too rapid for equilibration during vigorous exercise (see Fig. 7–3). At rest, the average time taken for a red cell to transverse a pulmonary capillary is about 0.75 sec, but in vigorous exercise, this drops to an average of 0.3 sec, and it is easy to envisage that in the shorter capillaries the residence time for a typical red cell will be much less than this.

Many physiology textbooks suggest that there is no problem with CO_2 equilibration, since carbon dioxide is very soluble in the aqueous film lining the lungs. The solubility augments D_M some 23-fold relative to oxygen, but the second term in the calculation of the carbon dioxide diffusing capacity (θVC) is as much as for oxygen, so that D_L for carbon dioxide is only 2 to 4 times that for oxygen. Moreover, the respective slopes of the oxygen and co_2 dissociation curves (λO_2 and λCO_2) are such that the effective blood solubility of CO_2 is at least 5 times that for oxygen. Thus, the critical ratio for equilibration at the pulmonary membrane ($\dot{D}L/\lambda\dot{Q}$, where $\dot{Q}$ is the cardiac output) is no larger for CO_2 than the oxygen, and in some forms of pulmonary disease, carbon dioxide may accumulate in the blood during vigorous exercise. Carbon dioxide buildup is also a problem when pulmonary ventilation is decreased by working at high gas pressures (submarine exploration).

LUNG FUNCTION TESTS

The pulmonary physiologist has developed a wide range of pulmonary function tests over the past 150 years. However, perhaps because the main limitation to gas transport lies in the cardiovascular rather than in the respiratory system, the healthy person shows only a modest relationship between lung function scores and the performance of endurance exercise.

Vital Capacity

The principal gas volumes of the lung are illustrated in Fig. 7-4. The vital capacity is the maximum volume which can be expelled following a maximal inspiration. At one time, vital capacity was used as a test of fitness for aircrew. There remains some logic in this, since the person who has a large gas volume within the chest cavity will sustain consciousness longer if there is a sudden drop in the partial pressure of oxygen (due, for example, to the explosive decompression of an aircraft).

Since vital capacity is a volumetric measurement, it tends to be larger in tall individuals. Normality of results must always be assessed relative to age and sex specific height standards (Table 7-2). Athletes who use the muscles of their shoulder girdles (such as paddlers) tend to have large vital capacities, even if the data is standarized for height or body mass (Table 7-3). This probably reflects the fact that the vital capacity can be increased a few hundred milliliters by forcibly altering the shape of the thoracic cage, a task more readily accomplished by those with powerful thoracic muscles.

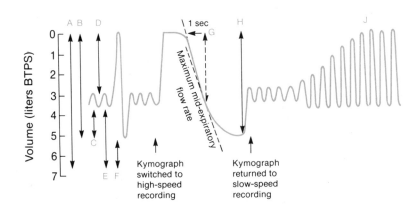

Figure 7–4 Subdivision of lung volume. A = total lung capacity, B = relaxed vital capacity, C = expiratory reserve, D = inspiratory reserve, E = functional residual capacity, F = residual volume, G = 1 sec forced expiratory volume, H = forced vital capacity, J = breathing pattern in vigorous exercise. (Note that tidal volume is increased at the expense of the inspiratory rather than the expiratory reserve).

TABLE 7-2   Equations for the Prediction of Lung Volumes

Variable	Sex	Height Coefficient ($m\ell$/cm or %/cm)	Age Coefficient ($m\ell$/yr or %/yr)	Constant ($m\ell$ or %)
Vital Capacity	F	54.5	−10.5	−5120
($m\ell$,BTPS)	M	56.3	−17.4	−4210
One second forced expiratory	F	40.0	−17.2	−3130
volume ($m\ell$, BTPS)	M	37.5	−35.0	−1290
$FEV_{1.0}/FVC\%$	F	−	−0.253	93.0
	M	−0.201	−0.400	129.0

In medium-distance swimmers, a large vital capacity offers some competitive advantage, since it increases thoracic buoyancy (although it does not support the legs, as fat would). A large vital capacity also facilitates breath-hold diving, since a dive must be terminated when the combined effects of increased hydrostatic pressure and gas absorption from the lungs reduce the chest volume to around residual volume (see section on Residual Volume).

The ordinary person becomes unpleasantly breathless when tidal volume equals 50 to 60 percent of vital capacity. The individual who is endowed with a large vital capacity is thus less vulnerable to breathlessness at any given rate of working. Subjects with ischemic heart disease tend to have small lung volumes because they are (or have been) heavy smokers.

Residual Volume

The residual gas volume is the gas volume which remains in the lungs after a maximal expiration. The influence of residual volume upon the tolerance of breath-hold diving has been noted above. Residual gas volume also has importance for the exercise physiologist in the context of the hydrostatic determination of body density; underwater weights must be corrected for the buoyancy of residual gas. The external hydrostatic force of the water tends to compress the residual gas volume by about 5 percent (unless measurements are made supine). Some authors thus advocate making residual volume determinations while the subject is submerged. However, the technical difficulties of measuring residual volume with sufficient accuracy are greatly increased by submersion. One option is to keep the head above water. Given also that there is unmeasured gas in the intestines, brassiere, and bathing cap (if worn), it is probably preferable to measure the residual volume by a helium dilution or nitrogen washout method while sitting in the comfort of a warm laboratory. In healthy young children, it is often better to assume that the residual volume is a fixed percentage (typically 28 percent) of the more easily measured vital capacity.

Maximum Voluntary Ventilation

The maximum voluntary ventilation (MVV) is arbitrarily defined by pulmonary physiologists as the maximum volume of air that can be respired within 15 seconds; the required technique requires breathing at a very rapid rate (about 100 breaths per minute). In a healthy young woman, typical MVV figures range from 100 to 150 ℓ per minute BTPS, and values as large as 200 ℓ per minute are sometimes observed in endurance athletes. Figures for male subjects are generally 20 to 25 percent larger than in females.

Under resting conditions, subjects experience difficulty in sustaining more than 50 percent of their MVV for 15 minutes. During exercise, a "warmup" of the chest muscles associated with the rise in body temperature, a catecholamine-related decrease of respiratory resistance, and an increased drive to the respiratory center allow 75 to 80 percent of the 15 second MVV to be sustained over a 15 minute period.

The physiological factors limiting the brief (15 sec) tests are essentially those of an anaerobic sprint—the ability of the chest muscles to convert chemical energy into ventilatory work and an uneconomic increase in the energy cost of pulmonary ventilation at the highest rates of chest movement and gas flow. Scores may also be influenced by technical factors (such as the choice of recording equipment, motivation, and the adoption of an optimal breathing frequency). Responses to a sustained 15 minute ventilatory effort can be substantially increased after a specific training

TABLE 7-3   Some Coefficients of Correlations Between Athletic Performance and Vital Capacity

Event	Coefficient of Correlation	
	Vital Capacity	Vital Capacity/kg
5000-m race	0.34	0.47
Rowing	0.71	0.47
White-water paddling	0.64	−
Middle-distance swimming	0.86	−

of the respiratory muscles, and physiotherapy for the chest muscles is an important facet of a modern training program for patients where the respiratory workrate is increased by chronic obstructive pulmonary disease. After conditioning of the inspiratory muscles, the 15-second MVV may be increased by about 14 percent; 96 percent of the increased MVV can be sustained over 15 minutes of activity. This reflects less ready fatigue, particularly in the accessory muscles of the neck and shoulders.

Forced Expiratory Volume

The 15 sec MVV test is exhausting for an elderly or sick subject, and if there is some lung pathology such as emphysema, structural damage may result from the repeated forcible ventilatory efforts inherent in the test procedure. It is thus more common to assess respiratory function in terms of the maximum volume that can be expelled in the first second of a single breath following a maximal inspiration (the "forced expiratory volume," or $FEV_{1.0}$). In a young and healthy adult, this volume amounts to 81 to 85 percent of the vital capacity, but in a 60-year old, the ratio of $FEV_{1.0}$ to vital capacity drops to about 70 percent.

The percentage of the total vital capacity expired in the first second is reduced by exposure to irritant vapours such as ozone and finely suspended particulates (such as tobacco smoke or industrial dusts).

The pattern of expiratory flow is revealed by a plot of screen flowmeter data. Usually this is presented as a flow–volume loop (Fig. 7-5). There is an early flow peak of about 10 ℓ per second (reflecting the strength of the respiratory effort), with a subsequent exponential fall of airflow. The latter has been attributed to a progressive collapse of the airways (Fig. 7-6). At the beginning of expiration, the pressure within the alveoli and small airways exceeds the pressures within the pleural cavity. The "equal pressure point" (where

pressure within the airway matches that in the pleural space) is not reached until the expirate is passing through the major airways (which are supported and held open by strong cartilaginous plates). However, the balance of forces shifts as expiration proceeds. The elastic forces drawing the small airways open diminish as lung volume declines, while at the same time the narrowing of the airways increases the rate of pressure drop along their length. The "equal pressure point" is thus displaced towards the small branches of the bronchial tree. These lack cartilaginous support, and collapse occurs rather readily. Thereafter, attempts at a more forcible expiration merely increase airway collapse and further limit expiratory flow (Fig. 7-6). Some authors thus divide the expiratory flow–volume curve into an early, "effort-dependent" section and a later "effort-independent" portion. At sea level, healthy young adults do not reach the conditions necessary for airway collapse until 60 percent of their vital capacity has been expired. However, collapse is likely if (1) the density of respired gas is increased, as in diving (since the pressure gradient along the airway is then augmented), (2) there is a weakening of the cartilaginous plates, (3) there is a decrease in the elastic recoil of the lungs, or (4) there is a spasm of the finer airways. Situations (2) and (3) are likely in old age, particularly if there is chronic obstructive pulmonary disease. Thus, while young subjects rarely develop airway collapse, even during vigorous exercise, an expiratory obstruction of airflow is not uncommon in an elderly person as maximum effort is approached. Nevertheless, some reports have suggested that there is less tendency to airway collapse during vigorous exercise than during performance of a forced vital capacity maneuver—in general, the expiratory effort is less powerful during exercise, and physical activity may also induce some bronchodilatation—particularly if it is pushed to the point of increased catecholamine secretion (Chapter 4).

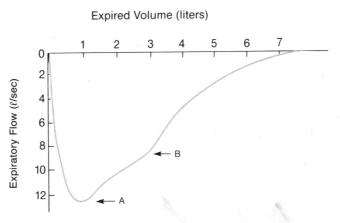

Figure 7–5 Expiratory flow-volume loop, initiated from point of maximum inspiration. *A*, is peak expiratory flow rate (the flow sustained for at least 10 msec). *B*, is the exponential, effort-independent part of expiration.

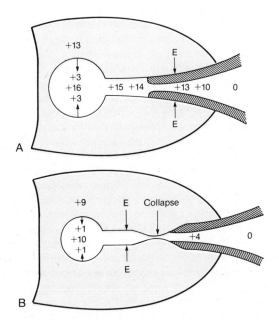

Figure 7–6 The basis of airway collapse during expiration: A. At the beginning of expiration, the intrapleural pressure is 13 kPa, and within the alveolar space the pressure is boosted to 16 kPa by the elastic recoil of the lungs. The pressure drops on passing along the airway toward the mouth, but does not reach the same figure as the intrapleural space until the point E in the major airways. Collapse of segments closer to the mouth is prevented by the cartilaginous walls. B. After expulsion of 60 percent of the vital capacity, the intrapleural pressure has dropped to 9 kPa. The airway is also narrower, so that pressure drops more quickly on moving towards the mouth, and the equal pressure point is reached before the zone of cartilaginous support.

WORK OF BREATHING

Mechanical work is performed pumping air in and out of the chest, and in vigorous exercise the oxygen demands of the respiratory pump can account for 5 to 10 percent of the total maximum oxygen intake. The total work demands include the storage of potential energy by the stretching of elastic tissues in the lungs and chest, viscous work developed against the resistance of gas and tissues, and inertial work performed against heavy but mobile viscera, particularly the liver.

Elastic Work

During inspiration, pressure is developed against the elasticity of the rib cage, lungs, alveolar fluid, and any external forces such as the difference between air and water pressure in a "snorkel" diver. Depending on the magnitude of the tidal volume, some of the resultant store of potential energy can be recouped during expiration.

Cells known as alveolar macrophages secrete a thin (5 nm) lipoprotein film ("surfactant") which lines the surface of the lungs and avoids development of a large surface tension at the air-tissue interface. If the surfactant were absent, the lungs would be vulnerable to collapse and would quickly fill with exudate. The deep inspirations of either pulmonary function testing or vigorous exercise increase surfactant reserves and reduce the tendency to alveolar collapse; for this reason it is sometimes interesting to compare a normal flow–volume curve (begun from full inspiration) with a partial flow–volume curve begun from a normal quiet inspiration.

The elasticity of the lungs and chest wall is usually expressed in compliance units (compliance = 1/elasticity). The relashionship of volume change to applied pressure is non-linear for both the chest and the lungs (Fig. 7-7). Over the middle range of tidal volumes, the compliance of the lungs (C_L) and of the chest (C_C) are each about 2 ℓ per kilopascal, so that the overall compliance ($C_{[C + L]}$) is given by $1/C_{(C + L)} = 1/C_C + 1/C_L$ (about 1 ℓ per kilopascal, or 100 mℓ per centimeter of water pressure.)

During exercise, several factors modify the average compliance, including (1) operation over a larger portion of the total pressure–volume curve (because tidal volume is increased), (2) the opening of previously collapsed alveolar units, owing to deeper inspiration, (3) a dependence of compliance on breathing rate (important only at very high respiratory frequen-

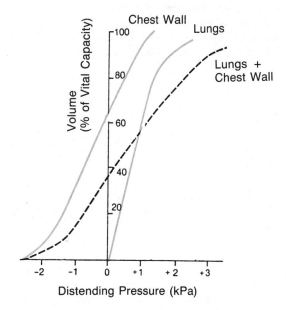

Figure 7–7 The relationship of volume change to applied pressure for the chest, the lungs, and a combination of the two structures.

cies), and (4) a stiffening of the lungs by an increase of pulmonary blood content. In practice, several of these influences tend to cancel one another out, and the main effect upon compliance being that which is due to an increase of tidal volume and thus operation over a larger part of the pressure-volume curve.

Because of the shape of the compliance curve, it is easier to resuscitate a patient by forced inflation (mouth-to mouth or arm-lift techniques) than by deflation of the lungs (forcible pressure on the back). Substantial force is nevertheless required even during inflation, since drowning and other emergencies cause pulmonary congestion, with a marked decrease in compliance of the lungs. When designing mannequins for the teaching of artificial respiration, it is important to simulate not only the characteristics of the normal chest, but also the way in which this is modified by drowning. If the lung is exceedingly stiff, mechanical respirators that are fitted with the safety device of an automatic blow-off valve may fail to deliver an adequate tidal volume before their cutoff pressure is reached.

Resistive Work

Airflow resistance includes components related to laminar, turbulent, and orifice flow. Flow is laminar (streamlined) in the small bronchioles, but on passing up the airway towards the trachea, a critical velocity is reached (often in the third or fourth generation branches of the bronchial tree). An irregular, turbulent pattern of flow then begins. The critical velocity F_C for the onset of this disturbance depends on gas viscosity (η), density (δ), radius of the airway (τ), and a dimensionless constant (the Reynold's number R, about 1,000 to 2,000 for a straight, smooth-walled tube, but substantially lower where the airway branches):

$$V_C = R\eta/\delta\tau$$

Generalized turbulence is usual in the air passages of the nose and throat, and more localized zones of turbulence may be anticipated at the proximal points of branching in the bronchial tree. Turbulence greatly increases the working of breathing. The pressure drop with laminar flow is approximately proportional to flow rate and gas viscosity; that for turbulent flow varies as the square of the flow rate. Physiologists often measure airflow resistance at an arbitrary flow rate of 0.5 ℓ per second, reporting a mouth to alveolar pressure gradient of about 0.2 kPa per liter per second gas flow; however, if the proportion of turbulent airflow is increased by a large respiratory minute volume, the pressure gradient becomes disproportionately increased relative to this estimate. The oral resistance may also be underestimated if the teeth have been wedged open by a large mouthpiece, and an additional resistance of some 0.2 kPa per liter per second is encountered if air is inspired via the nose.

During vigorous exercise, there is often some initial decrease of airway resistance, owing to (1) a secretion of catecholamines, (2) an opening up of collapsed airways, (3) an increase of mean alveolar gas volume, and (4) expectoration of mucus associated with deeper breathing. However, as effort continues, the inhalation of cold, dry air may provoke bronchospasm, especially in patients with a history of asthma. Spasm commonly appears a few minutes after a short bout of exercise, peaks over 10 to 15 minutes, and resolves some 40 to 60 minutes after activity has ceased. Occasionally individuals develop a serious and dangerous allergy to exercise, with hospital admission for total obstruction of the airway. There are several probable causes of exercise-induced bronchospasm, but one element is undoubtedly the release of histamine from mast cells in the bronchial walls. Attacks can often be avoided by warming and humidfying the inspired gas and by administering a prophylactic drug such as cromolyn sodium, which stabilizes the surface membrane of the mast cells and limits the liberation of histamine from these cells. Vigorous exercise bypasses the normal air-conditioning and filtering mechanism of the nose, so that the inhalation of particulate matter or irritant gasses may contribute to the exercise-induced bronchospasm. Other factors that increase airway resistance are carbon dioxide washout (for example, hyperventilation by a nervous athlete prior to competition) and inhalation of vomit (by a drowning or unconscious patient) or water (during involuntary hyperventilation on plunging into cold water).

Because of the increase of inspired gas density, the diver encounters a much higher proportion of turbulent airflow than a person breathing the same gas volume at sea level. The work of breathing may become sufficient to restrict maximum ventilation severely, with an accumulation of carbon dioxide in the active tissues. At great depths, the respiratory load can be reduced substantially by use of helium and/or oxygen mixtures (which have a much lower density). The main disadvantages of the helium mixtures are (1) an increase of laminar resistance (owing to the greater viscosity of helium relative to nitrogen), and (2) body cooling (owing to the greater thermal conductivity of helium).

During rest and light exercise, subjects tolerate a 4-fold increase of airway resistance before there are complaints of difficulty in breathing. Thus, substantial resistances are considered an acceptable feature of industrial respirators and facemasks. Military "gas masks" commonly add a resistance of up to 1 kPa at a steady flow of 85 ℓ per minute, but have remarkably little effect upon exercise performance.

The tissue resistance to respiration is fairly small (typically 50 to 100 Pa per liter per second) and it is correspondingly difficult to measure (usually it is estimated from the difference between airflow resistance and the total resistance to forced inflation). It arises in part from an incomplete relaxation of antagonist muscles (which are also acting on the thoracic cage in an opposing sense). this component of tissue resistance diminishes as exercise induces a rise of body temperature and muscle relaxation becomes more complete. A second component reflects the rigidity of joints in the thoracic cage; this component increases markedly with aging.

Inertial Work

A small amount of work is performed in accelerating gas molecules, the chest wall and heavy abdominal viscera. Figures of 1 Pa per liter per square second have been estimated for both pulmonary gas and visceral inertance.

Inertial effects are important not for their contribution to the overall work of breathing (which is generally quite small), but rather for their ability to damp "chatter" in the valves of any breathing equipment that is being used. The damping ratio (h) for breathing equipment can be calculated as $h = R/2 \sqrt{C/L}$, where R is the resistance of the system, C is its compliance, and L is its inertance. Ideally, h should be close to unity (Fig. 7–8). However, the human airway is underdamped (h is less than 1.0), and oscillation of the gas column is thus liable to develop. In order to avoid this problem, the damping ratio can be brought above unity by a reduction of inertance (breathing a low-density gas mixture such as helium), by an increase of compliance (e.g., breathing from an air-filled waistcoat),

or by an increase in resistance of the breathing line. The liability to "chatter" is worsened if gas density is increased (as in diving).

Overall Work of Breathing

The total work performed during the breathing cycle can be estimated from the area of a pressure-volume diagram for the chest (work = [force × distance] = [pressure × volume]). By having a subject make maximum inspiratory and expiratory efforts at various fractions of vital capacity, it is possible to draw a "static" maximum pressure-volume diagram (Fig. 7–9), indicating the limits to the mechanical work that can be performed by the respiratory muscles. During quiet breathing, only a very small part of the pressure-volume diagram is occupied. Even in maximum exercise, it is rare to use more than a quarter of the power output indicated by the static pressure–volume diagram. However, it is more appropriate to examine the required respiratory work-rate relative to a dynamic diagram, recorded during maximum ventilatory effort. In a dynamic situation, the area of the diagram is curtailed in comparison with static conditions, because of the inherent force–velocity relationship of the chest muscles (Chapter 4), and the fact that a substantial portion of the thoracic gas contents are expelled before maximum tension can be developed by the chest muscles. Nevertheless, there is little evidence that the area of the dynamic pressure–volume diagram limits the performance of physical work in a healthy young person.

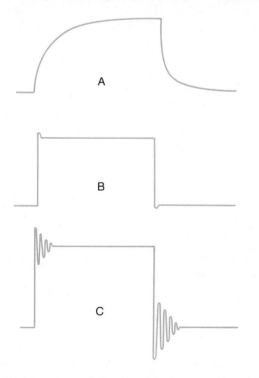

Figure 7–8 Responses of respiratory valves in *A*, overdamped system; *B*, optimally damped system, and *C*, underdamped system.

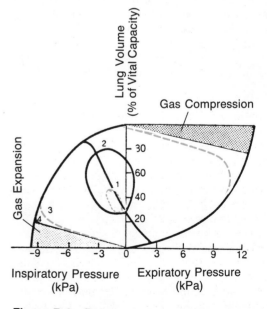

Figure 7–9 Pressure/volume diagram of the lungs. Solid line indicates "static" diagram, interrupted line curve developed under dynamic conditions Loop labeled (1) indicates area of the diagram occupied during rest, loop labeled (2) indicates area occupied during vigorous exercise.

Estimates of the mechanical efficiency of breathing have varied widely from 1 to 25 percent. In moderate breathing, the oxygen cost of respiration is probably only 0.5 to 1.0 ml per liter of ventilation, although it may rise to 4 to 5 ml per liter in vigorous effort because of (1) an increased proportion of turbulent airflow, and (2) operation over less favorable portions of the compliance curve. Given a maximum exercise ventilation of 100 ℓ per minute, the oxygen consumption of the chest muscles is thus likely to be 400 to 500 ml, 10 percent or more of maximum oxygen intake. Moreover, if an exercising subject hyperventilates, oxygen consumption is increased by 5 ml for every liter of unneeded ventilation. A point is soon reached where the greater ventilation not only fails to augment the overall oxygen intake, but oxygen delivery to the leg or arm muscles is actually decreased (Fig. 7–10). In a sedentary young woman, the crossover point of "diminishing returns" occurs at a ventilation of approximately 100 to 120 ℓ per minute, somewhat above the maximum value encountered in normal exercise. In athletes, a greater maximum cardiac output raises the crossover point, so that again there is generally some margin between the observed maximum exercise ventilation and the level of diminishing returns. However, problems are encountered in chronic obstructive pulmonary disease, where the work of breathing is increased as much as 10-fold (to 50 ml per liter). Cigarette smoking also increases the work of breathing substantially, partly by causing bronchitic changes in the respiratory mucosa; in such subjects, an apparently normal oxygen intake may mask the fact that a large part of the transported oxygen is being diverted to the respiratory muscles.

Use of Accessory Muscles

As respiratory minute volume is increased by the performance of external work, the ventilatory efforts of the diaphragm and intercostal muscles become supplemented by the activity of various accessory muscles. The internal intercostal muscles account for a large part of expiratory power when exercising at moderate loads, but as activity increases in vigor the transversus abdominis, internal obliques, and external oblique muscles are successively brought into play. The abdominal muscles make a significant contribution to

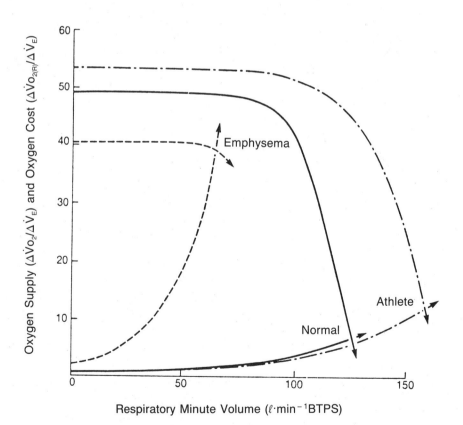

Figure 7–10 The concept of a critical cost of breathing, where the oxygen consumed by the respiratory muscles ($\Delta\dot{V}o_{2(R)}/\Delta\dot{V}_E$) exceeds the oxygen supplied by the additional ventilation ($\Delta\dot{V}o_2/\Delta\dot{V}_E$). Typical curves for normal sedentary male, endurance athlete and patient with emphysema. BTPS = body temperature and pressure, saturated with water vapor.

expiration when the rate of external working exceeds 50 W. At this stage, accessory muscles, such as the scalenes and sternomastoids, begin to contribute to inspiration, particularly if there is an external fixation of the shoulder girdle (as in cycling). However, the contribution of the thoracic muscles is never very large, and even if the chest is immobilized by a rigid binder, ventilation is only reduced by 20 to 30 percent.

TISSUE RESPIRATION AND ACID-BASE BALANCE

Tissue Respiration

Although respiration is often conceived in terms of movements of the chest and diaphragm, the ultimate site of respiration is within the tissues. During aerobic metabolism, substrate entering the mitochondrion is progressively broken down to CO_2 and hydrogen. The latter combines with the important cellular constituent nicotinamide-adenine dinucleotide (NAD+), its phosphorylated derivative NADP+ or, in one instance, flavoprotein. The resultant NADH or NADPH is then passed to the chain of cytochrome pigments on the inner surface of the mitochondrion (Fig. 7–11). Here, NAD^+ or $NADP^+$ is regenerated, together with two electrons and a proton (H^+). At the opposite end of the cytochrome pigment chain, protons and electrons interact with the oxygen delivered by the cardiovascular system to form water.

The difference of electrical potential between the two ends of the cytochrome chain is about 1.2 volts. In theory, each electron that is passed against this voltage should conserve about 115 kJ of free energy. In practice, 3 moles of ATP (equivalent to 138 kJ of energy) are reformed from ADP as one atom of oxygen, and two electrons pass through the system (an efficiency of about 60 percent).

Critical factors governing the rate of this reaction include (1) the availability of substrate (particularly NADH), and (2) the presence of oxygen, small amounts of ADP and phosphate. The ADP signal seems particularly important in increasing the rate of aerobic metabolism until phosphagen stores have been replenished.

The tissue usage of oxygen does not always match that measured at the mouth, at least on a minute-by-minute basis, since various small stores intervene. If the respiratory supply of oxygen is depleted, it is possible to decrease the oxygen content of the lungs, blood, and tissues, and these reserves must later be replenished.

Under steady-state conditions, the respiratory quotient (CO_2 output/O_2 intake) indicates the relative usage of carbohydrate and fat. Ignoring the fairly small contributions of protein and any alcohol that is being metabolized, a respiratory quotient of 0.70 reflects pure fat metabolism; a figure of 1.00 reflects pure carbohydrate usage. In rest and moderate activity, rather similar proportions of the two fuels are used, but as exercise becomes more vigorous, there is an increased

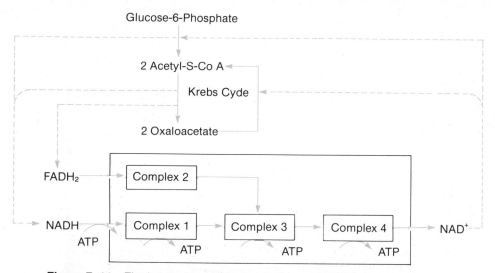

Figure 7–11   Final steps in aerobic metabolism within the mitochondrion. Nicotine adenine dinucleotide (NADH) and flavine adenine dinucleotide ($FADH_2$) generated by the breakdown of glucose-6-phosphate are passed through the four cytochrome complexes as shown, with the regeneration of NAD+:

$$NADH \rightarrow NAD^+ + H^+ + 2e^-$$

Passage of the electrons through the system provides energy to form ATP, and at the end of the cytochrome chain the electrons and protons react with oxygen to form water. The overall reaction is thus of the type:

$$NADH + \tfrac{1}{2}O_2 + H^+ \rightarrow H_2O + NAD^+$$

dependence upon carbohydrate. On the other hand, during prolonged sub-maximal exercise, there is a progressive decrease of respiratory quotient as reserves of glycogen are exhausted.

Carbon dioxide output reflects partly the metabolic production of carbon dioxide and partly the buffering of lactate. If activity is supported by anaerobic metabolism, glycogen is broken down partially to pyruvate, with an accumulation of hydrogen ions (H^+) and NADH; the NAD^+ needed for a continuation of the reaction is then reformed by conversion of the pyruvate to lactate:

$$\text{Pyruvate} + \text{NADH} + H^+ \underset{\xleftarrow{\hspace{2cm}}}{\overset{\text{lactate dehydrogenase}}{\xrightarrow{\hspace{2cm}}}} \text{Lactate} + \text{NAD}^+$$

Depending on the type of exercise that is being performed—particularly the size of the muscles that have been recruited, and the proportion of their maximum force that is being exerted, lactic acid begins to accumulate at 50 to 60 percent of maximum oxygen intake. The acid build-up is internal, reflecting the extent of the body's anaerobic metabolism, and it is thus described as a metabolic acidosis (in contrast with the "respiratory acidosis" imposed by the breathing of CO_2 or the use of respiratory equipment with a large dead space). The acidosis provides a strong stimulus to breathing, with a corresponding increase of CO_2 output. The respiratory gas exchange ratio (measured at the mouth, and to be distinguished from the metabolism-based respiratory quotient) may rise to 1.20 or higher when the lactate efflux from the working muscle is at its peak. The total CO_2 output in such circumstances reflects the sum of (1) aerobic metabolism, (2) the loss of CO_2 from body stores (body mass × change of mixed venous CO_2 pressure in torr, e.g., 60 kg × 5 torr = 300 ml, and (3) loss of CO_2 owing to lactate production (e.g., if a lactate concentration of 10 mmol per liter is distributed through 75 percent of body water (a volume of say 25 ℓ)—there is an accumulation of 250 mmol of lactate, equivalent on an equimolar basis to an output of 5.6 ℓ of CO_2.

Anaerobic effort is undesirable in endurance competition, partly because the metabolic efficiency is much lower than for aerobic work (Chapter 1), and partly because an unpleasant breathlessness develops when oxygen is diverted in excessive amounts to the respiratory muscles. In an event such as a marathon race, competitors thus choose a pace that is just below their personal anaerobic threshold. One of the characteristics of a well-trained marathon competitor is an ability to exercise close to maximum oxygen intake (85 percent or more) without an accumulation of lactic acid.

Acid-Base Balance

The regulation of tissue acid-base balance is important, since the activity of many enzyme systems (including those associated with glycolysis) is affected by pH. The limiting intramuscular value for the continued breakdown of glycogen is a pH of about 6.3, corresponding to a muscle lactate of 30 to 40 mmol per liter. With continuous, exhausting exercise, the corresponding limiting blood concentration of lactate (10 to 15 mmol per liter) is seen after a lag of 2 to 4 minutes. With an intermittent pattern of exercise, there is much more complete equilibration between muscle and blood, and the final blood lactate concentration may be as high as 30 mmol per liter.

The main buffers protecting the blood against an excessive change of pH are proteins (hemoglobin and plasma proteins), bicarbonate ions (HCO_3^-/H_2CO_3) and phosphate ions ($HPO_4^{2-}/H_2PO_4^-$). Of these several resources, hemoglobin is undoubtedly the most important buffer system. Within the red cell, the enzyme carbonic anhydrase facilitates the interconversion of CO_2 and carbonic acid (H_2CO_3). The resultant hydrogen ions react with hemoglobin, while the bicarbonate ions exchange with chloride ions in the plasma. Reduced hemoglobin is a weaker acid than oxyhemoglobin, so that the widened arteriovenous oxygen difference of vigorous exercise facilitates buffering and transport of CO_2 by the red cells. Buffering is further facilitated by an increase of phosphate radicals as the high-energy phosphagen bonds are broken down.

If lactic acid is produced, the pH of the blood initially falls somewhat ("uncompensated metabolic acidosis"), but as the disturbance is sensed by the respiratory control system, CO_2 elimination is augmented and pH is restored at the expense of some decrease of plasma bicarbonate ("compensated metabolic acidosis"). Over the next few hours, the normal bicarbonate content and buffering capacity of the plasma is restored by excretion of a more acid urine.

If a large dose of an "alkali" such as sodium bicarbonate is ingested, the converse situation of metabolic alkalosis arises. Initially, the pH of the blood is increased ("uncompensated metabolic alkalosis"), but within perhaps 30 minutes, a normal pH is restored by a diminution of ventilation and a retention of carbon dioxide ("compensated alkalosis"). In events where the main limiting factor is the accumulation of acid metabolites, some improvement of performance (up to 3 percent in a sprint event) is possible through a doping of athletes with carefully timed doses of sodium bicarbonate; the increase of plasma bicarbonate speeds transport of lactate out of the working muscle, allowing a greater total production of lactate.

Hyperventilation, whether deliberately undertaken prior to an athletic contest, or occurring as an unintended result of anxiety, leads to a respiratory alkalosis, with a diminution of plasma bicarbonate and an increase of blood pH. Metabolic CO_2 production usually restores a normal acid–base balance once vigorous exercise is undertaken, but if compensation remains incomplete, plasma bicarbonate can be restored by a decreased renal excretion of hydrogen ions.

The buffer status of the blood is often reported as the "standard bicarbonate" (the bicarbonate content of whole blood at 37 °C, when equilibrated with carbon dioxide at a partial pressure of 5.3 kPa). A figure of 24 mmol HCO_3^- per liter is anticipated at rest, but this drops to 17 mmol per liter during a brief period of exhausting exercise, and even lower readings may be encountered in the first few minutes of recovery, as additional lactate diffuses from the working muscles.

REGULATION OF BREATHING

In general, the respiratory minute volume is closely matched to the metabolic demand, to the point that a few observers have suspected that there are CO_2 detectors somewhere in the pulmonary circulation. Classical authors such as Haldane attributed the major regulation of respiration to the action of carbon dioxide upon medullary chemoreceptors. This was a reasonably plausible explanation in moderate exercise, since there was often a small increase of alveolar (and by inference, arterial) CO_2 pressure. However in more vigorous exercise, there may be a drop of arterial Pco_2, particularly as blood lactate rises, and it is then not possible to attribute regulation simply to the mean arterial CO_2 pressure.

Work with modern breath-by-breath recording apparatus suggests that the adjustment of ventilation to the needs of exercise proceeds in at least three phases, much as already described for the circulation. There is an early rise of ventilation, which accounts for perhaps a half of the steady-state increment of respiratory minute volume and occurs more or less simultaneously with the onset of activity. This has been attributed to cerebral influences; it may be a learned, conditioned response arising from the pre-frontal lobes of the cortex, or an irradiation of impulses from the motor cortex to the medullary respiratory centers. Once movement begins, this cortical drive is supplemented by impulses arising in the mechanoreceptors of the active muscles and joints. Over the next minute or so, one might anticipate an increased chemical drive, owing to oxygen usage and CO_2 elimination, but unfortunately the main changes of O_2 and CO_2 pressure occur on the venous side of the circulation, where there do not seem to be any appropriate sensing organs. It is quite difficult to show either an increase of CO_2 or a decrease of O_2 pressure on the arterial side of the circulation, (where it could influence carotid body and medullary chemoreceptors). One explanation (for which there is some support) is that other factors increase the O_2 and CO_2 sensitivity of either peripheral (carotid body) or central (medullary) chemoreceptors during exercise. Cunningham and his associates have also suggested that the response may reflect not the absolute CO_2 pressure, but rather the extent and timing of oscillations in gas pressures over the respiratory cycle. Some authors have argued for a significant input from chemoreceptors in the working muscles,

through fibers analogous to those that induce a rise of systemic blood pressure during exercise. If there is an arterial lactate accumulation, this induces a further dramatic increase of ventilation, as diffusion of CO_2 transmits the pH disturbance across the blood-brain barrier to the medullary chemoreceptors. With more prolonged exercise, ventilation may be further stimulated by an increase of core temperature and a secretion of catecholamines.

Following exercise, withdrawal of the cerebral drive leads to a rapid diminution of ventilation. There is then a slower phase of adjustment as metabolites are eliminated, body temperature cools, and catecholamine levels return to normal.

FURTHER READING

Asmussen E. Control of ventilation in exercise. Exerc Sport Sci Rev 1983; 11:24–154.

Bonsignore G, Cumming G. The lung in its environment. New York: Plenum, 1982.

Bouhuys A. Breathing. New York: Grune & Stratton, 1974.

Brooks CMcC, Kao FF, Lloyd BB. Cerebrospinal fluid and the regulation of ventilation. Oxford: Blackwell, 1973.

Caro CG. Advances in respiratory physiology. London: Arnold, 1966.

Cotes JE. Lung function. Oxford: Blackwell, 1965.

Cumming G, Hunt LB. Form and function in the human lung. Edinburgh: E. & S. Livingstone, 1968.

Cunningham DJC, Lloyd BB. The regulation of human respiration. Oxford: Blackwell, 1971.

Dempsey JA, Reed CE. Muscular exercise and the lung. Madison, Wisc: University of Wisconsin Press, 1977.

Garby L, Meldon J. The respiratory functions of the blood. New York: Plenum, 1977.

Gledhill N. Bicarbonate ingestion and anaerobic performance. Sports Med 1984; 1:177–180.

Haldane JS, Priestley JG. Respiration. Oxford: Clarendon Press, 1935.

Hornbein TF. Regulation of breathing. New York: Dekker, 1981.

Howell JBL, Campbell EJM. Breathlessness. Oxford: Blackwell, 1966.

Hultman E, Sahlin K. Acid-base balance during exercise. Exerc Sport Sci Rev 1981; 8:41–128.

Hutas I, Debreczeni LA. Respiration. New York: Pergamon Press/Akademiai Kiadó, 1981.

Jones NL, Ehrsaur RE. The anaerobic threshold. Exerc Sport Sci Rev 1982; 10:49–83.

Kovach AG, Dora E, Kessler M, Silver IA. Oxygen transport to tissue. Oxford: Pergamon, 1981.

Lin Y-C. Breath-hold diving in terrestrial mammals. Exerc Sport Sci Rev 1982; 10:270–307.

Nahas G, Schaefer KE. Carbon dioxide and metabolic regulations. New York: Springer Verlag, 1974.

Pengelly LD, Rebuck AS, Campbell EJM. Loaded Breathing. Don Mills, Ont: Longman, 1974.

Shephard RJ. Exercise and chronic obstructive lung disease. Exerc Sport Sci Rev 1976; 4:263–296.

Shephard RJ. Exercise-induced bronchospasm - a review. Med Sci Sports 1977; 9:1–10.

Torrance RW. Arterial chemoreceptors. Oxford: Blackwell, 1968.

Von Euler C, Lagercrantz H. Central nervous control mechanisms in breathing. Oxford: Pergamon, 1979.

Weibel ER. The pathway for oxygen. Cambridge, Mass: Harvard University Press, 1984.

West JB. Regional differences in the lung. New York: Academic Press, 1979.

Whipp BJ. The hyperpnea of dynamic muscular exercise. Exerc Sport Sci Rev 1977; 5:295–311.

Whipp BJ, Wiberg DM. Modelling and control of breathing. New York: Elsevier, 1983.

Widdicombe JG. MIT international review of science. Respiratory Physiology. London: Butterworths, 1974.

PERFORMANCE AND TRAINING

FITNESS AND ITS MEASUREMENT

CHAPTER 8

Physical fitness is central to discussions of exercise science by the physical educator and the sports physician alike. We shall here consider briefly some common concepts of physical fitness and their relation to performance. Distinction is made among anaerobic power, anaerobic capacity, and aerobic power. Laboratory and field tests of the various aspects of fitness (including strength, flexibility, percent body fat, and ECG appearances) are reviewed, and current standards of fitness are examined. A final section of this chapter will consider determinants of performance in prolonged exercise.

CONCEPTS OF FITNESS

The term physical fitness has had a somewhat checkered career—indeed, my Professor of Physiology thought it sufficiently vague that he proscribed its use. This was some years ago, and our understanding of human performance has now advanced to the point where it is useful to attempt a definition of fitness, recognizing that this is still not an easy matter. The task may be approached as an exercise in human ecology, ergonomics, or sports medicine, and it is facilitated by a breakdown of the concept in terms of the age and sex of the individual and the anticipated duration of activity.

Human Ecology

Fitness could be considered as the total matching of the individual to her or his environment. This might include not only physiological, but also psychological, sociological, and even theological matching of personal attributes to environmental demand.

Let us consider the situation of a 10-year old girl who is undertaking rigorous training 6 hours per day because her parents and coach hope for her future international success in a 100-meter swimming event. In terms of certain aspects of physiology, particularly the power and flexibility of her shoulder girdle, she may already have become an outstanding individual, at or above the 95th percentile on these two very specific criteria of fitness. However, in order to achieve such specialized development, she may have neglected opportunities for social contacts, hampering her psychological maturation, and she may also have learned to put an undesirable emphasis on competition rather than cooperation. Thus, in many aspects, she could be very unfit for the environment she must face as an adult. Even in physiological terms, the heavy emphasis on arm work has left her with a disproportionate development of the upper body musculature, so that she may remain relatively unfit in terms of leg performance.

Plainly, the ideal type of physical activity is one that encourages optimal development of all aspects of a person: physiological, psychological, sociological, and theological. In few instances do those preparing for competitive sports either seek or realize this objective.

Ergonomics

Some authors have considered fitness in the context of matching human capabilities to the machines that a person must operate—an excursion into applied ergonomics. For instance, the World Health Organization concluded after a week-long conference, that physical fitness was "the ability to perform muscular work satisfactorily."

While the duration of industrial activity is theoretically 8 hours, in practice an 8-hour shift is usually broken up by lunch and coffee breaks, maintenance of equipment, and other unscheduled interruptions, so that the usual work bout lasts 30 to 60 minutes. One important criterion of performance in such a situation is the level of the maximum oxygen intake; fatigue is likely if a person must use an average exceeding 40 percent of maximum oxygen intake. A further major consideration in heavy occupations is the ability to lift heavy objects. This criterion unfortunately places women at a substantial disadvantage in the labor market. One military survey found a need to lift to shoulder height loads of 36 kg occasionally, and 18 kg frequently.

Sports Medicine

A further group of investigators has approached fitness from the viewpoint of the sports physician. They may be attempting to identify potential talent, to analyse defects in the profile of a particular competitor, to optimize the training regimen so that "peaking" occurs at the time of a major competition, or to follow the course of rehabilitation following injury.

Tests of athletic performance are considered under three broad headings—physiological capability, neuromuscular skills, and psychological factors. The physiological tests must be sports specific, e.g., the use of a mill-race ("flume") or tethered swimming to measure the maximum oxygen intake of a distance swimmer. Neuromuscular skills determine how good is the use made of physiological characteristics; for instance, a highly trained swimmer moves through the water with at least four times the mechanical efficiency of a novice. Psychological factors may have a greater impact upon scores than either physiological attainments or neuromuscular skills, particularly under the stress of a major international competition. In a study of whitewater paddlers, for example, we found that anthropometric and physiological data (height, maximum oxygen intake, anaerobic power, isometric strength and percent body fat) provided an appropriate ranking of performance under conditions such as a regional competition, but the same information was quite misleading in the Olympic environment. Under the pressure of world-class competition, the paddler with the best physiological profile dissipated this advantage by hitting many of the slalom gates and accumulating a correspondingly large handicap of time penalties; in an emotionally-charged environment, psychological stability was of much greater importance.

Effects of Age and Sex

The types of fitness sought by the individual depend also upon age and sex. At the age of 25 years, fitness is commonly conceived in terms of a position on an athletic team. By the age of 35 years, many people have begun to accumulate a substantial excess of body fat, and now the urge is to find a form of fitness that will control a bulging waist-line. At 45 years, friends and peers are beginning to be affected by ischemic heart disease, and the desire changes to a form of fitness that will protect the individual against a "heart attack." Finally, in the sixth or seventh decade of life, the ordinary activities of daily living become fatiguing, and the search switches to a level of fitness (including muscle strength and flexibility) that will enable both occupation and leisure to be enjoyed, while allowing continued independence; ultimately, institutionalization may be needed because quadriceps strength is insufficient to rise from a toilet seat, or hip flexibility is insufficient to climb into a bath.

While the type of fitness needed for sports participation is highly specific, the control of obesity and protection against ischemic heart disease seem most likely through sustained endurance training of the type that is effective in developing maximum oxygen intake. A regimen that boosts maximum oxygen intake should also offer useful protection against fatigue in later life, since effort becomes tiring when the average oxygen cost of daily activities exceeds 40 percent of maximum oxygen intake.

When Bailey and I tested a large population in Saskatoon in 1973, we found that the men had a fairly precise perception of their personal fitness status in terms of their maximum oxygen transport, but that there was little relationship between the perceived fitness of the women and their maximum oxygen intake. We explained this observation on the grounds that the women were seeking something other than aerobic fitness from an exercise program—possibly a good figure, a good carriage, and an attractive appearance. Over the past decade women have become much more interested in fitness as the development of aerobic power, and it would be interesting to repeat these observations in 1987; however, a survey of a junior high school completed as recently as 1983 showed that some of the traditional gender differences in perceptions of fitness still persisted among many of the students.

Influence of Activity Duration

A further possible basis for the classification of fitness is the intended duration of physical activity (Table 8-1). Over the first 10 seconds of activity, key variables are reaction time, explosive muscular force, skill and flexibility, these various attributes being summarized in many of the common tests of anaerobic power (see section on Anaerobic Power). Between 10 and 60 seconds of exercise, such attributes still make a major contribution, but there is a growing dependence upon anaerobic capacity (see section on Anaerobic Capacity) muscular strength, (Chapter 5) and endurance. The limit of anaerobic effort is reached at about 1 minute, and thereafter the body depends on the aerobic replenishment of energy reserves. The key variable at this stage is thus the maximum oxygen intake, often expressed as a ratio to body mass. If the activity lasts longer than 1 hour, there is then a possibility that performance will be limited by depletion of fluid, difficulty in dissipating body heat, and exhaustion of glycogen reserves in the muscle and liver. Finally, if activity continues for more than about a month (as in a Cross-Canada race), body stores of fat become exhausted, so that a limitation is imposed by catabolism of muscle protein and the ability to ingest substantial amounts of food while exercising. Irrespective of the duration of exercise, motivation is of course highly important, as is the ability to use the physiological potential efficiently (Chapter 1).

Many types of athletic events involve quite brief periods of exercise, but as we have noted, the ordinary person is usually involved in bouts of activity lasting about 1 hour, a situation where the maximum oxygen intake per kilogram of body mass is the most significant variable.

Relation to Performance

Many authors have sought to establish correlations between physical performance and physiological test scores. Even for something as simple as the distance jogged in 12 minutes, reported coefficients of correlation with maximum oxygen intake have varied widely from 0.25 to 0.90. Much depends upon the range of variability of maximum oxygen intake seen in the sample, the allowance which is made for such simple covariates as age, height and body mass, the success in controlling environmental variables (wind, sun, rain, track conditions, altitude, turns), the motivation of the population, their experience of the test, and their ability to choose an appropriate running pace. Performance tests have been widely used in assessing the fitness of schoolchildren, although at least as far as the individual student is concerned, critics have pointed out that results are so heavily dependent on physical anthropometric variables that a better prediction of maximum oxygen intake could be obtained from a simple equa-

TABLE 8–1   Influence of Duration of Activity Upon the Determinants of Physical Performance

0 – 10 sec	10 – 60 sec	1 – 60 min	1 – 4 h	Very Prolonged (2 – 3 months)
Motivation	Motivation	Motivation	Motivation	Motivation
Reaction time	Anaerobic capacity	Maximum oxygen intake	Heat dissipation	Fat mobilization & body fat reserves
Anaerobic power	Muscle strength	Body mass	Glycogen reserves	Protein reserves
Explosive force	Muscle endurance	Strength	Fluid and mineral stores	Food intake
Skill	Skill		Maximum oxygen intake	Bone and joint injuries
Flexibility	Flexibility			

tion based upon age, sex, height, and body mass. Likewise, some samples of adults show very poor performance scores, despite at least average physiological results, largely because the individuals concerned have not had recent experience of the required gymnastic skills. The likelihood that athletic performance may differ from the physiological ranking when the performer is aroused or is overaroused by the excitement of a major event has already been noted.

ANAEROBIC CAPACITY AND POWER

Anaerobic Power

The absolute maximum of anerobic power is seen when a person makes a single maximum effort, as during a vertical jump and reach test. If the jump is made while the subject is standing on a force plate, the power output can be measured fairly precisely. C.T.M. Davies estimated that the average power output of women during this procedure was 2.3 kW, while that of men was 3.8 kW. Other investigators have reported figures of 2.2 kW for sprinting, 1.5 kW for weightlifting, and 0.45 kW for pole-vaulting, all of these values being measured in top competitors. Although there is a small contribution from tissue oxygen stores, the crucial factor in brief activities of this type is the rate at which energy can be transferred from creatine phosphate to ATP, and thus the actin–myosin interaction. There is an initial lag of perhaps 0.5 seconds, associated with enzyme activation, and then the limiting factor seems to be the maximum velocity of the reaction between creatine phosphate and ADP, catalyzed by the enzyme creatine phosphotransferase.

A second method of assessing anaerobic power is to have subjects run up a staircase as rapidly as possible, using the interruption of light beams to time the ascent from the fourth to the sixth steps. The power output during this maneuver is approximately 0.7 kW for a young woman, and 1.0 kW for a young man. Margaria assumed that the mechanical efficiency of effort during the climb was 25 percent, but this would only be true if account was taken of both phosphagen breakdown and the subsequent recovery process. During the actual ascent, phosphagen is not regenerated to any great extent, and the efficiency is probably about 40 percent, implying that the woman is using energy reserves at a rate of some 1.75 kW and the man is using about 2.50 kW. Approximately one-third of this power is lost by 60 years of age.

A third test possibility, advocated by Bar Or, is to have a subject pedal a cycle ergometer as hard as possible for 5 seconds, recording the power output that is developed. Success in this maneuver depends very much on the subject's knowledge of the technique and on an appropriate choice of loading for the cycle ergometer.

There is a rapid drop of anaerobic power output as the duration of activity is further extended. If we assume that the process has a simple exponential form, the half-time would be about 10 seconds.

In order to relate anaerobic and aerobic processes, it is helpful to translate the observed anaerobic power into an equivalent aerobic activity (Table 8–2). Here, an efficiency of 25 percent would be likely (as assumed by Margaria), so that the energy cost if a young woman were able to complete the staircase sprint aerobically would be 2.8 kW, corresponding to an oxygen consumption of 800 mℓ per minute (or if body mass is 60 kg, 133 mℓ per kilogram per minute). In a young man, an oxygen equivalent as high as 160 mℓ per kilogram per minute might be anticipated, while in an old person this would drop to about 90 to 110 mℓ per kilogram per minute. If the combined store of tissue oxygen and high-energy phosphagen molecules is exhausted within 8 to

$$\text{Creatine phosphate} + \text{ADP} \underset{}{\overset{\text{creatine phosphotransferase}}{\rightleftharpoons}} \text{ATP} + \text{creatine}$$

TABLE 8–2 Components of Oxygen Debt Accumulated in a Sedentary Subject

Component	Tissue Mass (kg)	Change of Concentration (mmol/kg or mℓ/kg)	Equivalent oxygen debt (mℓ)
Alactate Debt			
Depletion of O_2 stores			
Venous blood	4	100	400
Myoglobin	20	10	200
Tissue fluid	38	0.5	20
Creatine phosphate and ATP	20	30	600 mmol = 2180*
Lactate Debt			
Muscle	20	40	800 mmol = 5380*
		Total	= 8180

* The oxygen debt is larger than the oxygen equivalent of the corresponding anaerobic energy release, since the resynthesis of both phosphagen and glycogen is not 100 percent efficient. For the purpose of this calculation, it is assumed that phosphagen is reformed by the breakdown of glycogen with an efficiency of 60 percent, and that 90 percent of glycogen is reformed from lactate, using the energy content of the remaining 10 percent. Thus, 1 mol of ATP usage is equivalent to the breakdown of 1/37 mol of glucose-6-phosphate, a reaction that would require about 3.63 ℓ of oxygen under aerobic conditions. Likewise, 9 g of carbohydrate is metabolized for every mol of lactate that must be recycled, equivalent to an oxygen debt of about 6.73 ℓ.

10 seconds, the equivalent oxygen capacity of what Margaria has described as an "alactate oxygen debt" is no more than 1.5 ℓ in a woman and 2.0 ℓ in a man.

Anaerobic Capacity

The anaerobic capacity is set by an accumulation of lactic acid within the active muscles. During all-out effort, production of lactate continues for about 40 to 50 seconds. Exercise is usually halted when a blood lactate concentration of 10 to 15 mmol per liter has been reached (although intramuscular concentrations may by then be as high as 30 mmol per liter). The equivalent oxygen capacity of the lactate system is some 45 ml per kilogram. Margaria has calculated this equivalent oxygen delivery from the limiting blood lactate concentrations. The equivalent power, also expressed in oxygen transport units, is about 68 mℓ per kilogram per minute. The absolute size of the lactate oxygen debt varies somewhat with the lean tissue mass in which the lactate has been distributed. It is thus influenced by the mass of active muscle, being much less in situations where only the smaller muscles of the body have been activated (for instance, arm or forearm exercise).

Simple methods of measuring anaerobic capacity are (1) to time a treadmill run which is carried out at a speed and slope likely to cause exhaustion in about 45 seconds, or (2) to measure the maximum work that can be performed on the cycle ergometer over 30 to 45 seconds. It is also possible to measure the concentration of lactic acid in arterial or arterialized capillary blood 2 to 4 minutes following all-out effort. A final tactic is to examine repayment of the oxygen debt during the first few minutes of recovery from exhausting exercise. A semi-logarithmic plot of unpaid oxygen debt against time becomes linear from the second to the fifteenth minute of recovery. Extrapolation of

this relationship back to the ordinate indicates the magnitude of the initial lactate debt (Fig. 8–1). It is possible to make a second semi-logarithmic plot for the period 0 to 2 minutes of recovery, showing the unpaid debt in excess of the lactate component. Extrapolation of this line back to zero time in turn gives an estimate of the magnitude of the alactate debt. In practice, there are some difficulties in applying such a graphic approach. The oxygen consumption often fails to return to its initial resting value for a long time after exercise, because body temperature remains elevated, and there is continuing circulation of catecholamines; it is thus quite difficult to estimate what is the "excess" oxygen consumption used in debt repayment. Moreover, there is no absolute guarantee that all of the oxygen deficit accumulated by the performance of anaerobic work will be repaid in the form of an increased resting oxygen consumption. Some of the lactate that is produced during anaerobic effort is excreted in the urine and the sweat, and some of it may be metabolized, either during or following exercise, as part of the normal resting metabolism of other body tissues.

A formal analysis of the alactate and lactate debts is presented in Table 8–1. It is assumed here that muscle tolerates lactate to a concentration of 40 mmol per liter, that 20 kg of muscle is activated, and that 10 percent of the accumulated lactate is used to reconvert the remaining 90 percent to glycogen during the recovery period. On this basis, the breakdown of glycogen to 1 mole of lactate and its subsequent resynthesis requires the equivalent of 6.73 ℓ of oxygen. Likewise, if the resynthesis of phosphagen from glycogen proceeds with an efficiency of 60 percent, each mole of ATP usage is equivalent to the breakdown of 1/37 of a mole of glucose-6-phosphate, a reaction that would require some 3.63 ℓ of oxygen under aerobic conditions.

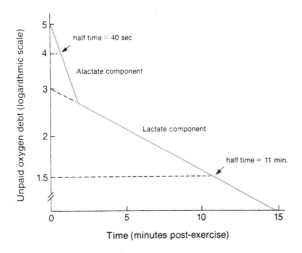

Figure 8–1 The "curve-stripping" approach to analysis of the oxygen debt. A semi-logarithmic plot of the unpaid debt between 2 and 15 min post-exercise is extrapolated back to the ordinate, indicating a lactate debt of 3 ℓ. The excess above this linear extrapolation for the period 0 to 2 minutes corresponds to repayment of an alactate debt of 2 ℓ. The half-time of these two processes is 40 sec and 11 min respectively.

AEROBIC POWER

The maximum oxygen intake, or aerobic power, provides an integrated measure of the individual's ability to pump oxygen from the atmosphere to the working tissues. As discussed in Chapters 6 and 7, in a healthy person the cardiovascular system limits this process more than does the respiratory system. The optimum approach to the measurement of maximum oxygen intake is to require the subject to carry out large muscle endurance exercise until exhaustion. However, in some circumstances, attempts are made to predict a corresponding score, using data obtained from submaximal exercise tests.

Direct Measurement

In theory, the maximum oxygen intake can be measured during any form of progressive exercise that involves the large muscles of the body. In practice, the highest scores are obtained during uphill treadmill running or walking (Table 8–3), and since the treadmill score cannot be materially exceeded by adding supplementary work (e.g., the maneuvering of ski poles or simultaneous arm cranking), it is usually considered the reference standard against which other types of measurement are judged.

TABLE 8–3   A Comparison of the Peak Oxygen Intake Determined With Three Different Types of Ergometry

	Maximum O₂ Intake		Maximum Heart Rate	Maximum Blood Lactate
	(ℓ/min)	(%)	(beats/min)	(mmol/ℓ)
Treadmill	3.81	100	190	13.6
Cycle ergometer	3.56	93	187	12.4
Bench stepping	3.68	96	188	11.7

Based on data obtained by International Biological Programme working party

There are many different treadmill protocols, but these cause only minor differences in maximal oxygen intake; if the test is of too short duration or increments of work-rate are too large, the peak oxygen consumption may not be defined with sufficient precision, and if it is too long, the subject may be exhausted before a true maximum oxygen intake is reached. The preferred procedure is a progressive uphill test, running for a young subject, and walking for an older person (Fig. 8–2). The optimum protocol begins with 3 minutes of exercise at no more than 70 percent of maximum aerobic power (a warmup of this type minimizes the risk of injuries and cardiac arrhythmias during the test, while also maximizing the peak oxygen transport). The slope of the treadmill is then adjusted to demand a power output which it is estimated will correspond to about 95 percent of the individual's maximum oxygen intake, and the slope is further increased by 1 to 2 percent at 2-minute intervals until the subject is exhausted or there are other indications to halt the test. The prime evidence of a good maximum oxygen intake test is the demonstration of an "oxygen plateau". This is defined as an increase in oxygen consumption of less than 2 mℓ per kilogram per minute (or 150 mℓ per minute) with a further increase of work-rate. Using modern, on-line devices for recording oxygen consumption, it has become relatively easy to ascertain whether subjects have reached a well-defined oxygen plateau. If an on-line device is not available, guidance can be obtained from the appearance of the subject. As exhaustion is approached, the color of the face changes from pink through a bluish hue to ashen grey, reflecting first a reduction of cutaneous blood flow and then a constriction of the peripheral veins. The gait may also become poorly coordinated, and the subject may show a confused response to questioning. The heart rate reaches a value close to the age-related maximum, the respiratory gas exchange ratio is at least 1.10, and in a young adult the peak blood lactate, collected from an arterialized capillary blood specimen 2 to 4 minutes after stopping the test, is 10 to 12 mmol per liter.

Under field conditions, a treadmill is rarely available. Maximum exercise may then be performed on a stepping bench. Typically, the observed maximum oxygen intake is about 96 percent of the value that would

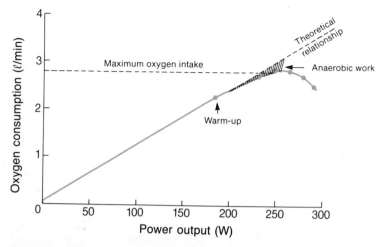

Figure 8–2 The measurement of maximum oxygen intake. An initial warm-up is performed at a treadmill speed and slope corresponding to approximately 70 percent of the subject's anticipated maximum oxygen intake. After 3 minutes at this loading, the slope is increased to 95 percent of the anticipated maximum, and is increased by a further 5 percent at 2-minute intervals until the subject is exhausted. The oxygen plateau shows an increase in consumption of less than 150 mℓ/per kilogram per minute with a further increase of power output. In theory, a linear relationship of oxygen consumption to power output would be anticipated. Departure from this line reflects the onset of anaerobic work.

have been seen during treadmill exercise. Another possibility is to use a cycle ergometer. The main objection to the cycle ergometer is that a large part of the required effort is borne by the quadriceps muscles, and many people find some difficulty in exercising to an oxygen plateau. Often, the test is halted by complaints of leg weakness and fatigue at a stage when the peak heart rate is less than the anticipated maximum figure, and the peak oxygen intake is only about 92 percent of the treadmill value. Such difficulties are compounded if exercise is performed in a supine position. Immobilization of the shoulders is most uncomfortable, and because the legs are above heart level, their perfusion is further restricted. Often supine subjects show a peak oxygen intake that is only about 88 percent of the treadmill score. During forearm cranking, the figure drops further to 70 percent of the treadmill value, partly because of the difficulty in perfusing small and strongly contracting muscles, and partly because of problems arising from a pooling of blood in the inactive lower limbs. If a cycle ergometer is modified by fitting drop handle-bars, a racing saddle and toe clips, values approach the treadmill result much more closely.

Many athletes quite rightly complain that treadmill exercise gives an unrealistic impression of their cardiorespiratory condition. In recent years, there has thus been a proliferation of sports-specific devices that allow a determination of the peak oxygen uptake while simulating the movements of rowing, canoeing, swimming, cycling and so on. In general, the aerobic power is still smaller than the score that the athlete can attain on a treadmill. However, a well-conditioned competi-

tor is distinguished by the ability to develop a large fraction of the treadmill oxygen intake during a sports-specific test.

Submaximum Prediction Procedures

There have been occasional attempts to predict maximum oxygen intake from the anaerobic threshold and from the progressive increase of respiratory gas exchange ratio as work-rate is augmented, but most prediction procedures still exploit the supposedly linear relationship between oxygen consumption and heart rate. A linear relationship would in fact only be anticipated if there were no changes of arteriovenous oxygen difference and stroke volume between rest and maximum effort, or if these two variables changed simultaneously and to a similar extent, but in opposite directions. Despite this insecure theoretical foundation, the heart rate–oxygen consumption line is in practice reasonably linear between 50 and 100 percent of maximum oxygen intake. A second major assumption in all heart rate predictions procedures is that the individual's maximum heart rate conforms to the population average. The widely used Åstrand nomogram makes the further assumption that the heart rate at 50 percent of maximum oxygen intake is 135 beats per minute in women and 128 beats per minute in men.

The Åstrand procedure requires only a single pair of data points (a heart rate between 122 and 170 beats per minute, and the corresponding oxygen consumption—or assuming a 23 percent net efficiency of cycling and a 16 percent net efficiency of stepping—

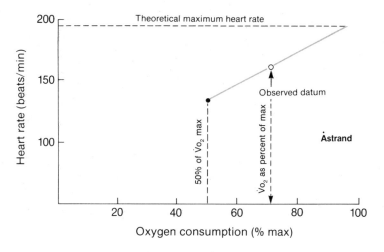

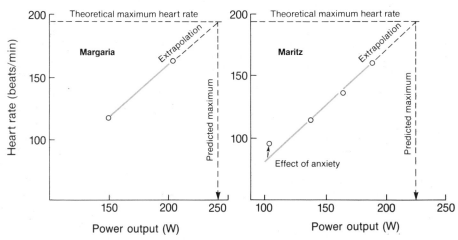

Figure 8–3   Three methods of predicting maximum oxygen intake from sub-maximum data. The Åstrand procedure is based on a single datum and a theoretical line; it thus converts an observed oxygen consumption or work rate to a percent of maximum. Margaria's procedure measures heart rate at two workrates. Maritz uses four pairs of data points; the first may show some increase of heart rate owing to anxiety.

the corresponding work-rate). In essence, the nomogram calculates a formula of the type $\dot{V}O_2$ max $= 2\dot{V}O_2$ obs $(203 - 138)/(P - 73)$ in women, and $\dot{V}O_2$ max $= 2\dot{V}O_2$ obs $(193 - 128)/(P - 63)$ in men (where P is the measured pulse rate at the observed oxygen consumption). The original 1954 nomogram ignored the substantial decline of maximum heart rate with age. In order to apply the nomogram to older adults it is thus necessary to "correct" the predicted maximum oxygen intake by a factor that varies with age (1.00 at 25 years, 0.87 at 35 years, 0.78 at 45 years, 0.71 at 55 years, and at 0.65 at 65 years).

Margaria developed a somewhat similar nomogram based on the heart rate observed at two specified rates of stepping, and Maritz, Wyndham, and associates suggested a linear extrapolation of four heart rate and oxygen consumption or work-rate measurements (Fig. 8–3). If four pairs of data points are used, the first pair

is inevitably measured at a rather modest work-rate, and perhaps because the slope of the heart rate–oxygen consumption line is strongly influenced by this first pair of readings, the Maritz extrapolation is not noticeably more accurate than either the Åstrand or the Margaria nomograms. Each of these three procedures predicts the individual's maximum oxygen intake with a coefficient of variation[1] of about 10 percent in a young adult (Table 8–4) and (because of interindividual differences in the rate of aging of maximum heart rate) 15 to 20 percent in older adults; this compares with a test-retest variation of about 4 percent for the direct measurement. Plainly, the submaximum predictions are sufficiently

---

[1] The coefficient of variation is given by the standard deviation of the discrepancy between the predicted and the directly measured value, divided by the directly measured value.

TABLE 8–4   Error of Sub-Maximum Predictions of Aerobic Power in Group of Young Men with Directly Measured Treadmill Maximum Averaging of 3.70 ℓ/min, on First and Fifth days of Repeated Testing

Mode of exercise	Error of prediction (ℓ/min STPD)					
	Åstrand prediction		Margaria prediction		Maritz prediction	
	Day 1	Day 5	Day 1	Day 5	Day 1	Day 5
Cycle ergometer						
Error	+ 0.30	+ 0.33	+ 0.18	+ 0.13	+ 0.19	+ 0.18
SD	± 0.31	± 0.35	± 0.27	± 0.35	± 0.28	± 0.34
Step test						
Error	− 0.18	+ 0.16	− 0.09	+ 0.12	− 0.03	+ 0.12
SD	± 0.46	± 0.25	± 0.39	± 0.28	± 0.36	± 0.28

Based on data of International Biological Programme working party

imprecise that it becomes difficult to counsel the individual concerning exercise and fitness on the basis of the test score; a supposed value of 40 mℓ per kilogram per minute would (on one occasion in twenty) reflect a very low level of fitness (32 mℓ per minute) or quite a high level of fitness (48 mℓ per kilogram per minute). However, in a large population survey, interindividual errors tend to cancel one another out, so that the average score still provides an appropriate estimate of fitness for a given community, often with little systematic error. The main advantages of using a submaximum procedure are that less motivation is required of the subject, and there is less danger that a cardiac emergency may be provoked by the test. Bruce noted that in his laboratory there was a threefold difference of risk between maximum and submaximum testing. The discrepancy between the directly measured and the predicted maximum oxygen intake remains reasonably consistent in any given individual from one day to another, so that the submaximum result may also be used to follow changes of physical condition (for instance, over the course of a training program). However, inaccuracies become likely in any situation where the heart rate is increased during submaximum effort (e.g., if the room is overheated and if the subject has had a recent meal, has been smoking, or is anxious). The effect of anxiety can sometimes be diminished by a deliberate repetition of the test—the process of negative conditioning or habituation. If oxygen consumption is estimated from work-rate, further problems arise in making day-to-day comparisons, since the subject becomes accustomed to carrying out the required form of exercise and learns to move in a mechanically more efficient manner.

Some authors have argued that given the various problems inherent in prediction procedures, it is better not to attempt an extrapolation of submaximum test results to a supposed maximum aerobic power. One alternative method of data treatment is to report a close interpolation of the plot of heart rate against work-rate or oxygen consumption e.g., the physical working capacity at a heart rate of 170 beats per minute (the

PWC$_{170}$), or the heart rate at an oxygen consumption of 1.5 ℓ per minute (the $f_{h,1.5}$). Such procedures suffer from many of the limitations noted for the other submaximal tests, but add the further problem that while the required effort is a fairly easy submaximal task for a young adult, it exceeds the aerobic tolerance of many older individuals.

A final possible approach requires that all subjects exercise at a consistent fraction of their personal maximum oxygen intake. Thus, in the Canadian Home Fitness Test (CHFT), subjects are set an age and sex specific rate of stepping which is designed to demand 70 percent of maximum oxygen intake from a person of average fitness (Table 8–5). Scores are determined from the time for which this work-rate can be sustained and the corresponding heart rate. The Home Fitness Test, as its name implies, was devised as a simple motivational tool, for use in the individual's home. The heart rate was to be palpated 5 to 15 seconds after ceasing exercise, as preliminary research had indicated that when the subject remained standing, the pulse count over this interval did not differ systematically from the heart rate recorded in the final 15 seconds of exercise. It was originally intended to report a three-category rating of fitness. However, subsequent investigators have used the CHFT for fitness surveys of large populations (for instance, the 20,000 subject Canada Fitness Survey). Keys to accurate interpretation of the CHFT score are maintenance of the required stepping rate (facilitated by walking the steps with the subject or testing several people at the same time) and accurate counting of the heart rate (preferably by an ECG or a reliable pulse counter). Assuming these two criteria are satisfied, the prediction of maximum oxygen intake seems about as accurate as that obtained with other submaximal step tests. The data can be fitted into the Åstrand nomogram, or alternatively, a prediction equation developed by Jetté can be used:

$$Vo_2 \text{ max} = 42.5 + 16.6(E) - 0.12(M) - 0.12(f_h) - 0.24(A)$$

(where E is the energy cost of the age and sex-specific

TABLE 8–5 Stepping Rates and 10-Second Recovery Pulse Counts for the Canadian Home Fitness Test*

Age (yr)	Required Stepping Rate		Duration of Test Required Recovery Count and Fitness Category		
			First 3 min (Undesirable)	Second 3 min	
	F	M		(Minimum)	(Recommended)
15 – 19	120	144	≥30	≥27	≤26
20 – 29	114	144	≥29	≥26	≤25
30 – 39	114	132	≥28	≥25	≤24
40 – 49	102	114	≥26	≥24	≤23
50 – 59	84	102	≥25	≥23	≤22
60 – 69	84	84	≥24	≥23	≤22
Warm-up for 60 – 69	66	66	–	–	–

* All subjects climb a double 8-inch (20.3 cm) step, starting with 3 minutes at a rate appropriate for a person years older, and continuing for a further 3 minutes at the age- and sex-specific rate. The test is designed to demand about 70 percent of maximum oxygen intake, irrespective of age.

stepping rate, in ℓ per minute; M is the body mass in kg; f_h is the heart rate in beats per minute and A is the age in years). The Jetté formula depends much less upon heart rate than does the Åstrand nomogram. Perhaps for this reason it is less vulnerable to artifacts of habituation.

Field Tests

The original field tests of aerobic power proposed for children were the 300-yard (274-meter) run in Canada, and the 600-yard (549-meter) walk-run in the United States. These distances were originally selected on grounds of safety. In more recent years it has been recognized that running is a natural, safe activity for a child, and there has been a tendency to use longer distances of one mile (1,606 meters) or 1½ miles (2,409 meters) to estimate aerobic fitness. The longer running distances provide a more thorough evaluation of aerobic characteristics in well-motivated young adults, but in young children there remain uncertainties regarding an appropriate choice of running pace and difficulties in sustaining motivation for 12 or more minutes. The largest coefficients of correlation with the directly measured maximum oxygen intake in young children are thus observed over distances of 800 to 1,000 meters. In elderly subjects, there are also risks in proposing an all-out run without a thorough preliminary medical examination.

A rough parallel can be drawn between the distance covered in 12 minutes and the directly measured maximum oxygen intake in young adults (Table 8–6). However, mechanical inefficiencies of running technique lead to substantially higher oxygen costs and thus shorter 12-minute distances in both young children and older subjects.

STRENGTH AND FLEXIBILITY

A full report on the muscular strength of an individual would discuss isotonic, isokinetic, and isometric strength and endurance of muscle groups about each of the major joints in the body. Plainly, constraints of cost and time allow the testing of only a few joints on any one person. Laboratory methods of measuring isotonic, isokinetic, and isometric strength have been discussed in Chapter 5. Each can be measured for a single, maximal effort, or the drop-off in scores can be examined with a specified number of repetitions. Isokinetic tests can also be performed at fast and slow speeds, to examine the performance of fast and slow-twitch fibers respectively. Some types of dynamometer and tensiometer can be taken into the field. The explosive strength can also be measured quite simply by such performance test items as a jump and reach or a standing broad jump, although the scores depend in part on the size and the body mass of the individual under investigation. A combined index of muscular strength and endurance is obtained from scores on such gymnastic items as speed sit-ups, push-ups, and the en-

TABLE 8–6 Approximate Relationship Between Distance Run in 12 Minutes and Maximum Oxygen Intake*

Distance (km)	Maximum Oxygen Intake (mℓ/kg min STPD)
< 1.6	< 28.0
1.6 – 2.0	28.0 – 34.0
2.0 – 2.4	34.1 – 42.0
2.4 – 2.8	42.1 – 52.0
> 2.8	> 52.0

* Young children and older adults are not able to cover as great a distance. Based on data of K. H. Cooper.

durance of a flexed arm hang. These items all require sustained isometric contractions, and because of the associated rise in systemic blood pressure, they should be avoided in coronary-prone adults.

In theory, the assessment of static and dynamic flexibility also requires an examination of many joints, but again, in practice, time permits the making of only one or two representative measurements. The commonest presently used test is the Dillon sit and reach procedure, which in essence measures how far a person can reach beyond the toes while the knees remain extended (Fig. 8–4). It has been suggested that scores on this test are adversely affected in subjects who have a substantial limb to trunk length ratio.

BODY FAT

Methods of determining the percentage of body fat were discussed in Chapter 3. The simplest assessment relates the standing height to actuarial tables of body mass. However, if the total body mass is excessive, a distinction must be drawn between muscle and fat. In general, if additional mass has been accumulated since the age of 25 years, it can be assumed that this is fat, and indeed in older adults even the maintenance of body mass is usually an indication that muscle has been replaced by fat (Table 8–7).

Skinfold calipers are now sufficiently inexpensive that they should form part of the armamentarium of any physician or fitness assessor. Several skinfolds should be measured, since the distribution of body fat between the trunk and the limbs varies with sex, ethnic group, and nutritional status. Given uncertainties in the relationship between skinfolds and total body fat, some investigators have suggested that it is desirable to interpret the skinfold data in their own right. The main argu-

TABLE 8–7 Influence of Age on Body Mass (Excess Relative to Actuarial Tables) and Average Thickness of Eight Skinfolds. Data for Average Torontonians

Age (yr)	Females		Males	
	Excess Body Mass (kg)	Skinfold (mm)	Excess Body Mass (kg)	Skinfold (mm)
25	8.3	16.2	1.7	11.2
35	1.4	13.5	6.4	16.1
45	6.8	17.3	9.3	14.0
55	4.9	18.2	8.8	15.2
65	4.5	22.5	5.1	15.4

Note: The excess body mass decreases in the older age categories, although skinfold thicknesses are still increasing; the decrease of mass is thought to reflect a loss of lean tissue.

ment for attempting a conversion to percentage body fat is that the amount of lean tissue can then be estimated.

More sophisticated methods of estimating body fat, such as hydrostatic weighing, are also discussed in Chapter 3. On average, a fit young woman should have about 18 percent body fat, while the normal figure for a young man is about 14 percent. In some types of athlete, much lower readings (10 percent in women, 5 percent in men) are seen; however, there is continuing debate on the wisdom of such extensive depletion of body fat stores.

ELECTROCARDIOGRAPHIC APPEARANCES

At one time, it was customary to comment on electrocardiographic appearances when subjects performed an exercise test with an electrocardiogram. In a statistical sense, the risk of a future cardiac attack is increased several-fold if the ECG shows substantial ST depression, but nevertheless, if the person is symptom-free, the risks of a false-positive relative to a true diagnosis of myocardial ischemia are as large as two to one (Chapter 6). It is thus best to reserve any attempts at ECG prognostication for a "high risk" group of individuals characterized by cigarette smoking, a high systemic blood pressure, and an adverse lipid profile. The mathematics of prognosis (as described by Bayes theorem) are such that the success rate of adverse predictions is about ten times greater in such a population (Chapter 6).

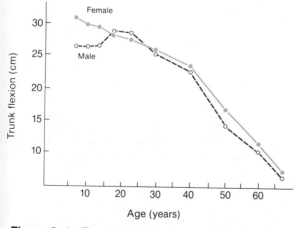

Figure 8–4 Trunk flexibility is measured by Dillon's "sit and reach" test. Based on Canada Fitness Survey data of 1981. Note: score = 25 cm if subject is able to reach board with finger tips while knees are kept extended.

CURRENT STANDARDS OF FITNESS

Although there is periodic lamentation about the poor levels of fitness in most industrialized nations, it

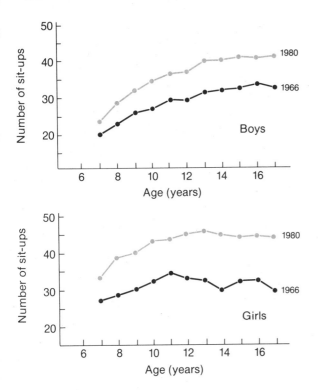

Figure 8–5 The gain on physical performance test scores between 1966 and 1980. Data for two random samples of Canadian schoolchildren tested by the Canadian Association for Health, Physical Education and Recreation (CAHPER).

is hard to obtain objective information on this point.

Various random samples of schoolchildren around the world have completed a series of six to seven gymnastic performance tests. In the original comparisons, European children substantially outperformed their North American counterparts; although this probably indicated that the Europeans were more fit, the contribution from a recent practice of the specific skills tested was highlighted by the superior performance of North American students on a softball throw (an activity that is uncommon in Europe). The original surveys have now been repeated several times. At the first repetition, both American and Canadian children showed a considerable improvement in test scores (Fig. 8–5) and it was tempting to infer that this reflected an improvement of physical condition, attributable to the investment of government funds in fitness programming. However, a more probable explanation for much of the improvement in scoring was that the students had been repeatedly exposed to the tests by their classroom teachers over the intervening period.

With regard to most fitness tests, a plethora of results has been published, but unfortunately few authors have examined a randomly selected population sample. Indeed, it is very difficult if not impossible to obtain such a sample in a free society. Attempts to test a representative sample of the adult population in Canada have recruited no more than one-third to one-half of the populations contacted. It then becomes rather unlikely that the scores reported are representative of the total national population. Several authors have demonstrated that there is a selective recruitment of the more active individuals when a fitness test is offered to a company or a city. The Canadian Association for Health, Physical Education and Recreation were able to recruit a random sample of children aged 7 to 17 years, carrying out a physical working capacity (PWC_{170}) test in 1968 and again in 1983. Their data suggest that there was some improvement in the fitness of Canadian schoolchildren over the intervening period, gains being particularly obvious among the older girls (Table 8–8).

Information on the maximum oxygen intake of adults goes back to Dr. Sid Robinson, who evaluated a university population at the Harvard Fatigue Laboratory in 1938. The sample was non-random, and some of the subjects may not have reached our current definition of an oxygen plateau. The results that he reported were not grossly different from those which are observed at the present time, although at most ages his sample was a little fitter than current Canadian men are (Table 8–9). Robinson also tested some endurance athletes, and it does not seem that this earlier generation of competitors, who trained for relatively few hours per day had much smaller figures for aerobic power than current endurance performers.

One other piece of evidence concerning historical trends in physical condition is provided by the national per capita consumption of food. This showed a decrease of 1.3 MJ per day from 1930 to 1965, with a gradual recovery thereafter (Table 8–10). It is unlikely that wastage of food decreased from 1930 to 1965, and allowing also for the secular trend to an increase of stature, one might have anticipated that the daily energy intake would have increased by 0.4 to 0.5 MJ per day

TABLE 8–8   Physical Working Capacity at a Heart Rate of 170 beats/min (PWC_{170})

Age (yr)	Girls 1968	Girls 1983	Boys 1968	Boys 1983
7	1.6	1.9	2.0	2.2
8	1.8	1.8	2.1	2.2
9	1.7	2.0	2.1	2.3
10	1.7	2.0	2.1	2.3
11	1.7	2.0	2.2	2.3
12	1.7	1.8	2.2	2.2
13	1.5	1.8	2.3	2.3
14	1.4	1.8	2.3	2.5
15	1.4	1.8	2.1	2.5
16	1.4	1.8	2.2	2.5
17	1.4	1.9	2.2	2.4

Results for random samples of Canadian girls and boys, tested in 1968 and in 1983, expressed in watts/kg. Based on data of Canadian Association for Health, Physical Education and Recreation.

TABLE 8–9   Comparison of Robinson's Data for Maximum Oxygen Intake (U.S. Males, Tested at the Harvard Fatigue Laboratory in 1938) with More Recent Canadian Data

Age (yr)	Robinson (1938)	Toronto (1966)	Saskatoon (1973)	Canada (1981)
25	48.7	47.0	40.1	46.4
35	43.1	39.5	37.1	44.4
45	39.2	34.7	33.8	38.5
55	37.6	33.0	32.3	32.6

if exercise habits had remained constant. The most reasonable explanation of the observed decrease in food consumption is that there was an accompanying decrease in various types of daily physical activity over the intervening years. It is also a reasonable assumption that this would have led to some decrease of endurance fitness. The increase of food consumption over the past decade has been associated with an increase in expenditures on recreation durables; this suggests that the fitness movement has spawned an increase of habitual physical activity in at least a substantial segment of the community.

International comparisons of both fitness and activity patterns are hampered by the absence of true random samples. Taken at their face value, the fitness scores obtained on near random samples of the Canadian population seem of the same order to figures reported for other developed countries. This is logical, for in most of the countries concerned there has been not only much automation in industry and the home, but also a recent concern for the promotion of fitness.

A substantial number of "primitive" populations were tested as part of the International Biological Programme. Again, the results in most instances were quite similar to those observed in North American city dwellers. Often, those tested had abandoned their habitual active lifestyle, and indeed at the time of examination many had already adopted the worst lifestyle habits of the "white" person. Further, in some cases the scores of those living in underdeveloped societies were depressed by chronic diseases affecting lung function (for instance, tuberculosis) or hemoglobin levels (parasitic infections such as malaria, and schistosomiasis). However, a few examples were found where

TABLE 8–10   Daily Per Capita Food Consumption in the United States (based on data from U.S. Year Books)

Year	Energy Value (MJ)	Year	Energy Value (MJ)
1930	14.4	1965	13.1
1940	14.0	1970	13.8
1950	13.6	1975	13.6
1960	13.1	1977	14.1

health was good and traditional pursuits still demanded a high level of physical activity (for example, Canadian Inuit hunters, and the Tarahumara Indians in Mexico who run distances of up to 150 km). In such subjects, fitness levels were higher than in the city dwellers of the western world. It could be argued that the advantage of the Inuit reflected a genetic endowment rather than a training response. However, we had opportunity to repeat our studies in the arctic after the indigenous peoples had become acculturated to a western way of life for a period of 10 years. The results unhappily demonstrated a substantial decrease of both aerobic power and muscular strength, with an increase in the percentage of body fat; the 10 years of "civilization" had brought a proud and a fit people to the sad level of physical condition anticipated in a Canadian city dweller (Table 8–11).

FITNESS FOR PROLONGED EXERCISE

Blood and Tissue Glucose

The resting blood glucose concentration is 3.9 to 5.0 mmol per liter (70 to 90 mg per deciliter). A peak concentration of 7 to 8 mmol per liter is reached 30 to 60 minutes after ingesting a sugar-containing meal, and occasionally the renal threshold for excretion of glucose (8.9 to 9.5 mmol per liter is surpassed. Given a blood volume of perhaps 5 ℓ, the total carbohydrate content of the blood is at most 40 mmol, equivalent to about 115 kJ of work. Moreover, only one-half of this reserve can be used before symptoms of hypoglycemia appear.

The likelihood that hypoglycemia will impair prolonged exercise performance has been debated extensively. In marathon running, where the exercise task is distributed over the large muscles of the body, relatively normal blood glucose values have been observed a few minutes after completion of a race (possibly because of a rebound release of glucose from the liver). In contrast, glucose levels as low as 1 to 3 mmol per liter have been observed in exhausting cycle ergometer exercise, perhaps because a high proportion of the activity is sustained by a single muscle group (the quadriceps); intravenous glucose and/or saline infusions have also been needed by some competitors after 3 to 4 day paddling marathons. It has been suggested that a falling blood glucose may have an adverse effect on cerebral performance in pursuits such as orienteering and dinghy sailing, where much thought must be given to forward tactical planning, including the choice of an appropriate route. Blood glucose also falls in team sports where muscle glycogen is exhausted by frequent stops and starts (e.g., ice-hockey and soccer); in such situations, a low blood-sugar concentration may lead to a deterioration of teamwork and loss of scoring skills, and both performance and muscle carbohydrate reserves can be conserved by ingesting appropriate fluids during competition.

TABLE 8–11   Change of Fitness Levels in Canadian Inuit with 10 Years of Acculturation to North American Life Style

Variable	25-yr-old Female		25-yr-old Male	
	1970	1980	1970	1980
Skinfold thickness (average of 3, mm)	8.6	11.9	5.5	6.9
Knee extension force (N)	664	533	870	754
Maximum oxygen intake (mℓ/kg min STPD)	48.1	42.0	58.6	52.7

Based on data of Rode & Shephard

Some endurance athletes ingest strong solutions of glucose (1.7 to 2.3 mol per liter) while they are exercising, in an attempt to counteract hypoglycemia. In distance running and cross-country skiing, a lack of carbohydrate certainly seems to impair competitive times (particularly over the final few kilometers of a race (Fig. 8–6). However, the ingestion of concentrated glucose solutions also has a number of adverse consequences, including a slowing of both gastric emptying and fluid absorption, a depression of fat mobilization, and a depression of glucagon secretion. Many of these difficulties can be avoided or minimized if glucose is replaced by a glucose polymer with a high molecular weight and thus a low osmotic pressure at any given concentration. Depression of glucagon secretion inhibits the hepatic uptake of glucose-forming metabolites (lactate, glycerol and alanine). Initially, much of the glucose that the liver contributes to the blood comes from its glycogen stores (equivalent to 550 mmol of glucose), but after 4 hours of moderate activity, as much as 45 percent of the continuing glucose output has been recently synthesized in the liver. The process of hepatic gluconeogenesis is important to the survival of certain tissues that can only metabolize glucose (for instance, the brain and red cells). Once local intramuscular reserves of glycogen have been depleted, the contracting muscles also depend on glucose drawn from the blood stream to sustain any periods of vigorous anaerobic activity.

Glycogen

The glycogen-storing capacity of the muscles averages about 83 mmol per kilogram, or in a subject with 28 kg of muscle, the equivalent of 2.3 mol of glucose. Levels in a localized area of muscle can be assessed by needle biopsy. Adding to the intramuscular total the 550 mmol of glycogen stored in the liver, the total reserve of complex carbohydrate is about 2.84 mol, sufficient to perform some 8.5 to 8.6 MJ of work. During the first hour or so of vigorous activity, at least 75 percent of energy needs are supplied from carbohydrate. The endurance competitor usually holds the intensity of competitive activity around the anaerobic threshold. It is thus unusual to find an energy expenditure higher than 60 kJ per minute. If 75 percent of this need were satisfied from an 8.6 MJ store, exercise would deplete the glycogen reserve in 193 minutes. Some subjects show signs of glycogen deficiency sooner than this. One obvious explanation is that in most forms of exercise not all of the 28 kg of muscle are active. While stored glycogen can be utilized within the working muscle, there is little possibility that it can be mobilized and used elsewhere in the body. A second factor is that even within a given muscle, fiber recruitment is far from uniform. One fiber may thus be depleted, while another is not.

Once glycogen stores have been exhausted, the muscle fiber must use as its fuel for the resynthesis of phosphagen, glucose that is produced in small amounts by gluconeogenesis plus free fatty acids that are transported from the adipose tissue depots. These twin resources provide a reasonable basis for continuing aerobic activity (e.g., cycling on the flat), but the negotiation of a slight rise or cycling against a headwind quickly brings to light the state of glycogen depletion.

Athletes have shown considerable interest in extending their endurance performance through an artificial boosting of their glycogen stores (the process of supercompensation). The optimum regimen for this purpose seems to adopt a high fat diet for several days; a bout of glycogen-depleting exercise is then followed by several days on a high carbohydrate diet. Normal

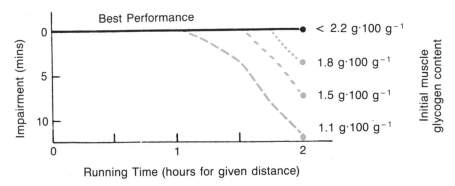

Figure 8–6   Impairment of running times over a 30 km race in relation to initial intramuscular stores of glycogen. All data are plotted relative (based on an experiment of B. Saltin).

glycogen levels are restored in the first 24 hours after the exhausting activity, and at the end of 2 to 3 days of high carbohydrate intake the store may have increased to 0.16 mol per kilogram in the muscle (more in fast- than in slow-twitch fibers) and 0.32 mol per kilogram in the liver. The disadvantage of prolonged carbohydrate feeding is that it induces enzyme changes which encourage the metabolism of carbohydrate rather than fat during the exercise bout itself.

There is a water storage of about 3 g for every gram of glycogen that is stored. Thus, on beginning a bout of severe dieting, the bound water is released, and there is a gratifying early weight loss of 1 to 2 kg. Likewise, during a marathon race, the water is released as glycogen stores diminish, and this process can make a useful contribution to the maintenance of body hydration under adverse thermal conditions.

Fluids and Minerals

Problems associated with a progressive depletion of plasma fluid and minerals are discussed further in Chapter 12. Testing is based on keeping records of body weight, supplemented where necessary by mineral analyses of plasma and urine. A progressive cold dehydration can be an important factor contributing to deterioration in the condition of a mountaineer after a prolonged period at very high altitudes. In the heat, a person may produce as much as 14 ℓ of sweat over a working day. However, if we accept that the maximum practicable rate of fluid replenishment is about 600 mℓ per hour, and that the maximum desirable dehydration is equivalent to a 4 kg decrease of body mass, then the total desirable sweat production is 8 to 9 ℓ, accumulated over the course of an 8-hour working day. With maximal sweating of 2 ℓ per hour, this limit would be surpassed in 4 hours or less.

The tissues contain substantial reserves of most minerals, so that problems of mineral depletion are unlikely to arise with a single bout of exercise in a hot environment. However, repeated heat exposures can give rise to cumulative deficiencies of several important mineral ions. Lack of sodium can cause a secondary depletion of plasma volume, and loss of calcium and magnesium can interfere with muscular contraction (e.g., the "stoker's cramps" once observed on coal-fired steamships).

Heat

Factors influencing the accumulation of heat within the body are discussed in Chapter 12. Monitoring is best based on rectal thermometer readings. Under adverse conditions (a warm day with a high radiant heat load), the core temperature can reach a dangerous level (41°C) as a result of 30 minutes of fast running. Equally high temperatures are common after participation in marathon events, even when the day does not appear particularly warm to the bystanders. If the temperature is near freezing, slower marathon runners can also develop hypothermia over the final few kilometers of their event.

Body Fat and Injury

Occasionally, subjects engage in very prolonged bouts of exercise, such as walking or running across Canada (a distance of about 8,000 km). If the time available is relatively short (e.g., because of a limited vacation), distances of 80 to 100 km may be attempted regularly for a period of 80 to 100 days. There is then little opportunity or inclination for an adequate intake of food, and performance becomes limited by the available reserves of body fat. The techniques for measuring body fat have been discussed. A person who has trained heavily in preparation for such a feat may begin the run with less than 10 percent body fat, not all of which is available for immediate metabolism. In fact, there is a need for 8 to 10 kg of surplus fat at the beginning of such an event. Once the fat reserves (perhaps 150 MJ in a thin person) are exhausted, the major remaining source of fuel is the breakdown of muscle protein. At this stage, the runner becomes very vulnerable to musculoskeletal injuries.

FURTHER READING

Alexander JF, Serfass RC, Tipton CM. Physiology of fitness and exercise. Chicago: Athletic Institute, 1972.

American College of Sports Medicine. Guidelines for graded exercise testing and exercise prescription. Philadelphia: Lea & Febiger, 1975.

Andersen KL, Shephard RJ, Denolin H, Varnauskas E, Masironi R. Fundamentals of exercise testing. Geneva: W.H.O. 1971.

Appenzeller O, Atkinson R. Health aspects of endurance training. Medicine and Sport 1978; 12:1–208.

Burke EJ. Towards an understanding of human performance (2nd Ed.) Ithaca, NY: Mouvement Publications, 1980.

Burke EJ. Exercise science and fitness. Ithaca, NY: Mouvement Publications, 1980.

Cureton TK. Physical fitness appraisal and guidance. St. Louis: CV Mosby, 1974.

Franklin BA. Exercise testing, training and arm ergometry. Sports Med 1985; 2:100–119.

Franks DB. Exercise and fitness, 1969. Chicago: Athletic Institute, 1969.

Hammond HK, Froelicher VF. Exercise testing for cardiorespiratory fitness. Sports Med 1984; 1:234–239.

Hollmann W. Zentrale themen der sportmedizin. Berlin: Springer Verlag, 1982.

Hollmann W, Hettinger T. Sportmedizin—arbeits und trainingsgrundlagen. Stuttgart: Schattauer Verlag, 1976.

Larson LA. Fitness, health and work capacity. New York: MacMillan, 1974.

Léger L, Mercier D. Gross energy cost of horizontal treadmill and track running. Sports Med 1984; 1:270–277.

Mellerowicz H, Smodlaka VN. Ergometry. Basics of medical exercise testing. Baltimore: Urban & Schwarzenburg, 1981.

Milvy P. The marathon: physiological, medical epidemiological and psychological studies. Ann NY Acad Sci 1977; 301:1–109.

Pollock ML, Wilmore JH, Fox SM. Health and fitness through physical activity. New York: John Wiley, 1978.

Sharkey BJ. Physiology of fitness. Champaign, Ill: Human Kinetics 1979.

Shephard RJ. Frontiers of fitness. Springfield, Ill: CC Thomas, 1972.

Shephard RJ. Endurance fitness (2nd Ed.) Toronto, Ont: University of Toronto Press, 1977.

Shephard RJ. Tests of maximum oxygen intake. A critical review. Sports Med 1984; 1:99–124.

Shephard RJ, Lavallée H. Physical fitness assessment. Principles, Practice and Applications. Springfield, Ill: CC Thomas, 1978.

Weiner JS, Lourie JA. Practical human biology. New York: Academic Press, 1981.

RESPONSES TO TRAINING

CHAPTER *9*

BODY FAT

Exercise and Fat Loss
Exercise and Lipid Profile

CENTRAL NERVOUS SYSTEM

Learning
Habituation

TYPES OF TRAINING

Endurance Training
Interval Training
Sprint Training
Sports Participation
Calisthenics
Circuit Training
Weight Lifting
Isometric Training
Eccentric and Isokinetic Training
Prescribing for a Sedentary Person
Prescribing for an Athlete

THE TRAINING PROCESS

OVERTRAINING

This chapter considers the physiological effects of training and its converse (bed rest). It also looks at the various techniques of training and suggests an optimum regimen for specific categories of individual.

LOSS OF PHYSICAL CONDITION

Most people experience occasional unavoidable loss of physical condition through such circumstances as intercurrent infection or injury to a leg. Study of recovery from deliberate bed rest thus yields information on the training process, and also provides guidance concerning necessary modifications of exercise prescriptions immediately following illness or injury.

Deliberate Bed Rest

H. L. Taylor observed a 17 percent loss of maximum oxygen intake when healthy subjects were given 3 weeks of deliberate bed rest. There was a complete recovery of physical condition 36 days after resumption of normal activity. Saltin carried out a similar experiment on five healthy students, finding 27 percent loss of maximum oxygen intake over 20 days of bed rest; in his study there was a parallel reduction of stroke volume, cardiac output, and maximum oxygen intake during the period of immobilization. Following the resumption of normal activity, there was a progressive restoration of normal function. He noted a 30 percent gain of maximum oxygen intake over 3 weeks, and when reconditioning was continued to 8 weeks, the final figure for the sedentary members of the group was 63 percent above that observed at the end of bed rest.

Leg Injury

After industrial injury that required immobilization of one leg in plaster, Fried and Shephard noted that the maximum oxygen intake of their subjects was 5 percent below the sedentary normal, while skinfold thicknesses averaged 4 to 5 mm greater than the anticipated figure; there was also weakness and wasting of the quadriceps muscles (Table 9–1). A 4-week program of endurance training yielded a 13 percent gain of maximum oxygen intake, a decrease of subcutaneous fat, and a 4 percent gain of knee extension strength. In those with leg injuries, specific quadriceps training gave larger (15 percent) gains of local muscular strength. However, the cross-sectional area of the thigh muscles as assessed by soft-tissue radiography increased by only 1 percent, showing that the increase of muscular strength reflected a lesser inhibition of all-out effort or a better coordination of the extensor muscles rather than a true muscle hypertrophy.

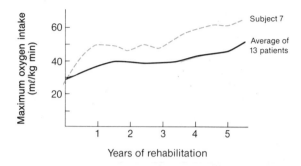

Figure 9–1 Course of gains in maximum oxygen intake with sustained and progressive rehabilitation. Results for group of 13 subjects and one specific individual who prepared themselves for marathon running following myocardial infarction (based on data of Kavanagh and Shephard).

Myocardial Infarction

Kavanagh and Shephard found that on admission to a postcoronary rehabilitation program, middle-aged men had only 70 percent of the normal aerobic power for their age. However, after participation in a program of progressive endurance training (fast walking progressing to jogging), the group reached a directly measured treadmill maximum oxygen intake that was 112 percent of the anticipated sedentary value. The aerobic condition of many patients peaked after 1 to 1½ years of moderate endurance training, but some continued to improve their maximum oxygen intake for as long as 3 to 4 years after infarction, and 50 subjects progressed to the point of running more than 300 marathon distances. In the best-trained members of this elite group, maximum oxygen intake had increased from an initial figure very typical of postcoronary patients attending rehabilitation programs (26 to 27 mℓ per kilogram per minute) to over 60 mℓ per kilogram per minute (Fig. 9–1), and one man was able to complete a marathon event in 3 hours 17 minutes.

Space Travel

A loss of physical condition owing to the absence of gravitational forces is a problem that has plagued

TABLE 9–1 Gains of Condition When Workmen's Compensation Injury Cases Given Vigorous Endurance Rehabilitation

Factors Measured	Before Training	After 4 weeks of Training
Maximum oxygen intake (mℓ/kg · min STPD)	36.5	41.1
Skinfold thickness (mm) (average of 8 folds)	17.1	12.8
Leg extension strength (N)	636	664

Based on data of Fried and Shephard

astronauts. In extended space missions (real or simulated), there is progressive loss of aerobic power with associated hemolysis, muscle wasting, obesity, decalcification of bones, and a danger that calculi ("stones") will form in the kidneys. Muscle weakness and a loss of proprioceptive coding are sufficient to cause some problems of balance on emerging from the space capsule, while a loss of venous tone leads to postural hypotension.

Submersion

Submersion for more than 6 hours (for example, a very long distance swim) causes some of the difficulties noted during space travel (including hypotension and a loss of balance).

Preventive Measures

Regular exercise offers the best overall prospect for the prevention of these various problems. If the limb is immobilized in plaster, isometric contractions of the muscles remain a possible method of maintaining lean tissue, and contractions can also be induced by faradic stimulation; the latter approach has recently been proposed to reverse muscle wasting in paraplegia. In a space capsule, an ergometer can be used to maintain aerobic power, although a simulation of weight-bearing seems necessary to prevent calcium loss from the bones.

EFFECTS OF ILLNESS

The aerobic component of physical fitness is adversely affected by various diseases that attack links in the oxygen transport chain. Advanced tuberculosis, for example, may impair gas exchange and thus limit oxygenation of arterial blood, and malaria and bilharzia can both cause a severe anemia and thus a poor oxygen transport for each liter of blood that is pumped. While anemia persists, the working capacity remains poor, but once the hemoglobin level has been restored to normal, there is a substantial increase of maximum oxygen intake. In the heavy smoker who has developed chronic obstructive pulmonary disease, a large part of the available maximum oxygen intake may be used in the respiratory muscles.

CONSTITUTION VERSUS ENVIRONMENT

Genes Versus Training

While some indication of potential training responses can be obtained by comparing well-trained athletes with sedentary individuals, much uncertainty remains as to how far the advantage of the typical athlete is attributable to a favorable genetic endowment. P.O. Åstrand believed genes to be the major factor, suggesting that the aspirant to success in international competition needed to have inherited superior ability from his or her parents.

The issue of genes-versus-training has obvious practical importance for the coach—should time be devoted to identifying potentially well-endowed subjects through a battery of simple field tests, or should the prime focus be upon the improvement of existing talent by a vigorous training regimen?

Twin and Sibling Studies

It might be thought a simple matter to determine the relative importance of constitutional factors by comparing training responses in monozygous and dizygous twins. However, in practice, estimates of "heritability" seem very unstable. One report suggests that more than 90 percent of the advantage in a variable such as maximum oxygen intake is inherited, but a second analysis carried out on an apparently similar population shows almost no constitutional component. Complications of the twin approach are that monozygous twins sometimes experience a more similar environment than dizygous twins, and that constitution may influence the willingness or the ability of a subject to train.

Empirical Estimates

Taking again the example of maximum oxygen intake, a simple empirical approach is to look at the difference in aerobic fitness between a sedentary young woman and a top female endurance athlete (35 versus 70 ml per kilogram per minute). There is a 20 percent coefficient of variation of maximum oxygen intake among the sedentary population. Thus, one woman in a hundred has a maximum oxygen intake of 49 ml per kilogram per minute, and one in a thousand a figure of 56 ml/kg • min; a full search of the national population might even bring to light a woman at the forth standard deviation above the average for her age (63 ml per kilogram per minute). This might suggest that with respect to this variable, 80 percent of the difference between the athlete and the average woman is inherited. However, a part of the 20 percent variation in the supposedly sedentary general population is due to differences of habitual activity rather than constitution. If there is a 30 percent difference (10 ml per kilogram per minute) between the least and the most active of those who are poorly endowed, then that proportion of the 35 ml per kilogram per minute difference between a sedentary woman and the superb female athlete which is due to training would rise to (7 + 10) ml per kilogram per minute, or almost 50 percent.

Certainly, a poor choice of parents is not an insuperable obstacle to competitive success. The sports history books provide details of quite a number of international competitors who apparently had a poor constitutional endowment (the "wrong" body build or the wrong physiological characteristics for their event), yet by dint of hard training went on to international success.

LONGITUDINAL TRAINING STUDIES

Design of Longitudinal Studies

Because of uncertainties about inheritance and other factors of initial selection, most modern training studies adopt a longitudinal design. In some instances, sports enthusiasts are studied as they resume training after an "end of season" vacation. Good motivation to vigorous and progressive activity is then likely, but details of the conditioning regimen may not be clearly documented.

Alternatively, the subject may be invited to the laboratory to perform standardized bouts of exercise on a standardized training device such as a treadmill or a cycle ergometer. This is time-consuming for all concerned, and there is often a high drop-out rate, particularly if the study is continued for longer than 8 to 10 weeks. The volunteers for such a program may have an above-average interest in fitness when they are first recruited, and it is important to include a check of their initial habitual activity patterns (see Chapter 2) in the experimental design. Note must also be taken of changes in lifestyle induced by the training regimen—for example, distance running might encourage a cessation of smoking. Finally, the drop-out process tends to leave a residual sample that is atypical of the population from which subjects were recruited.

Effects of Learning and Habituation

In any longitudinal training design it is important to distinguish the effects of learning and habituation from those due to training. A subject who is anxious may initially carry out laboratory exercise in a tense manner. As the activity is repeated, more economical movement patterns are learned, with a decrease in physiological responses such as oxygen consumption and heart rate at any given power output. Habituation further diminishes the heart-rate response to any given metabolic stress; in one-quarter of subjects, a lessening of anxiety decreases the heart-rate response to moderate endurance exercise by as much as 10 to 15 beats per minute.

Regulatory Versus Dimensional Change

Holmgren has distinguished regulatory from dimensional responses to training. Examples of a regulatory response include an increase in tone of the peripheral veins (leading to a greater central blood volume and thus stroke volume) and an increase of muscle strength through a more effective activation of the anterior horn cells. Such changes occur over the first few weeks of conditioning. Dimensional changes include hypertrophy of skeletal and cardiac muscle. These responses are much more difficult to elicit and may not be completed for months or even years.

PATTERN OF TRAINING

Specificity of Training

It is now well accepted that training is relatively specific to the particular form of exercise used in conditioning. The various possible types of training are detailed in section II of this chapter. A program of isometric or isotonic muscle training does little to improve the condition of the cardiovascular system, and hard cardiovascular endurance training may lead to some loss of muscle strength (for example, a loss of lean tissue from the arms in a distance runner).

The various methods of cardiorespiratory and muscular training are themselves moderately specific with respect to the region trained and the intensity of effort adopted (power versus endurance). For instance, training by forearm cranking does little to increase the maximum oxygen intake as tested by leg exercise on a cycle ergometer. However, approximately one-half of the increase in aerobic power developed by cycle ergometer training is available to improve aerobic performance on a forearm crank ergometer. In the latter situation, we may hypothesize that a fair part of the improvement in function reflects a training of the heart. However, conditioning by arm cranking apparently reflects largely a local reaction to a strengthening of the active muscles—possibly a lesser local neuromuscular drive to the cardiorespiratory centers, a lesser local accumulation of metabolites at any given work-rate, or a more ready perfusion of the working muscles because their strength has been increased.

Optimum Pattern of Aerobic Training

There is still much discussion on the optimum duration, frequency, and intensity of aerobic training sessions for both the athlete and the sedentary, middle-aged subject. With the serious competitor, training is often pushed close to the point of injury, but there is much to commend alternating light and heavy days of training. The light days allow opportunity for a replenishment of glycogen reserves and for the repair of any minor injury to the active muscles. The busy business executive is more interested in the minimum amount of exercise that will achieve a reasonable level of aerobic condition. A multiple regression analysis suggests

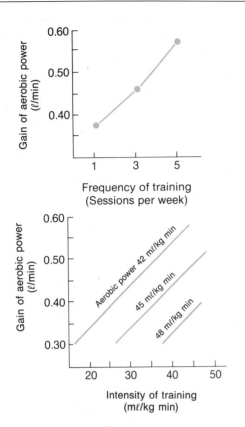

Figure 9–2 Influence of intensity of training, initial fitness, and frequency of training on gains of aerobic power. Based on data of Shephard. The results can be represented by the equation:

$$\dot{V}O_2\text{max} = 1.27 + 0.0132(I) + 0.0502(F) - 0.0359 (\dot{V}O_2\text{max})$$

where I is the intensity of training (ml/kg · min), F is the frequency of training sessions per week and $\dot{V}O_2$max is the maximum oxygen intake, measured in ml/kg · min.

that in a sedentary person, the gain of aerobic power over a given period of training ($\Delta\dot{V}O_2$ max) can be represented by an equation of the type

$$\Delta\dot{V}O_2 \text{ (max)} = a \text{ (initial fitness)} + b \text{ (intensity)} + c \text{ (frequency)} + d \text{ (duration)} + e \text{ (total work)} + f$$

where f is a constant. Of the five independent variables, the most important are the first two—the level of initial fitness and the intensity of physical activity that is undertaken (Fig. 9–2).

Karvonen is generally credited with the concept of an aerobic training threshold. He had university students undertake regular 30-minute bouts of exercise on a treadmill, finding a response when the training heart rate was 153 beats per minute, but not when it was 135 beats per minute. These observations have since been reported (or misreported) as indicating an aerobic training threshold at 60 percent of maximum heart rate (117

beats per minute), or 60 percent of the way from rest to maximum heart rate (145 beats per minute). It has further been assumed that Karvonen's observations can be extended to people of differing ages, with differing initial levels of fitness.

In contrast to Karvonen's study, Durnin found an improvement of cardiovascular condition when soldiers undertook repeated 10 to 30 km walks. He did not monitor the heart rate on these excursions, but argued that it was unlikely to have exceeded 120 beats per minute. Certainly, it seems logical that in the average city dweller (where a 24-hour heart rate recording rarely shows a heart rate as high as 120 beats per minute), the intensity of exercise demanded by fast walking will provide some aerobic training stimulus. Indeed, in some successful cardiac rehabilitation programs, the initial training heart rate after myocardial infarction is no higher than 100 to 110 beats per minute. Details of the interactions between intensity and duration of exercise have still to be worked out, but some authors find aerobic training with as little as 5 minutes of very vigorous activity per day. Nevertheless, it is generally thought that the optimum prescription for a sedentary person is 30 minutes of exercise at 60 percent of maximum oxygen intake, carried out 4 to 5 days per week.

Time Course of Aerobic Training

There have been reports that the half-time of aerobic training is as short as 10 days, with no additional response if conditioning is continued beyond 3 months. However, if the intensity of the prescription is increased periodically in order to keep the heart rate within the appropriate training range, gains of cardiovascular condition may continue for several years (Fig. 9–1). Certainly a steady, continuing improvement of physical condition is characteristic of both postcoronary patients and top-level endurance competitors.

Magnitude of Aerobic Training Response

A typical response to aerobic training is a 5 to 30 percent increase of maximum oxygen intake. If there is an associated decrease of body fat, the gain will be larger in relative units (ml per kilogram per minute) than when expressed in absolute terms (ℓ per minute).

Roskamm has further suggested that with moderate-intensity endurance training, the gain of fitness is larger in a submaximal than in a maximal test—an example of an intensity-specific pattern of response.

Particularly large changes occur in such measures of conditioning as the treadmill endurance time. If the task initially demands 95 percent of maximum oxygen intake, gains of aerobic power with training are likely to reduce the relative cost of the same speed and slope combination to 75 percent of the individual's maximum oxygen intake. There is then little accumulation of lactate in the blood during a test, and the endurance time may increase from perhaps 10 minutes to near infinity.

Impact on Oxygen Debt

After aerobic training, a larger power output can be sustained before the anaerobic threshold is reached; this reflects not only an increase of maximum oxygen intake, but also an increase of anaerobic threshold expressed as a percentage of maximum oxygen intake. The size of the accumulated oxygen debt is also augmented, especially if the training plan has included interval work. Factors contributing to a larger oxygen debt include increases of (1) motivation, (2) muscle mass, (3) blood volume, (4) myoglobin content of the muscles, (5) tissue enzyme activity, and (6) possibly alkaline reserve.

CARDIOVASCULAR RESPONSES

Heart Rate

After aerobic training, the heart rate is decreased at rest and in submaximal effort. Some authors have also suggested a small decrease of maximal heart rate (5 to 10 beats per minute). Possible explanations of the training bradycardia include (1) an alteration of the balance between sympathetic and parasympathetic discharge, (2) an increased secretion of acetylcholine for a given rate of vagal discharge, (3) a passive effect of the increase in stroke volume (a lower heart rate being necessary for a given cardiac output), and (4) possibly a reflex from stretch receptors in the hypertrophied atria (although the normal response to atrial stretching is an increase rather than a decrease of heart rate).

Stroke Volume

Aerobic training increases the stroke volume of the heart both in rest and in exercise, this change reflecting (1) an increased myocardial contractility, (2) a general increase of blood volume, and (3) an increase of venous tone with a resultant increase of central blood volume. In older subjects, training also seems to counteract the tendency for stroke volume to decrease as maximum effort is approached.

Heart Volume

Chest radiographs have shown substantial enlargement of the heart shadow in endurance athletes, some male competitors reaching estimated volumes of 1,000 to 1,100 mℓ, compared with perhaps 550 and 700 mℓ in sedentary women and men respectively. Cardiac hypertrophy seems to be a response to prolonged aerobic training rather than an effect of selection, since if the athletes concerned stop training their heart volumes regress to normal sedentary values over the next 5 to 10 years.

The elongated electrical conduction path through the hypertrophied myocardium may give rise to various unusual electrocardiographic features—particularly a mild, right bundle branch block (Fig. 9–3). The increase of stroke volume and faster cardiac emptying may cause turbulent blood flow in the aorta, with a systolic murmur that is increased by exercise; this sign can be distinguished from a pathological murmur (due to blood flow through a ventricular septal defect), since the latter usually becomes less obvious with exercise.

Increased loading of the ventricle owing to a pathological stenosis of the pulmonary or aortic valve can also induce a massive hypertrophy of the corresponding ventricle, although in this case the myocardium is responding to a stress which has been imposed 24 hours per day. Where sedentary subjects undertake more moderate endurance exercise (e.g., 1 hour per day at a heart rate of 150 to 160 beats per minute), there is sometimes no evidence of cardiac hypertrophy even after 2 to 3 years of training. Bouchard has suggested that a critical factor is the individual's genetic susceptibility to the conditioning regimen.

In experimental animals, prolonged endurance training increases the dimensions of the coronary vessels, opening up new collateral anastomoses. However, this type of response has yet to be demonstrated in humans. The long-term health benefit of cardiac hypertrophy is also debated. Some authors have suggested than when training ceases, the thickened ventricular wall has a poorer coronary vascular supply and thus an above average vulnerability to myocardial ischemia.

Hemoglobin

The hemoglobin level is increased in some types of athlete, particularly in muscle builders who are using anabolic steroids. However, in the typical endurance competitor, a normal or low-normal figure is more likely, and indeed many endurance athletes suffer from an insipient anemia, as shown by an undesirably low percentage iron saturation (less than 20 percent) of the carrier protein transferrin. In part, the endurance athlete's anemia is an artefact, due to an expansion of plasma volume. The total hemoglobin content of the body may still be normal or increased, but it is diluted by the greater volume of plasma in which the red cells are suspended.

Specific causes of a low hemoglobin reading include (1) the iron needs of tissue hypertrophy, (2) iron loss in sweat (up to 1 mg per day), (3) inhibition of iron uptake by a diet that is high in animal fat, (4) reduced synthesis of red cells, and (5) increased hemolysis, either in the spleen or in the capillaries of the active limb (for instance, in the feet when running).

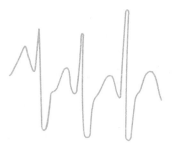

Figure 9–3 Appearance of CM-5 ECG lead in subject with partial right bundle branch block.

Arteriovenous Oxygen Difference

The arteriovenous (a-v) oxygen difference is increased from perhaps 140 mℓ per liter to as much as 160 mℓ per liter with endurance training. At one time, the widened a-v difference was attributed to an increased oxygen extraction in the working muscles, but it is now known that during maximum endurance exercise, oxygen extraction is relatively complete in the active muscles even in sedentary subjects. A more convincing explanation of a widened a-v difference is that the well-trained person directs less of the total cardiac output to regions of the body where oxygen extraction is poor (for instance, the skin and the viscera). Less skin flow is needed in the endurance-trained individual because (1) sweating occurs sooner and in greater quantities, cooling the skin and increasing heat transfer per unit of blood flow, and (2) there is less superficial fat after training, so that heat transfer through the subcutaneous tissues is less dependent on blood flow.

Cardiac Output

Aerobic training increases the maximum cardiac output. However, the gain in cardiac performance is less than the increment of maximum oxygen intake, part of which is attributable to a widening of the arteriovenous oxygen difference.

Blood Pressure

The resting blood pressure is reduced by about 1 kiloPascal (kPa) (5 to 10 mm Hg) as a consequence of endurance training. Although the change is quite small, it may have substantial therapeutic value in patients with mild hypertension. In assessing the decrease of blood pressure, it is important to assess artefacts arising from (1) habituation, and (2) an improved fit of the sphygmomanometer cuff as subcutaneous fat is reduced. Since hypertension is linked to obesity, part of the decrease in blood pressure is probably due to the fat loss induced by regular endurance exercise.

The larger stroke volume of a well-conditioned endurance performer generally causes an increase of pulse pressure. During a given exercise bout, an improvement of myocardial contractility may allow a trained person to develop a higher blood pressure than would be possible in a sedentary individual, particularly as exhaustion is approached. Thus, in the Toronto Rehabilitation Centre postcoronary program, Kavanagh and I found that the maximum systolic reading was 2 kPa higher after 3 years of progressive endurance training.

RESPIRATORY SYSTEM

Static Lung Volumes

Static lung volumes are not greatly influenced by most types of training. In the adult, there may be a small increase of vital capacity reflecting the ability of strengthened chest muscles to compress the thorax further and expel blood from the pulmonary vessels. Training in preadolescence may also increase the dimensions of the rib cage.

Dynamic Lung Volumes

Exercise that involves the chest muscles—either directly (deliberate isotonic or endurance regimens for the respiratory muscles), or incidentally (e.g., swimming or paddling) can increase the maximum voluntary ventilation (MVV) by 10 to 20 percent. Nevertheless, care must be taken to distinguish a learning of the MVV technique from a true training of the chest muscles. The latter can have substantial value in the rehabilitation of patients with chronic obstructive pulmonary disease.

Exercise Ventilation

The endurance athlete has a much larger respiratory minute volume than the sedentary subject (perhaps about 130 to 140 ℓ per minute BTPS in a top female competitor, compared with 70 ℓ per minute BTPS in a sedentary young woman). However, endurance training also decreases the respiratory rate, both in rest and in submaximum exercise. The decrease of breathing frequency is particularly marked with participation in sports that require a tight control of breathing (e.g., swimming and rowing).

The ventilatory equivalent for submaximal exercise (normally 30 to 35 ℓ respired per liter of oxygen intake) drops to 25 to 30 ℓ per liter in an endurance competitor. An increase of mechanical efficiency and strengthening of the active muscles allow a lesser accumulation of lactate in the trained person during moderate work. There is thus an increase in the anaerobic threshold, and a lesser ventilation for a given oxygen consumption.

Diffusing Capacity

Aerobic training increases the diffusing capacity of the lungs, especially during exercise. The increase of central blood volume and the greater pulmonary blood flow lead to an increase of pulmonary blood flow and coverage of an increased fraction of the pulmonary membrane by a film of venous blood. Diffusing capacity thus increases roughly in parallel with the increase of maximum oxygen intake.

MUSCULOSKELETAL SYSTEM

Bone

A regular weight-bearing exercise program reverses the normal 2 percent annual loss of calcium from bones and can actually increase their calcium content. One exception to this generalization is the young woman who is exercising to the point of inducing amenorrhea. In such a person, the altered hormone balance may favor calcium loss unless the dietary intake of calcium is deliberately increased (Chapter 4). A second possible exception is the old person who undertakes a jogging program while on a calcium poor diet; in such an individual, calcium may be transferred from the arm to the leg bones.

Specific sports may also induce a strengthening of local bone architecture; for instance, strong and well-buttressed bones can be seen in the serving arm of a top tennis player.

Ligament and Cartilage

As a result of the local training of a limb, ligaments become thicker, stronger, more flexible, and less easily torn from their insertions into bone. The hyaline cartilage is also thickened and becomes more resistant to compression. However, if the articular surface is damaged by exercise-related trauma leaving areas of exposed bone, the person thus affected becomes vulnerable to osteoarthritis. Spikes of bone grow out from the bare areas, mechanically restricting movement and causing considerable local pain.

Particular care must be taken to avoid musculoskeletal injuries when setting an exercise prescription for a middle-aged person. Some aerobic conditioning programs have been marred by injury rates as high as 50 percent over the first 6 months of training. Methods of reducing injury include (1) a thorough warm-up, (2) a gradual progression of training (so that the subject is no more than pleasantly tired on the day following an exercise session), (3) avoidance of exercise on hard surfaces such as concrete floors with vinyl covering, and (4) care if the exercise prescription is changed (e.g., a change from jogging to rope skipping on moving indoors at the onset of winter).

Muscle

It is now generally agreed that any increase of muscle dimensions reflects hypertrophy with some splitting of existing fibers. Hyperplasia (the growth of new fibers) is not possible, at least in adult subjects.

Rhythmic, endurance activity leads to only a minor degree of skeletal muscle hypertrophy in the active limbs. Isotonic or isokinetic training with overload improves the strength and endurance of the moving limb, while isometric training gives a more specific increase of isometric strength and endurance with a substantial increase of muscle bulk. The capillary supply to the trained muscle is also increased, but there is a decrease of fat and connective tissue within the muscle belly.

Biopsies show substantial increases of enzyme activity in response to various types of training. Endurance training augments the aerobic, mitochondrial enzymes involved in the Krebs cycle, while anaerobic and specific muscle-building training augments the activity of the enzymes involved in glycolysis. The time required to induce changes in enzyme activity is only 1 to 2 weeks. The fact that tissue responses to endurance training outpace any gains in aerobic power is one important argument in favor of a circulatory rather than a peripheral limitation of maximum oxygen intake. The main function of the greater aerobic enzyme activity in the endurance-trained athlete is probably to allow a preferential metabolism of fat; this would spare the limited intramuscular reserves of glycogen during prolonged exercise.

Other changes observed at needle biopsy are an increase of adenosine triphosphate, creatine phosphate, myoglobin, and glycogen stores in well-trained muscles.

BODY FAT

Exercise and Fat Loss

Contrary to the view of some nutritionists, regular endurance activity is an effective method of reducing the amount of body fat. In one group of elderly retirees, Sidney and I were able to decrease skinfold thicknesses by an average of 3 mm over a 3-month period of aerobic training (Table 9-2). The loss of adipose tissue included about three-quarters of the subcutaneous fat that had accumulated over adult life. Furthermore, the required pattern of exercise was not unrealistically heavy for middle-aged or elderly individuals—the subjects merely participated in lunchtime exercise classes for about 1 hour, 3 to 4 times per week, without dietary restriction. The site of fat loss was sex specific; women trimmed fat from the thighs and men from the abdomen.

The negative attitude of some health professionals to fat loss through regular endurance exercise reflects a misunderstanding of the process of fat loss. Dieticians and their supervising physicians often seek a reduction

TABLE 9-2   Changes of Skinfold Thickness and Estimated Percentage of Body Fat with 7 and 14 Weeks of Vigorous Training

Training Pattern	Change Over 7 Weeks		Change Over 14 Weeks	
	Average Skinfold (mm)	Predicted Body Fat (%)	Average Skinfold (mm)	Predicted Body Fat (%)
Low frequency, low intensity	-0.8	-0.8	-1.4	-1.9
Low frequency, high intensity	-1.4	-1.1	-1.9	-2.4
High frequency, low intensity	-1.5	-0.9	-2.9	-2.0
High frequency, high intensity	-2.4	-1.6	-3.1	-2.7

Based on data of Sidney and Shephard for subjects enrolled in preretirement exercise programme.

of body mass, but if this occurs, it usually reflects a loss of both fat and lean tissue (muscle protein). The end result of enhanced activity is much more satisfactory—there is then a loss of fat plus an increase of lean tissue, often with no overall change of body mass.

Exercise and Lipid Profile

Programs of endurance exercise can also improve the lipid profile. Resting serum triglycerides are decreased, and particularly if there is a decrease of body mass, there may be some drop in serum cholesterol. Some endurance athletes show a substantial increase of the valuable scavenger HDL proteins, so that HDL cholesterol is augmented. However, a substantial weekly volume of exercise (for instance, a jogging distance of 18 to 20 km per week) seems necessary to increase the HDL fraction.

The optimum regimen for reducing body fat involves a substantial daily energy expenditure—a 1-hour walk is of greater benefit than 5 minutes of more intensive exercise. This reflects not only a greater total increase of energy expenditure, but also the higher proportion of fat that is metabolized during moderate exercise. Cold exposure (probably by stimulating catecholamine release and increasing total energy usage) seems to help fat mobilization.

CENTRAL NERVOUS SYSTEM

The responses of the central nervous system to various types of training include learning and habituation. Learning involves the development of neural loops between the premotor cortex and the cerebellum, with the storage of information on appropriate gamma-loop settings for a particular activity within the cerebellum.

Learning

Reaction time is decreased with learning of a particular motor skill, and in general, mechanical efficien-cy is improved. However, in some activities such as high-speed sprinting, the process of learning involves a decrease of mechanical efficiency as a technique is developed for forcing the limb to move faster than its most economical (ballistic) speed. Cardiovascular adjustments, both to the onset of physical activity and also in response to a change of posture, occur faster after a period of endurance training.

Habituation

Habituation reflects an adjustment to the circumstances of exercise and competition, particularly a lesser emotional tachycardia. The prefrontal cortex is necessary to this response.

After isotonic or isometric muscle training, a greater performance may also be possible because there is less inhibition of maximal effort.

TYPES OF TRAINING

Endurance Training

The general principles of cardiovascular endurance training have been discussed above. Nevertheless, it remains quite difficult to set an exercise prescription that is exactly 60 percent of maximum oxygen intake for any given individual because of the wide range of potential activities, differences in the mechanical efficiency of performance, and differences in the speed of movement from one person to another.

Many aerobic exercise programs now use tables of MET equivalents (ratios to basal metabolism). The advantage of this approach is that a similar relative effort can be demanded of people who differ widely in their body mass (Table 9-3). Cooper's aerobic points scheme is a somewhat similar tactic designed for popular use, although it seems that different activities in his tables yield the same number of points for rather divergent rates of energy expenditure.

Any prescription for cardiovascular conditioning does no more than approximate the required intensity of exercise. There are thus advantages to the teaching of self-monitoring techniques; these allow a subject to fine-tune the vigor of her or his activity to a level appropriate for moderate, progressive conditioning. The intensity should be sufficient to generate a moderate sweat, leaving the individual able to engage in normal conversation. Such indications can be checked against the heart rate, determined by light carotid palpation during the first 15 seconds following activity. In post-coronary patients, the symptoms associated with myocardial ischemia and premature ventricular contractions can also be taught, and the intensity of the prescribed exercise can be kept below this threshold.

Interval Training

The proportions of aerobic and anaerobic effort developed during interval training can be regulated by an appropriate adjustment in the length of active and recovery phases (Table 9–4). With a 30-second/30-second ratio, a substantial cardiovascular stimulus is accompanied by little anaerobic activity (much of the energy demand over the brief work intervals can be met from the alactate resources, stored oxygen and phosphagen). With a 60-second/60-second ratio, lactate begins to accumulate, and this is much more obvious with a 2-minute/2-minute or 3-minute/3-minute rhythm.

While interval training can yield a substantial increment of maximum oxygen intake, the improvement of performance is relatively specific to high intensities of effort, and in more moderate activity, larger gains result from continuous endurance training. On the other hand, interval training is more effective in increasing tolerance of anaerobic activity.

Sprint Training

Repeated accelerations to maximum speed over 6 to 10 seconds are helpful in developing reaction speed, explosive force, and anaerobic power.

Sports Participation

Participation in various types of sport can be helpful in sustaining the motivation of middle-aged people, although it is often difficult to regulate the intensity of such activity. Moreover, although the intrinsic interest of a sports pursuit is usually greater than a deliberate jogging program, organizational factors (cost, facilities, and the need for a partner or a team) may actually reduce the frequency of participation relative to a simpler form of exercise such as walking or jogging.

Athletes must be careful that involvement in a second type of sport does not impede their competitive performance—an inappropriate group of muscles may be developed with an increase of overall body mass, and there may be a negative transfer of skills (e.g., enjoyment of badminton playing may lead to a loss of competitive technique in tennis).

Calisthenics

Many people anticipate that calisthenics will form part of an exercise prescription and, particularly in a group situation, rhythmic exercises provide a useful basis for warmup. Flexibility can also be improved by gentle stretching routines, but over-vigorous twisting can increase the toll of joint injuries. In general, the aerobic cost of calisthenics is rather low, but if a vigorous rhythm is set, cardiovascular training can occur. Large group gymnastic exercises appeal more to the extrovert than to the introvert.

Circuit Training

Circuit-training is a popular method of maximizing the use of various types of weight-training equipment. It is intended mainly for muscle training, although it is possible to include cardiovascular "stations" within the training circuit.

Weight Lifting

For a period, weight-lifting programs were heavily criticized by exercise physiologists. It was argued that (1) heavy shoulder muscles were developed without any strengthening of the heart that would have to carry them, (2) there was a large rise of systemic blood pressure as the weights were lifted, and this might provoke ventricular fibrillation, and (3) lifting caused a serious toll of musculoskeletal injuries.

There is some truth in the first criticism—if a mass of 50 kg is lifted through a height of 2 meters 30 times in 15 minutes, the power output is only about 33 Watts. Plainly, the prescription must include some cardiovascular endurance training to assure a well-balanced development of fitness. However, the rise of blood pressure is unlikely to be marked unless the glottis is closed (Valsalva maneuver) and the load is supported for a long time. Likewise, if the mass is increased progressively as condition improves, and twisting movements are avoided, the injury rate is not particularly high.

A typical prescription notes the number of sets (e.g., three), the number of repetitions per set (e.g., ten), and the load (e.g., 50 percent of the single lift maximum).

Increasingly it is recognized that a pure cardiovascular training plan can lead to muscle weakening. Thus, when it is essential for the subject to perform some type of heavy muscular work, the weakened muscles are forced to contract at a high percentage of their maximal force. This restricts perfusion, increasing blood pressure and cardiac work-rate to the point that ventricular fibrillation may be provoked. Ultimately, the pure cardiovascular trainee may thus be at as great a risk as the pure weight lifter. Plainly, the best answer is moderation with both types of training.

TABLE 9–3 Energy Cost of Selected Activities, Expressed as an Oxygen Consumption (ml/kg • min) and as a Ratio of Actual to Basal Metabolic Rate (METs)*

Oxygen Consumption (ml/kg • min, STPD)	METs	Activities	
5	1.4	Desk work Driving car Standing	Walking (1.6 km/hour) Motorcycling Flying
9	2.6	Washing car Woodworking Fishing Walking (3.2 km/hour)	Shooting Power-boating Riding Lawn mowing
10	2.9	Housework Janitorial work Light welding Power-saw operation Driving heavy truck Walking (4.8 km/hour)	Cycling (8 km/hour) Billiards Bowling Horseshoe pitching Horseback riding (walk) Canoeing (4 km/hour)
12	3.4	Stocking shelves Assembly line (lifting) Wheelbarrow (90 kg)	Archery Ice-boating Sailing (handling boat)
14	4.0	Painting Masonry Paper hanging Garage mechanic Carrying trays, dishes Farm work Lawn mowing (power mower)	Walking (5.6 km/hour) Cycling (10 km/hour) Golf (no cart) Baseball Volleyball Softball Waltzing Canoeing (5 km/hour)
18	5.1	Carpentry Handyman work Carrying (15–25 kg) Walking (6.4 km/hour)	Cycling (13 km/hour) Gardening Lawn work Level cross-country skiing

TABLE 9-3 Continued

Oxygen Consumption (ml/kg • min, STPD)	METs	Activities	
21	6.0	Operating pneumatic tools Handsaw or axe Carrying (25–30 kg) Shovelling light earth Hand lawn mowing Cycling (15 km/hour)	Cross-country hiking Hunting Water skiing Snowshoeing (4 km/hour) Fishing (wading)
23	6.6	Skating (14 km/hour) Square dancing	
25	7.1	Carrying (30–35 kg) Run or walk (8 km/hour) 5 BX exercises (level 1A) Cross-country skiing (6.5 km/hour)	Rhumba Horseback (trotting) Canoeing (6.5 km/hour) Badminton Tobogganing Scuba diving
28	8.0	Carrying (35–45 kg) Pushing Cycling (19 km/hour)	Breast-stroke swimming (40 m/min) Tennis Touch football
32	9.1	Shovelling (moderate load) Cycling (21 km/hour) Running (9.6 km/hour)	Skiing Horseback (gallop) 5 BX exercises (level 2A)
35	10.0	Running (11.2 km/hour) Swimming crawl (50 m/min) Cross-country skiing (8 km/hour) Snowshoeing (5.5 km/hour)	Squash Fencing Gymnastics Mountain climbing
42	12.0	Shovelling (heavy load) Hockey Soccer Basketball (competition)	Wrestling Handball 5 BX exercises (level 3A–4A)
45	12.9	Running (12.8 km/hour)	
49	14.0	5 BX exercises (level 5A–6A)	
53	15.1	Very heavy shovelling Running (14.4 km/hour)	

* Note: The cost of many activities depends on the speed with which they are performed. (Based in part on data collected by the Committee on Public Health of the Ontario Medical Association)

TABLE 9–4   A Comparison of Responses to One Hour of Intermittent or Continuous Exercise

Type of Exercise	Length of Work Bout (min)	Length of Rest Phase (min)	O_2 Intake (ℓ/min STPD)	Resp. Minute Volume (ℓ/min BTPS)	Heart Rate (beats/min)	Blood Lactate (mmol/ℓ)
Intermittent						
(Power output	½	½	2.9	63	150	2.2
360W in	1	1	2.9	65	167	5.0
active phase)	2	2	4.4	95	178	10.4
	3	3	4.6	107	188	13.3
Continuous						
180W	60	--	2.4	49	134	1.3
360W	9	--	4.6	124	190	16.7

Based on data of I. Åstrand

Isometric Training

Hettinger and Muller have claimed that very brief isometric contractions (1 to 2 sec duration at maximum force) are sufficient to induce substantial gains of muscle strength. Later papers have described training following 4 to 6 sec contractions at two-thirds of maximum force. However, the response has been specific to a particular joint angle, and often there has been no immediate increase of muscle bulk. Critics have thus suggested that part of the apparent gain in strength results from using the same equipment to both test and train the subjects. Other factors are probably a decrease of central inhibition and an increase of anaerobic power.

Eccentric and Isokinetic Training

During eccentric training, the subject usually exercises against gravity, lowering weights or running downhill. It seems at least as effective as other analogous forms of muscle and endurance training, but in some subjects can provoke severe enzyme release and muscle soreness.

Isokinetic training devices such as the Cybex dynamometer allow exercise of the muscles about a specific joint at a predetermined speed of 30 to 360 degrees per second. Although sometimes used for the rehabilitation of top athletes, the cost of the equipment precludes its widespread use.

Prescribing for a Sedentary Person

The average sedentary person is seeking to reduce body fat and improve cardiac condition. The safest approach is a gradual but progressive increase over current activity, such that there is no more than pleasant tiredness the next day. If there are no cardiac risk factors or other symptoms, a specific medical clearance is not essential to the introduction of such a regimen. The intensity should be increased progressively until sessions are reaching a little below the anaerobic threshold. In practical terms, the exerciser shows some breathlessness, but this is not enough to prevent talking while she or he is exercising.

The main long-term problem is loss of motivation over 3 to 6 months of renewed activity. The feedback of improving scores on the Canadian Home Fitness Test may help to sustain the subject's interest.

As condition improves, cardiovascular training may be supplemented by exercises to restore flexibility (gentle stretching) and muscle strength (rhythmic isotonic exercise). Safety is enhanced if exercise is taken in pairs rather than alone. In older individuals, due account must also be taken of poorer balance, slower reflexes, more brittle bones, and a heavier body mass.

Prescribing for an Athlete

Given the specificity of training, the optimum prescription for the sports enthusiast might seem the endless repetition of the athlete's competitive event. However, such a training plan quickly leads to a loss of motivation in all except the most determined individuals. In the case of runners, the distribution of training time between speed work, the development of anaerobic capacity, and aerobic training can be related to the competitive distance (Fig. 9–4). A suitable yearly regimen might allow a 1-month vacation following a major competition. During the vacation period, the emphasis should be upon competitive endurance sports, guarding against any negative transfer of skills. The next 3 months are allocated to the development of aerobic power and strength, and then follow 4 months of more specific preparation (e.g., speed work). Over the final 4 months there will be a series of major competitions, and training schedules are tapered to ensure a peaking of physiological condition for these specific dates.

THE TRAINING PROCESS

The nature of the training process is still unclear. As noted in Chapter 12, there is some interaction between heat exposure and cardiovascular training, suggesting an element of hypothalamic control. Oxygen

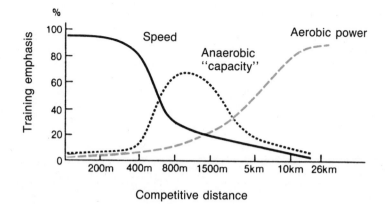

Figure 9–4 Relationship between competitive distance and training emphasis to be recommended to a runner.

lack does not seem to be a factor, since the response to aerobic training is no greater when conditioning is undertaken at altitude. Moreover, the absolute response to both cardiovascular and muscular training is reduced in old age (where the tissue oxygen supply is generally poor). Even the role of the various anabolic hormones in the hypertrophy of cardiac and skeletal muscle is doubtful. While a deficiency of thyroid and pituitary hormones can affect overall growth, animals still show a training-induced hypertrophy after a pituitary hypophysectomy—if growth hormone is implicated in the conditioning process, it serves mainly as a linear amplifier of hypertrophy induced by other means. One essential feature both in cardiac and skeletal muscle seems to be an overload of the active fibers. In some way that is still poorly understood, the local increase of tension apparently encourages an increased synthesis of protein.

The learning processes that are inherent in the regulatory phase of training probably involve an accumulation of specific chemicals at synapses within the brain. There may also be a growth of new anatomical connections between the cerebellar neurons.

The characteristics of the muscle fibers are influenced by their pattern of innervation. Some authors have suggested that a "trophic" chemical passes along the axis of the motor nerve, but it is more likely that the cue to an appropriate development of a given muscle fiber is the pattern of electrical impulses passing down the corresponding motor nerve.

The output of androgens is probably adequate for the training response of a young person, but some authors believe that a hormonal supplement may help the course of muscle hypertrophy in some older individuals, particularly after immobilization by injury.

OVERTRAINING

Following a bout of heavy exercise such as a marathon run, there is often muscle soreness and a leakage

into the plasma of enzymes such as creatine kinase (CK). This process reaches its peak 1 to 3 days after the event. Histological examination shows an alteration in the appearance of the overworked muscle fibers. Although some authors have dismissed this as an "artefact of fixation," there must be some underlying reason why there is a different fixation response following overexertion.

The leakage of cellular contents suggests that there has been an impairment of membrane function, but it is uncertain whether this reflects local hypoxia, a deficiency of glycogen, or both. In some fibers, the cellular damage may be sufficient to be considered a subclinical injury.

It has been proposed that the serum CK of athletes should be plotted on a regular basis to ensure a peaking of condition at the time of competition. However, repeated biochemical analyses are hardly possible for every competitor. It is thus to be hoped that information obtained on limited samples of athletes will enable generalizable recommendations to be made for the peaking of training. Other useful advice is (1) to moderate training if severe soreness is developing, and (2) to alternate heavy- and light-training days to allow repair of subclinical injuries.

FURTHER READING

Appenzeller O, Atkinson JR. Health aspects of endurance training. Basel: Karger, 1978.

Arnheim DD. Modern principles of athletic training. St. Louis: Times Mirror/Mosby, 1985.

Atha J. Strengthening muscle. Exerc Sport Sci Rev 1981; 9:1–74.

Barnard RJ. Long term effects of exercise on cardiac function. Exerc Sport Sci Rev 1975; 3:113–134.

Booth FW, Gould EW. Effects of training and disuse on connective tissue. Exerc Sport Sci Rev 1975; 3:84–112.

Bouchard C, Malina RM. Genetics for the sport scientist: selected methodological considerations. Exerc Sport Sci Rev 1983; 11:275–305.

Bouchard C, Malin RM. Genetics of physiological fitness and motor performance. Exerc Sport Sci Rev 1983; 11:306–339.

Clarke DH. Adaptations in strength and muscular endurance resulting from exercise. Exerc Sport Sci Rev 1973; 1:74–102.

Cohen MV. Coronary and collateral blood flows during exercise and myocardial vascular adaptations to training. Exerc Sport Sci Rev 1983; 11:55–98.

Daniels JM, Scardina N. Interval training and performance. Sports Med 1984; 1:327–334.

Dowell R. Cardiac adaptations to exercise. Exerc Sport Sci Rev 1983; 11:99–117.

Fox EL, Matthews DK. Interval training. Philadelphia: WB Saunders, 1974.

Gollnick PD, Hermansen L. Biochemical adaptations to exercise: anaerobic metabolism. Exerc Sport Sci Rev 1973; 1:1–45.

Gonyea WJ. Muscle fiber splitting in trained and untrained animals. Exerc Sport Sci Rev 1980; 8:19–40.

Greenleaf JE, Kozlowski S. Physiological consequences of reduced physical activity during bed rest. Excer Sport Sci Rev 1982; 10:84–119.

Heck H, Hollman W, Liesen H, Rost R. Sport: Leistung und Gesundheit. Koln: Deutscher Arzte-Verlag, 1983.

Hollman W, Hettinger TH. Sportmedizin-arbeits-und trainingsgrundlagen. Stuttgart: FK Schattauer Verlag, 1976.

Holloszy JO. Biochemical adaptations to exercise: anaerobic metabolism. Exerc Sport Sci Rev 1973; 1:46–73.

Howell ML, Morford WR. Fitness training methods. Toronto: CAHPER, 1965.

Matoba H, Gollnick P. Response of skeletal muscle to training. Sports Med 1984; 1:240–251.

Morgan RE, Adamson GT. Circuit training. London: G. Bell, 1961.

Newell KM. Knowledge of results and motor learning. Exerc Sport Sci Rev 1977; 4:195–228.

Oscai LB. The role of exercise in weight control. Exerc Sport Sci Rev 1973; 1:103–125.

Pollock ML. The quantification of endurance training programs. Exerc Sport Sci Rev 1973; 1:155–188.

Saltin B, Blomqvist G, Mitchell JH, Johnson RL, Wildenthal K, Chapman CB. Response to exercise after bed rest and after training: a longitudinal study of adaptive changes in oxygen transport and body composition. Circulation 1968; 38 VII:1–78.

Schmidt RA. Control processes in motor skills. Exerc Sport Sci Rev 1977; 4:229–262.

Shephard RJ. Endurance fitness (2nd ed). Toronto: University of Toronto Press, 1977.

Shephard RJ. The fit athlete. Oxford: Oxford University Press, 1978.

Taylor AW. Training: scientific basis and application. Springfield, Ill: CC Thomas, 1972.

Taylor AW. The scientific aspects of sports training. Springfield, Ill: CC Thomas, 1975.

Tipton CM. Exercise, training, and hypertension. Exerc Sport Sci Rev 1984; 12:245–306.

Vrbova G. Influence of activity on some characteristic properties of slow and fast mammalian muscles. Exerc Sport Sci Rev 1979; 7:181–213.

EFFECTS OF AGE AND GENDER

CHAPTER *10*

SEX- AND GENDER-RELATED DIFFERENCES IN WORKING CAPACITY

GROWTH AND PHYSICAL ACTIVITY

Secular Growth Trends

Realization of the individual's growth potential depends on an optimization of environment. In the past, there have been substantial differences of size between children from urban and rural areas and between the offspring of professional families and those coming from working class homes (Fig. 10–1). With the general improvement of socioeconomic conditions in developed nations during the present century, a large part of these differences has now disappeared in Western Europe and North America (Table 10–1), although there remain substantial gradients of stature within economically less-well-established nations. Perhaps, for this reason, the general trend to an increase of adult size (about 1 cm per 10 years) has now slowed or stopped in many developed countries.

Historically, many interpopulation differences of body size have been attributed to a quirk of inheritance. However, with the better and more varied nutrition that has accompanied adoption of a "western" lifestyle, a number of traditionally small "primitive" groups such as the African pygmies and the Arctic Inuit have shown a rapid increase of adult size, so that their adult height now approaches that found among people of the technically advanced nations. Moreover, any residual differences of size probably reflect as much economic as genetic factors.

Plainly, it is necessary to allow for secular trends of body size when comparing performance data from one generation to another (Table 10–2).

Basis of Data Standardization

Allowance for discrepancies of size is particularly important when comparing physical performance of children of differing stature. Around puberty, two children of the same calendar age may differ substantially in both maturity and body dimensions. The basis of standardization is thus quite critical—for instance, if maximum oxygen intake is expressed relative to the third power of stature (H^3) or per unit of body mass, boys show little change of score throughout the period

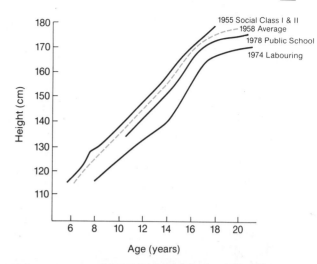

Figure 10–1 Influence of social class upon growth. Note that in the 1870s, children of the laboring classes in Britain were some 10 cm shorter than those attending "public" school, and much of this difference was conserved as an adult. By the 1950s, the difference between the two highest social classes and the British average had been reduced to 2 to 3 cm, with little discrepancy in the final adult height (based on observations collected by Tanner).

of childhood. However, if the appropriate basis for the standardization of aerobic power is to divide scores by H^2, as some have argued, then maximum oxygen intake would appear to increase steadily as the child becomes older (Fig. 10–2).

Von Dobeln and others have argued that linear measurements (including stride length and leverage) should be expressed relative to stature, that measurements such as muscle force depend on cross-section and should thus be proportional to H^2, and that volumes such as vital capacity should be proportional to H^3. Particular difficulty arises when dealing with measurements that include the dimension of time (e.g., the rate of working, or maximum oxygen intake). Von Dobeln argued that height could be substituted for distance; thus the product of force and distance was proportional to $H^2 \times H$, while power output, as work/time, was proportional to H^3/H or H^2. In practice, the growth of

TABLE 10–1 Secular Trend to an Increase of Height (cm) in the Average Belgian School Child*

Age (years)	Girls					Boys				
	1840	1924	1929/30	1960	1971	1840	1924	1929/30	1960	1967/68
6	103.1	109.2	109.5	113.5	116.7	104.7	109.7	110.3	114.0	116.3
9	119.5	124.5	126.1	129.0	131.7	121.9	124.8	126.3	130.0	132.0
11	129.9	134.8	135.3	139.5	142.7	133.0	134.1	134.8	140.0	141.4
13	140.3	145.8	147.2	151.5	150.6	143.9	143.0	143.8	149.5	149.1

* Note: The increase in size of the average child has now largely eliminated differences between rich and poor and between urban and rural students. Based on data of Hebbelinck & Vajda.

TABLE 10–2 Development of World Athletic Records From 1900 to 1975, With an Analysis of the Theoretical Effects of Body Size on Performance

Event	Improvement in World Records: 1900–1975 (%)	Theoretical Effect of Stature	Optimum Size
Running			
100-yard run	11	Speed = independent Acceleration = 1/H	Small
1-mile run	9	Air resistance = $1/H^2$	
1-hour run	12	Lifting work = $1/H^3$ Aerobic power = H^2	Small
Jumping			
Long jump	19	Body mass = H^3 Leverage = H Muscle force = H^2	Independent or tall
High jump	17	As long jump, also center of gravity = H	Tall
Throwing			
Shot-put	49	Leverage = H	
Discus throw	83	Ejection = H	Tall
Hammer throw	48	Muscle force = H^2	
Javelin throw	91		

physiological function does not seem to conform very closely with these theoretical predictions (Table 10–3); for example, as children grow, both their strength and their maximum oxygen intake increase as approximately $H^{2.7}$ to $H^{3.3}$.

Normal Growth

The general process of growth develops rapidly from 0 to 2 years, continues moderately from 2 to 10 years, and shows a final pubertal spurt during the early teens (1 to 2 years earlier in girls than in boys). In order to study growth in detail, it is necessary to make repeated measurements of stature over each year of life,

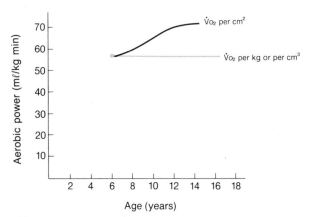

Figure 10–2 The influence of the method of data standardization upon aerobic power is shown. If data for a boy are expressed per unit of body mass or per cm^3 of stature, the score changes very little throughout childhood. However, if data are expressed per cm^2 of height, the maximum oxygen intake increases steadily as the child becomes older. In girls, accumulation of body fat depresses aerobic power per kg of body mass from the time of puberty.

plotting graphs that show both the velocity and acceleration of the growth process (cm/year and cm/$year^2$ respectively). When comparing data from one child to another, it is now common practice to align physiological data relative to the peak velocity of growth (Fig. 10–3); it can then be assumed that two individuals are being compared at the same stage of maturation, and often seemingly large interindividual differences of performance disappear if this adjustment is carried out.

The various regions of the body each have a characteristic growth curve. In the head, growth is 90 percent completed over the first year of life, and is 100 percent completed at 10 years of age. The major openings in the skull of an infant (the anterior and posterior fontanelles) close at about 18 months, and the various suture lines of the cranium unite by 10 years of age. Thereafter, growth is only possible by an eating away of bone from the inside of the skull, with the deposition of fresh bone on the exterior. The thymus, which has an important role in the development of immune function, reaches twice its adult size at puberty, and thereafter shows a gradual regression. The reproductive tissues lie largely dormant until puberty and then

TABLE 10–3 Observed Height Exponents for the Growth of Various Measures of Physical Performance

Variable	Girls	Boys
Maximum oxygen intake (ℓ/min, STPD)	2.66	3.21
Handgrip force (N)	3.16	3.29
Leg extension force (N)	2.96	2.80
Vital capacity (ℓ BTPS)	2.68	2.71
45.4 m (50 yard) run (sec)	−0.87	−1.04
274.3 m (300 yard) run (sec)	−0.84	−0.95

Data of Shephard and Lavallée for children of Trois Rivières, followed from 6 through 12 years of age.

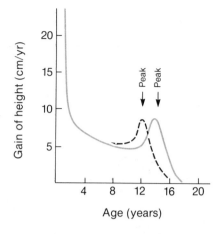

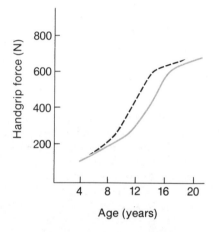

Figure 10–3   The need to align physiological data in terms of peak height velocity is illustrated. In the upper panel, one boy has a peak rate of growth at 14 years, and in a second boy it is at 12 years. The latter shows a larger handgrip force throughout adolescence (lower panel). However, if the two graphs had been realigned to give a common peak height velocity, there would be little difference of grip force between the two subjects.

show a period of rapid growth. Within the limbs, the extremities mature more rapidly than the proximal parts; thus in the growing child the foot is nearer to adult size than is the thigh, and the hand is nearer to its adult dimension than is the upper arm.

Assessment of Maturation

In a longitudinal study, the simplest method of controlling for interindividual differences of maturation is to displace the calendar age of individual students until they all share a common peak height velocity (Fig. 10–3). If local regulations of exposure to x-irradiation permit, it is possible to make a fairly accurate assessment of maturity from the number of centers of ossification seen in the small bones of the wrist and fingers (Table 10–4). A skilled reader can assess maturation to within 3 to 4 months around the period of puberty.

Alternatively, an x-ray film of the jaw allows an assessment of developmental age based upon dental maturation; this also has a precision of 3 to 4 months. If roentgenograms are not available, a simpler assessment can be based on an inspection of the mouth for tooth eruption (Table 10–5). Around puberty, a further source of information is provided by the development of the secondary sex characteristics (Table 10–6).

Control of Growth

The initial differentiation of the sexes depends upon chromosome structure—a double x chromosome leads to typical female development, and an xy chromosome to normal male development. Occasionally, variants with more than one y chromosome are seen; these are thought to have an excess of normal male aggressiveness, and these individuals may gravitate to the more violent contact sports. Sex determinations at athletic competitions are based upon chromosome characteristics, as observed in smears of the buccal mucosa. A fetus with xy chromosomal characteristics shows an enhanced androgen production from the twelfth week of intrauterine life. A normal level of thyroid hormone also seems important to growth (particularly brain growth) during the intrauterine period.

After birth, the pituitary growth hormone assumes an important role, facilitating the incorporation of amino acids into protein; if there is a deficiency of pituitary hormones, sexual maturation is delayed, and slow growth continues to approximately 30 years of age. Normal levels of thyroid hormone also remain important for growth after birth, and in hypothyroid dwarfs, skeletal age lags far behind calendar age.

At puberty boys show a sudden surge of androgen production, development of their secondary sex characteristics being accompanied by a rapid increase of muscle force and an increase of hemoglobin concentrations

TABLE 10–4   As Assessment of Skeletal Age, Based on Maturation of the Wrists and the Long Bones

Skeletal Age (years)	Ossification of Carpals	Other Bones Showing Centers of Ossification
1	Os magnum (capitate)	Head of femur
2	Unciform (hamate)	Lower epiphysis of radius, tibia, and fibula
3	Cuneiform (triquetral)	Patella, head of humerus
4	—	Lower epiphysis of ulna, upper epiphysis of fibula and greater trochanter
5	Trapezoid, Semilunar	Upper epiphysis of radius
6	Scaphoid	Centers in head of humerus coalesce
10	—	Upper epiphysis of ulna Tuberosity of os calcis
12	Pisiform	—

TABLE 10–5 The Use of Tooth Eruption in the Assessment of Developmental Age

Age	Teeth Erupted
Deciduous ("milk") teeth	
6–9 months	Lower central incisors
8–10	Upper incisors
15–21	Lower lateral incisors and first molars
16–20	Canines
20–24	Second molars
Permanent teeth	
6 years	First molars
7	Two central incisors
8	Two lateral incisors
9	First premolars
10	Second premolars
11–12	Canines
12–13	Second molars
17–27	Third molars

to the adult level. The adolescent growth spurt seems to be held in check by the hypothalamus and is triggered by an increased output of gonadotropins.

Environmental Factors

The important contribution of socioeconomic factors to the growth process has already been noted. In 1870, the son of a British laborer was, on average, 10 cm shorter than an office worker's boy of similar age, and in 1950 there was still a 3-cm difference related to social class. Among the environmental constraints responsible for this large discrepancy, investigators commented upon nutrition (the total quantity of food that was available, the amount of high-quality protein and the proportion of refined carbohydrates), psychological stresses, the level of habitual activity, and the general organization of the home (reflected in such items as the incidence of chronic infections, the regularity of meals, and the adequacy of sleeping arrangements). Lack of food in Germany during the Second World War caused a 3-cm diminution of stature relative to immediate prewar statistics. However, this was a delay rather than a permanent limitation of development, and the children concerned showed rapid catch-up growth as adequate amounts of food once again became available. Widdowson showed the importance of psychological factors to growth in a crossover experiment at an orphanage. By chance, a rather forbidding matron exchanged the supervision of floors in the orphanage with a second more motherly individual; both children showed a slow rate of growth while exposed to the adverse psychological environment, with more rapid development while supervised by the other individual.

Secular Trend

For several decades, most western nations have experienced a secular trend to an increase of stature, amounting to about 1 cm per decade. In Japan, the recent rate has been as large as 3 to 4 cm per decade, and in some of the circumpolar populations, figures of 1 to 2 cm per decade have been reported. The age of

TABLE 10–6 Assessment of Maturation from Development of the Secondary Sex Characteristics

Stage of Maturation	Pubic Hair	Axillary Hair	Breast Development (Female)	Genital Development (Male)
1	No greater than on abdomen	None	Elevation of papilla only	Child-size testes, scrotum, and penis
2	Sparse growth of long, slightly pigmented downy hair, only slightly curled, mainly at base of penis or along labia	Slight mound	Elevation of breast and papilla as small Enlargement of areola diameter	Enlargement of scrotum and testes
3	Darker, coarser, more curly hair, spreading sparsely over junction of pubes—visible in black and white photo	Adult quantity	Further enlargement and elevation of breast and areola	Enlargement of penis; further growth of testes and scrotum
4	Adult-type hair, but area smaller than in adult—no spread to medial aspect of thighs		Areola and papilla forming secondary mound above level of breast	Increased size of penis, growth in breadth of glans, further growth of testes and scrotum, darkening of scrotal skin
5	Adult in quantity of type		Projection of papilla, but recession of areola to breast contour	Adult size and shape genitalia

Based on schema of Tanner.

menarche has also advanced by about 0.35 years per decade during the present century.

In addition to improvements of nutrition, the conquest of disease, and greater genetic hybridization may be factors that have contributed to these secular trends. In some countries such as the United States and Germany, the process now seems to have halted, and it is arguable that growth has reached its maximum potential; in others, including Holland and Canada, adult size is still increasing.

The increase of body size is one factor that has led to a progressive development of athletic records over the present century (see Fig. 10–2). Other considerations are a greater searching of national populations for appropriate competitors, better methods of training and preparation, the development of equipment and facilities, and in some sports the abuse of steroids and/or blood doping.

Exercise and Growth

Most authors have found that a deliberate increase of physical activity has only a very limited impact upon growth. In a longitudinal study of primary students, Lavallée and associates found than an additional required hour of physical activity per day did not alter the dimensions of primary school students over the age range 6 to 12 years. Roentgenograms of the jaw suggested that maturation of the teeth had been accelerated by 1.5 months relative to control students, but in the wrist (which was more directly affected by some of the gymnastic exercises that were undertaken) there was a 3.6 month delay of maturation.

Hyperplasia and Hypertrophy

The muscle fiber number seems set soon after birth, and thereafter no hyperplasia is possible. Likewise, the fat cell number is established in the first year of life. However, the dimensions of a muscle can be increased by (1) hypertrophy of fibers, (2) splitting of fibers, and (3) lengthening of fibers by addition of further sarcomeres.

Some authors have argued that the high levels of growth hormone and androgens seen during adolescence favor an exceptional training response at this stage in life. However, any hormonal advantage of the adolescent is usually offset by a higher initial level of fitness than would be anticipated in a sedentary adult (and therefore a lesser "trainability"); thus training responses are often quite small. In the controlled trial undertaken by Lavallée and his associates, a required school program of 1 hour of endurance-type activity per day enhanced strength, maximum oxygen intake, and physical performance by 10 to 20 percent relative to sedentary controls, apparently with some associated improvement of academic performance. However, there was little change of percentage body fat in those of the sample

who were initially obese; presumably any fat-consuming effect of the additional physical activity was offset by an increased intake of food on returning to their homes.

Menarcheal Abnormalities

Some female students who engage in very intensive training show a delay of menarche. This cannot be attributed simply to the selection of late maturers for particular types of competition.

Frisch suggested that menstruation was inhibited if the combined energy demands of exercise and growth brought the body fat below a critical value of some 12 percent (Table 10–7). While her data show a gradient of body water and thus estimated body fat with menstrual regularity, all figures appear to correspond with more than 12 percent fat. Others find no consistent relationship between body fat and menstrual irregularities and attribute any disturbance of the menstrual cycle to exercise-induced hormonal changes (Chapter 4).

Physical Activity and Bone Injury

One important reason for caution when recommending exercise to a growing child is that the epiphyses of the long bones are still unclosed. There is thus a danger that the carriage of excessive loads (more than 15 kg in girls, 20 kg in boys) will deform both the long bones and the pelvis.

A greenstick fracture of a soft bone in an arm or a leg (if poorly reduced) can lead to a permanent deformity of the limb. On occasion, the fracture line may pass through the epiphyseal region, and in about 10 percent of such cases, the normal maturation of the bone disturbed.

A further source of difficulty in young children is that the repeated application of strong forces to a developing epiphysis can lead to a traumatic epiphysitis

TABLE 10–7 The Relationship Between Body Water (as a Percent of Total Body Mass) and Menstruation in the Young Athlete*

Body Water/ Total Mass (%)	Estimated Body Fat (%)	Menstrual Pattern
59.5	18.5	Primary amenorrhea (over 16 years)
58.9	19.3	Primary amenorrhea (under 16 years)
58.3	20.1	Secondary amenorrhea
57.7	21.0	Irregular menstruation
56.6	22.5	Regular menstruation

* Based on data of Frisch. Note that lean tissue contains about 73% water; a high ratio of water to total mass thus implies a low percentage of body fat.

(for example, baseball pitcher's elbow is caused by an excessive traction on the medial epicondyle of the humerus, and a corresponding lesion of the tibial tubercle is seen in children who train too hard for jumping events).

Physical Activity and Psychological Stress

It has finally been argued that the exposure of young children to major league competition gives rise to excessive psychological pressures, with adverse effects on long-term mental health. In some major competitions it has been noted that children became too excited to sleep or to eat. However, such excitement is generally short-lived, and classroom studies have not indicated any adverse effects upon long-term psychological development—indeed, the improvement of self-image resulting from competitive success has sometimes given the student an advantage over her or his peers.

PHYSIOLOGICAL DEVELOPMENT OF THE CHILD

Movement Patterns

A typical timetable can be drawn up for the appearance of reflex, rhythmic, voluntary conditional, and symbolic movements (Table 10–8). The appearance of the various movements is delayed if a child is mentally retarded, but it is also important to stress that a substantial range of maturation rates are compatible with normal mental health.

TABLE 10–8   Landmarks in Psychomotor Development

Landmark	Months
Reflex and rhythmic movements decrease	0–4
Head raising, progressing to sitting	4–8
Leg movements and walking	8–14
Conditional and symbolic movements (e.g., speech)	14–24
Walking, one foot on board*	27.6
Standing, both feet on board*	31.0
Attempting to step on board*	32.8
Alternating feet, part way along board*	38.0
Alternating feet, full length of board*	56.0
Length covered in 6–9 sec	59.5
Length covered in 3–5 sec	66.0
Length covered in less than 3 sec	80.0

* Board 2.5 m long, 6 cm wide and 10 cm high
Based in part on observations of Bayley (1935)

Performance Tests

Over the school years, a variety of performance-type tests can be used to evaluate the development of motor skills. In the 1950s, many American children were tested using the Brace test, which included 20 stunts that evaluated agility, motor control, balance, and flexibility.

The girls of this era showed little improvement of performance beyond the age of 12 years, and after the onset of puberty were better than the boys only on tests of body position and static balance. The scores for the boys improved on most tests from 6 through 16 years of age, although there was a tendency for them to become more clumsy between 12 and 16 years of age. The item causing test failure in the largest number of students was a lack of flexibility, leading to an inability to touch the toes with the knees extended.

More recent performance test batteries developed by the American Alliance for Health, Physical Education, Recreation and Dance and its Canadian homologue have shown girls with a slightly inferior performance to boys prior to puberty. In the original surveys (conducted 20 to 30 years ago), the performance of the girls plateaued at 12 to 13 years, but this was thought to be partly a reflection of cultural values. With the greater habitual physical activity of the current generation of adolescent girls, this picture has shown some improvement. In the boys, a large increase of muscular strength and endurance items is seen at puberty, and the scores for most performance items continue to increase until the age of about 17 years.

Aerobic Power

Until recently, the aerobic power has averaged about 37 to 41 mℓ per kilogram per minute in girls, and 48 to 50 mℓ per kilogram per minute in boys, although there have been occasional reports of higher figures in active populations such as the Canadian Inuit. During the last few years, the greater popular interest in physical activity has apparently pushed figures up to about 46 mℓ per kilogram per minute in girls, and 53 mℓ per kilogram per minute in boys.

If the aerobic power is expressed relative to body mass, it tends to remain fairly constant throughout childhood, although the girls inevitably show some decrease of maximum oxygen intake with the accumulation of body fat at puberty, and this tendency is often reinforced by a culturally determined decrease of habitual physical activity in the later teen years. Most reports describe a maximum heart rate of only 195 to 200 beats per minute in the preadolescent child, but this may be partly a question of difficulty in motivating the youngster to perform exhausting work. For the same reason, it is often difficult to demonstrate a satisfactory oxygen consumption plateau when a direct measurement of maximum oxygen intake is made in the young child. Nevertheless, P. O. Åstrand was able to record heart rates as high as 210 to 215 beats per minute in some of the children that he tested.

The blood lactate at exhaustion is typically about 9 mmol per liter (80 mmol per deciliter) compared with 11 to 13 mmol per liter in a young adult. Some authors have suggested that the anaerobic capacity of the preadolescent child is limited by lesser reserves of glycogen and a lesser activity of key glycolytic enzymes. However, the ratio of muscle mass to blood volume is also smaller in the child than in an adult, and due account must finally be taken of problems of motivating a young performer to undertake all-out anaerobic exercise.

Submaximum Exercise

During submaximum work, the cardiac output of a child is said to be "hypokinetic." In other words, the blood flow per unit of oxygen consumption is less than in the adult because of (1) more ready heat dissipation (less subcutaneous fat, and a greater relative body surface), (2) a lesser visceral mass, and (3) possibly a greater oxygen extraction from blood perfusing the active muscles. On the other hand, the ventilatory equivalent (typically 35 to 40) is greater in a child than in an adult.

Submaximum exercise tests are quite satisfactory in a school-aged child (coefficient of variation about 10 percent). When a Canadian national sample of children was tested in the mid-1960s, typical values for the physical working capacity (PWC$_{170}$) were 1.8 watts per kilogram in girls and 2.3 watts per kilogram in boys. However, the girls showed a 10 to 20 percent improvement of score when a similar random sample was tested in 1983 (see Table 8–8).

The hemoglobin content of the young child is only about 12 g per deciliter. However, with maturation this increases to 13.8 to 14 g per deciliter in the female and 16 g per deciliter in the male. There is a parallel increase of red cell count, from about 4.6×10^6 per cubic millimeter to 5.4×10^6 per cubic millimeter.

Muscle Strength

Girls show little gain of isometric muscle force after puberty, but again this seems partly culturally determined. In populations where a high level of physical activity is demanded of teenage girls (e.g., traditional Inuit who carry children on their backs through deep snow), the teenage years are marked by an increase of both lean mass and muscle strength.

In boys, there is a surge of strength at puberty, but the growth of height precedes the growth of strength by about a year. There is thus a period in which the boys outgrow their strength during adolescence.

FUNCTIONAL LOSS WITH AGING

The ever increasing average age of the population in most developed nations, the demand in many countries for an abandonment of compulsory retirement, and the possibility that enhanced physical activity might reduce the needs of the elderly for expensive institutional care have all helped to create a growing interest in interactions between physical activity and the aging process.

Theories of Aging

The very nature of aging remains something of a mystery. One simple but effective description, applicable to both the body and the individual cell, is an "increased probability of death" (Fig. 10–4). A second characteristic of an elderly person is a poor tolerance of environmental challenge; heart failure becomes more likely during a heatwave; hypothermia is more probable during exposure to severe cold, and vigorous bouts of exercise seem progressively more likely to provoke ventricular fibrillation.

It can be argued that there is an evolutionary need for death in an environment with finite resources, and it has thus been suggested that cells are capable of only a finite number of divisions before they "run out of program." For example, hyperplasia or cell replacement does not seem possible in the central nervous system after birth, and in some tissue cultures the process of cell division is halted after as few as 50 cell divisions have been completed. The most likely explanation of the loss of reproductive capacity and eventual death is that individual cells lose their normal functional capability through errors in protein copying ("transcription"). There should be a precise copying of the templates used in protein synthesis immediately prior to cell division, but a buildup of oxidants, irradiation, or the development of autoimmunity could all lead to sufficient malformation of genetic proteins that one or both of the products of cell division lack this essential information and are no longer viable. Associated phenomena include a cross-linkage between individual molecules (for instance, the long collagen molecules

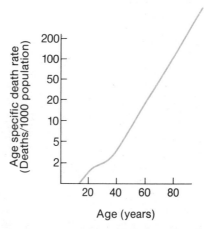

Figure 10–4 The concept of aging as an increased probability of death is illustrated. Note that the age-specific death rate is expressed on a logarithmic scale.

of fibrous tissue develop cross-linkages limiting their flexibility), and an accumulation of waste products (particularly "age pigments" such as lipofuscin) within the cells.

As a substantial number of cells die, partial or complete organ failure develops, and once a critical loss of organ function has occurred, death becomes very likely (although the precipitant of the ultimate catastrophe is often some minor intercurrent infection).

Various tactics whereby the rate of cell aging might be slowed have been suggested: (1) reducing the rate of metabolism through inactivity and rigid dieting (thus avoiding exhaustion of enzyme supplies), (2) avoidance of excessive natural radiation, and (3) administration of antioxidant substances such as Vitamin E. As yet, there is no proof to support the value of any of these tactics.

Biological Age

It is increasingly recognized that old age is not a single entity. Three categories of old people are commonly recognized—the "young old" who are healthy and fully able to care for themselves, the "middle old" who face some restrictions of their activities, and the "old old" who require full institutional care. Commonly, these three categories correspond to age ranges of 65 to 75, 75 to 85, and over 85 years.

Nevertheless, there is wide interindividual variation in the rate of aging, and it is thus useful to calculate an estimate of a person's biological age. This calculation may consider many variables including appearance features such as pigmentation, wrinkling of the skin, and the greying of the hair, along with physiological data such as maximum oxygen intake, muscle force, and renal function.

THE INTERPRETATION OF DATA ON AGING

Sources of Bias

There are several important problems of data interpretation when examining the aging of physiological function. Firstly, as many as 50 percent of any elderly population which is examined may have some chronic medical abnormality, and in perhaps one-half of these individuals the condition will adversely affect the functional variable under consideration. It is thus necessary to make some arbitrary circumscription of an elderly sample. One possible decision is that all of those who are well enough to work (or in a retired population, can care for themselves) will be included in the test sample. There is next the problem of volunteer bias. Many of those who volunteer for exercise-related projects have an above-average interest in physical activity, a healthy lifestyle, and life-long abstinence from

cigarettes. Moreover, even in such a sample, the aging process tends to become confounded with the effects of declining physical activity, since for both sociological and medical reasons aging is associated with a decrease of habitual exercise. Finally, if the analysis is based on cross-sectional data for a very old population, results become biassed by the progressive elimination of the least fit members of the population through death.

Problems of Statistical Analysis

Data are often presented in the form of linear regression equations, showing (for example) a 25 ml per year reduction of vital capacity between the ages of 20 and 65 years. However, the relationship between biological function and age is usually curved rather than linear. In the female, many biological functions peak around the time of menarche rather than at 20 years of age, although it is less clear whether further development would occur in a different sociocultural environment. Likewise, the male vital capacity peaks at 24 or 25 years of age rather than at 20 years, and there is an accelerating rate of functional loss as the retirement years are reached. The fitting of a linear regression equation to data extending from 20 to 65 years of age can thus give a rather misleading impression of the course of the aging process (Fig. 10–5).

AGING AND OXYGEN TRANSPORT

Overall Oxygen Conductance

Aging leads to a progressive deterioration in each of the various links in the oxygen transport chain. The overall consequence is a decrease of maximum oxygen intake from the value of perhaps 45 ml per kilogram per minute found in an adolescent girl to about 25 to 28 ml per kilogram per minute in a woman at the age of 65 years. Since both figures are expressed relative to body mass, a part of the deterioration in aerobic power is attributable to an accumulation of body fat. However, the main explanation is a reduction of both maximum ventilation and maximum cardiac output.

Respiratory System

A combination of thoracic ankylosis (a fusion of the joints in the chest cage) with increasing bronchitis and emphysema reduces vital capacity and thus increases the work of breathing. The maximum exercise ventilation shows a 25 percent reduction by the age of 65 years, and as much as a 50 percent loss at 75 years.

Furthermore, the effectiveness of this ventilation in terms of oxygen transport is reduced by an increase in the anatomical dead-space, an impaired matching of ventilation and perfusion, and a reduction of pulmonary diffusing capacity.

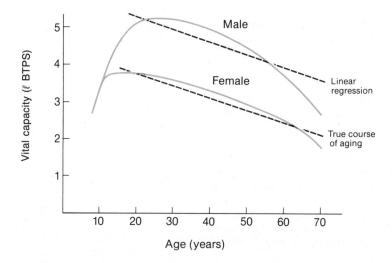

Figure 10-5 An illustration of the errors which may arise when a linear regression equation is fitted to data with a curvilinear aging curve.

Cardiovascular System

The maximum cardiac output is progressively diminished with aging. Some authors have suggested that the maximum heart rate of an elderly person can be calculated as 220 − (age in years). This equation probably exaggerates the true effect of aging, but nevertheless the maximum heart rate at the age of 65 years commonly drops to about 170 beats per minute. A youthful heart rate cannot be restored by administration of oxygen, so ischemia does not seem to be responsible for this change; it probably reflects a loss of myocardial compliance and slow ventricular filling. Older subjects also seem to find difficulty in sustaining their stroke volume at the high systemic blood pressures encountered during maximum effort, probably because of a lesser myocardial contractility (Fig. 10-6).

Oxygen delivery is further reduced by a narrowing of the maximum arteriovenous oxygen difference from perhaps 140 ml per liter to 120 ml per liter. Obesity and a decreased sweating response increase the need for skin blood flow during vigorous exercise, while a combination of weaker muscles and less capillarization of the individual muscle fibers leads to a lower maximum muscle flow. Together, these changes inevitably reduce the maximum arteriovenous oxygen difference.

In some older people, the situation is compounded by anemia. However, a low hemoglobin is not a necessary accompaniment of aging. It generally reflects internal bleeding, pathological changes in the gastric mucosa, or poor nutrition owing to poverty and loneliness.

Systemic Blood Pressure

The resting blood pressure generally shows some increase with age. The systolic reading increases more than the diastolic value, reflecting the combination of an unchanged resting stroke volume with a loss of elasticity in the vessel walls.

During exercise, poor myocardial contractility may lead to a lower ceiling of blood pressure than in a younger individual. Reflex adjustments of pressure to a sudden change of posture are also impaired, reflecting a low level of cardiovascular fitness, a poor response of the capacity vessels, impairment of cardiovascular reflexes, and often pathological changes such as varicose veins. Older people are thus vulnerable to a loss of consciousness from postural hypotension. This is a particular hazard when emerging from the water after swimming or an aqua-fitness class, since the capacity vessels have been in almost a "zero gravity" situation while submerged.

Electrocardiogram

The exercise electrocardiogram shows a progressive increase in abnormalities with aging, and by 65 years about 30 percent of both women and men show either ST segmental depression or frequent premature ventricular contractions during near maximal effort.

The similar proportion of electrocardiographic abnormalities in the two sexes is somewhat puzzling in that the incidence of myocardial infarction (Chapter 13)

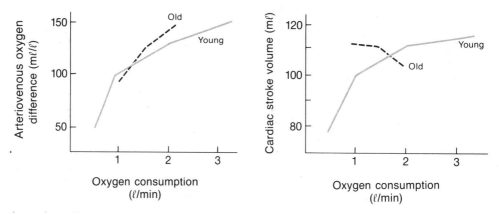

Figure 10-6   A comparison of cardiovascular responses to exercise in 25 and 65 year old subjects (based on experiments of Niinimaa and Shephard).

in women is only about one-third of that seen in men. It may be that older women have as much atherosclerosis (Chapter 13) as men, but that a lesser frequency of excessive effort or a lesser proportion of cigarette smokers gives rise to a smaller proportion of cardiac catastrophes in the course of daily activities. Alternatively, weakening of the heart muscle of a woman may produce ischemic changes in near maximal effort, despite a lesser relative degree of atherosclerosis.

Physicians who are not accustomed to viewing exercise electrocardiograms from the elderly sometimes prohibit exercise for such patients on the basis of an abnormal tracing. However, if a senior citizen is symptom-free and wishes to exercise, there seems no reason to forbid this. Health will probably be improved rather than worsened. But even if the activity were to shorten life somewhat, it is important to take account of the quality as well as the quantity of the remaining years of life; 2 years of pleasure may well match 3 years of a severely restricted existence.

AGING AND OTHER BODY SYSTEMS

Musculoskeletal System

Muscle force remains at a plateau value through early adult life to the age of perhaps 45 years. It then begins an accelerating decline, so that by the age of 65 years, values are no more than 70 percent of the young adult figure. The loss of strength reflects partly a greater inhibition of maximum effort in the older subjects, and partly a loss of active lean tissue, especially from the thighs. The type II (fast-twitch) fibers seem affected more than the slow-twitch component, probably reflecting the decreased inclination of elderly people to undertake heavy muscular tasks.

The peak blood lactate following exhausting exercise is often only about 7 mmol per liter. This reflects in part the reduction of muscle mass and in part a lesser degree of motivation to exhausting effort.

Joints such as the knees show a progressive loss of cartilage from the articular surfaces with development of osteoarthritic growths from the bone (exostoses) that are painful and increasingly limit the scope of daily activities. Deterioration in the molecular structure of collagen and elastic tissue also leads to a progressive decrease of flexibility at most of the major joints. By the age of retirement, scores on the "sit and reach" test of flexibility are 18 to 20 percent poorer than in a young adult.

A combination of compression of the intervertebral discs and a bowing of the back (kyphosis) leads to a steady diminution of standing height after the age of 50 years. Loss of stature is particularly marked where there has been frequent exposure to severe vibration (for instance, the daily driving of agricultural tractors). This complicates the standardization of physiological data on the basis of standing height.

There is a progressive loss of both calcium and organic matter from the bones (the conditions of osteoporosis and osteomalacia respectively), and these changes leave the older person vulnerable to fractures as the result of minor falls.

Body Fat

Most adults show an accumulation of 8 to 10 kg of fat over the span of adult life. After the age of 50 years, body mass may diminish again, but measurements of skinfold thickness show that this is due to a loss of lean tissue rather than a reduction in the amount of body fat.

Control Systems

There is a progressive deterioration in the function of all of the various sense organs with aging. Loss of sight and hearing progressively restrict the potential for sport participation. A deterioration of balance, together with poor vision and a liability to postural hypotension cause an increased risk of falls during vigorous movement. The normal reflex adjustments to exercise are less effective in the elderly; the on-transients of ventilation and heart rate increase are lengthened and there is often difficulty in executing a smooth, well-damped pattern of movement without oscillation of the limbs.

In many instances, the normal hormonal response to exercise is impaired—for example, there may be less than the expected growth hormone output during vigorous activity. Less fat is thus mobilized, and more protein is broken down. Regulatory adjustments necessary to exercise in a hot or cold environment also proceed less effectively than in a younger person.

Employment Potential

The physical capacity of an older person is such that questions are commonly raised about the ability to sustain physically demanding work. It is generally accepted that fatigue is likely when the 8-hour average oxygen consumption exceeds 40 percent of an individual's maximum oxygen intake. In a woman with a maximum oxygen intake of 1.5 ℓ per minute (a typical value at age 65 years), the 40 percent standard corresponds to an oxygen consumption of 0.6 ℓ per minute, or an energy consumption of about 12.5 kJ per minute. Given the anticipated standard deviation of oxygen transport, at least one 65-year-old woman in 40 will have a maximum oxygen intake 20 percent smaller than this (corresponding with an energy expenditure of around 10 kJ per minute), and some men also will have a working capacity of only 13 to 14 kJ per minute at retirement. Given that light work demands an energy expenditure in the range 8 to 14 kJ per minute, and moderate work demands 14 to 20 kJ per minute, it is surprising that there are not more complaints of fatigue among workers who are nearing retirement. It may be that fear of dismissal keeps some from making com-

TABLE 10–9 Values for Track and Field Events at Various Ages as Percent of World Records

Age (years)	Shot Put	Discus	200 m	Marathon
10	61	60	79	68
20	91	90	98	94
30	100	100	99	100
40	98	95	93	96
50	76	78	84	88
60	49	53	74	76

Based on an analysis of D. H. Moore.

plaints, and the physical demands of heavy work may also help to conserve fitness. Other possible explanations are that the elderly employee (1) reduces the energy cost of work through experience and knowledge of technique, (2) adopts a slower pace, with frequent rest, (3) solicits help from younger workers, and (4) bids successfully for the least demanding components of a task on the basis of seniority.

Tactics to increase the employability of the elderly through an increase in their O_2 transport include (1) a cessation of smoking, with clearance of perhaps 5 percent carboxyhemoglobin from the blood, a rightward shift of the oxygen dissociation curve back to its normal position, and a reduction in the oxygen cost of breathing, (2) a decrease of obesity and thus the energy cost of body movement, and (3) an increase of cardiovascular performance and/or muscle strength through deliberate leisure-hour training.

Age and Athletic Performance

The age of optimum physical performance depends very much on the cardiorespiratory and muscular demands of a task, relative to the needs for skill and experience. In gymnastic and speed events, performance commonly peaks during the mid or late teens, in endurance activities such as cycling and distance running the best times are recorded in the mid-twenties (Fig. 10–7 and Table 10–9), and in events where endurance must be combined with experience (e.g., soccer or tennis) the top players may be in their late twenties. In some activities such as riding, sailing, golf, and bowling, there is a heavy reliance upon experience, and the best performances may not be seen until the mid-thirties. In general, professional players continue to compete longer than amateurs.

Age and Trainability

It is difficult to decide whether the elderly are more or less trainable than those who are younger. When matching for initial fitness, it is probably wise to express condition as a percentage of age-related normal values, but this begs the question as to whether the aver-

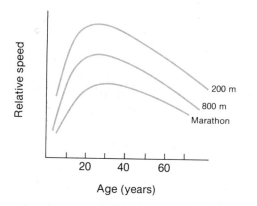

Figure 10–7 Relative speed records by age for 200 m, 800 m, and marathon distances (based on data collected by Moore, for male athletes).

age older person is less fit than someone who is younger.

It is also unclear how the gains that result from training should be expressed. For instance, in absolute terms, the increase of maximum oxygen intake that is seen in a 65-year-old individual is less than that which would be observed in a younger person who undertook endurance training at a similar relative intensity. However, if the conditioning response is expressed as a percentage of the base value, the 10 to 20 percent improvement is about what might have been expected in a young adult. In older people who elect a high-frequency, high-intensity endurance training regimen, the increments of maximum oxygen intake can be as large as 10 mℓ per kilogram per minute over 7 weeks. However, many of the more feeble elderly subjects cannot begin training in this fashion, and it is thus encouraging that a response can be observed with regular participation in much milder intensities of physical activity (Fig. 10–8).

In addition to the increment of aerobic power, an increase of physical activity improves the health of the senior citizen through a substantial decrease of skin-readings (as much as 3 mm per fold over 3 months of endurance exercise), some reversal of the loss of lean tissue, and at least a halting of the demineralization of bone.

Exercise and Aging

There is little evidence that an increase of physical activity will extend lifespan or alter the rate of the inherent aging process. Studies in rats suggest that there may be a small extension of lifespan if an endurance exercise program is begun before the age of 400 days (corresponding to an age of about 40 years in a human), but in older animals the commencement of a vigorous exercise program may even have a small adverse effect upon life-expectancy.

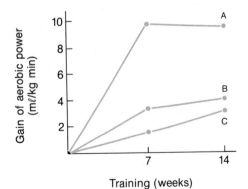

Figure 10–8 The influence of intensity and frequency of training of an elderly subject. *A,* 3.3 sessions per week, pulse 130–140 beats/min. *B,* 1.3 sessions per week, pulse 130–140 beats/min. *C,* 3.3 sessions per week, pulse 120 beats/min (based on data of Sidney and Shephard).

The slope of the aging curve for most biological functions is similar in athletes and nonathletes (Fig. 10–9), although athletes have an important advantage in that their line is set at a higher level at all ages. Thus, if a certain minimum of maximum oxygen intake is necessary to independent living, it takes 8 to 10 years longer before the function of a continuing athlete drops to this critical stage (Fig. 10–9). Although the lifespan of the individual may not have been extended by the exercise program, much has been added to the quality of those last remaining years, and the vast social cost of prolonged institutional care seems likely to have been minimized.

SEX- AND GENDER-RELATED DIFFERENCES IN WORKING CAPACITY

We may first note the use of the words sex and gender. A sex difference is constitutionally determined (e.g., the secretion of estrogen and progesterone versus testosterone), while a gender difference has a sociocultural basis (for instance, much of the deterioration in physical condition of the female seen in late adolescence).

General Considerations

There are a number of obvious sex differences between women and men that have implications for physical performance. Many of these differences have already been noted in earlier chapters. The adult stature of the female is shorter than that of the male, and because of the development of breast tissue, the percentage of body fat is higher. There are specific sex differences in the secretion of several hormones, and in the female the output of both estrogen and progesterone vary over the menstrual cycle. Finally, pregnancy makes major demands upon the cardiovascular system and thus has considerable implications for endurance performance. At the same time, sociocultural conditioning has compounded the inevitable impact of many of the underlying constitutional differences; for instance, females of postpubertal age were, until recently, encouraged to adopt a rather inactive lifestyle as an expression of "femininity." Current demands for equality of employment opportunities have heightened interest in assessing the true physiological potential of the female.

Maximum Oxygen Intake

Although there is little difference of aerobic power (mℓ per kilogram per minute) between girls and boys in the prepubertal period, women are at a substantial (15 to 20 percent) disadvantage to men during most of their working careers (Table 10–10). Only in retirement do the two sets of values come together again. Some 6 to

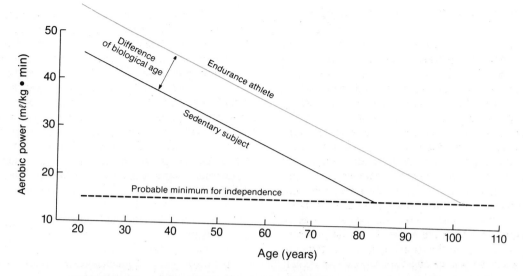

Figure 10–9 The gain from endurance training is shown. In a sedentary subject, the maximum oxygen intake drops to the minimum required for independent living (about 14 mℓ/kg per minute) by the age of 80 to 85 years. In a continuing athlete, the slope of the aging process is similar to that of a sedentary individual, but it is set at a higher level. It thus takes many more years before this critical limit is reached; usually, death from some inter-current disease occurs over this interval, so that the expense of extended institutional care is less likely.

7 percent of the female handicap can be attributed to the mass of metabolically inert fat carried in the breasts.

It is unclear how much of the residual difference is cultural in origin. A comparison of endurance athletes reveals up to a 20-percent difference of maximum oxygen intake between men and women in many sports, but this does not prove that there is an equally large inherent limitation in the females, since the intensity of selection for female participants is still smaller than for men. Moreover, in most types of competition, female scores seem to be progressively overtaking those for male participants.

If aerobic power is tested on a peripherally-limited device such as a cycle ergometer, the women are at a further disadvantage, since they generally have a smaller muscle mass and are more likely to stop exercising because of leg fatigue. The maximum heart rate is at least as high in young women (198 beats per minute) as in men, but probably because of the smaller mass of active muscle, most female subjects are exhausted at a lower maximum blood lactate reading. When data are expressed per kilogram of body mass, the aerobic power of most women peaks at or just before puberty, with some decline thereafter, as fat accumulates in the breasts and around the hips. This is in contrast with the findings in young men, where aerobic power usually continues to increase until about 20 years of age.

Submaximal Exercise

At any given submaximal power output, a woman is using a larger fraction of her total aerobic power than a man. In consequence, the heart rate and respiratory minute volume of the woman are larger, and there is a greater relative production of lactate.

Anatomical and sociocultural factors also give rise

TABLE 10–10 Sex Differences of Maximum Oxygen Intake (mℓ/kg · min STPD)

Sport	Maximum Oxygen Intake		
	Female	Male	Percent Difference
Alpine skiing	61	68	11.5
Swimming	57	67	17.5
Running (400–800 m)	56	68	21.4
Normal young adult (Toronto)	38	48	26.3
Cross-country skiing	63	82	30.1
Orienteering	59	77	30.5
Table tennis	43	58	34.9
Fencing	43	59	37.2
Speed skating	53	78	47.2

Based in part on data of Åstrand for Swedish national champions.

to appreciable sex- and gender-related differences in the mechanical efficiency of most activities. Thus, when walking, men produce less rotation of their hips and a greater vertical displacement of their center of mass, leading to a poor mechanical efficiency. When swimming, men are also at a considerable disadvantage; a lesser amount of subcutaneous fat exposes them to a greater degree of cold stress, while a lesser total amount of body fat reduces their buoyancy. In particular, a relative deficiency of fat in the thighs plus heavier long bones cause the legs of the male swimmer to droop; the male competitor must thus overcome more drag than the female.

Heat Exposure

When exercising in a hot environment, it might be thought that a greater amount of subcutaneous fat would place women at some disadvantage relative to men. Wyndham and his associates found that 92 percent of women were unable to complete a standard heat exposure test, whereas 50 percent of men tolerated the same set of conditions. He noted further that while women apparently had a larger number of active sweat glands than men, they produced less sweat. Man "is a prolific sweat waster, whereas the female adjusts her sweat rate better to the required heat loss."

Despite this research, the relative capacity for heat loss in the two sexes remains debatable. There is a substantial interaction between fitness and heat tolerance, but nevertheless, many of those making comparisons have had difficulty in equating either fitness levels or work–rates between the two sexes. For example, if subjects are matched for initial aerobic power, the women who are tested will be fitter than the men. However, if all subjects are required to operate a cycle ergometer at 100 W, or to climb a 40-cm bench, this is a harder relative work–rate for a woman than for a man.

Oxygen Conductance

The various links in the oxygen transport chain all have smaller maximum values in a woman than in a man. Static lung volumes are some 20 to 25 percent smaller in the female, with a corresponding difference in maximum exercise ventilation. The heart volume, stroke volume and maximum cardiac output are also smaller in a woman; also a lower average hemoglobin level (13.8, versus 15.6 g per deciliter in a man) inevitably reduces oxygen transport per liter of cardiac output. Finally, the weaker skeletal muscles of a woman must contract at a higher percentage of their maximum voluntary force, increasing the difficulty in perfusing the active limbs.

Muscle Force

In girls, there is a tenfold increase in the number of muscle cells from the age of 2 months to 16 years, compared with a 14-fold increase in boys studied over the same timespan. Moreover, girls do not show the hypertrophy of the large muscles that is observed in boys in the years immediately following puberty. Part of this difference in development is attributable to the relatively small amounts of androgen secreted by the female, part is due to a lesser sociocultural interest in muscle-building activity among women; and part reflects a concentration of investigations upon muscles where males have a large advantage (females come much closer to male strength figures for the thighs than for the arms).

For many muscle groups, the maximum muscle force that an average woman can develop is only about 60 percent of that observed in a man. Asmussen has pointed out that at least one-half of this apparent handicap is attributable to the smaller size of the female. Indeed, if one accepts that strength is proportional to height^3 rather than height^2, then 30 percent of the 40 percent differential is due to size.

Skeletal Structures

The female anatomy is characterized by a greater angle of pelvic tilt, and the femoral axes are also more oblique in women than in men. A woman's arms also have a greater carrying angle. These characteristics are a disadvantage in some sports. However, most women have good flexibility and a wide range of motion at the joints, leading to excellence in pursuits such as gymnastics.

Bone strength and density are less in a woman than in a man, so that fractures are more likely if bones are subjected to an equal mechanical stress. The interaction between amenorrhea and bone mineral loss has already been noted.

Training Response

If appropriate allowance is made for the differences in initial fitness levels, the response to cardiorespiratory training seems very similar in women and in men. However, even a strenuous weight training program seems to induce relatively limited muscle hypertrophy in the female.

Performance During the Menstrual Cycle

Hormonal variations during the menstrual cycle seem to have only a limited impact upon the physiological responses to vigorous physical activity. Some authors have described an earlier onset of sweating during menstruation; others have noted somewhat higher core temperatures during the luteal phase of the cycle. Body mass is inevitably increased by water retention during the premenstrual phase, but this has only a minor effect—mainly upon activities where body mass must be displaced. The related discomfort may lead to some deterioration in all-out or skilled efforts, while increasing both maximal muscle force and the risk of accidents. The temporary rise of intraocular pressure may have an adverse effect upon vision in some subjects.

Very strenuous training may either retard the on-set of menstruation (primary amenorrhea), or stop normal cycles (secondary amenorrhea). At one time this was attributed to an inadequate energy intake, but most authors now believe that the main effect comes from some alteration of hormonal balance; for example, one hypothesis has suggested that an exercise-induced secretion of prolactin has an inhibitory effect upon the secretion of pituitary gonadotrophins. Normal menstrual cycles are restored quite quickly when the intensity of training is moderated. There is no evidence that temporary amenorrhea has any harmful consequence, other than a tendency to bone demineralization that can be countered quite simply by increasing the dietary intake of calcium. Recent research suggests that a similar pattern of pituitary inhibition can develop among male endurance athletes, with a drop in the secretion of testosterone and a temporary reduction of spermatogenesis.

Exercise During Pregnancy

The energy cost of all body movements is increased during pregnancy. This is due partly to an increase of body mass (ultimately, a gain of at least 10 kg), and in part to a displacement of the center of mass of the body (leading to an awkward and unaccustomed pattern of movement).

A substantial fraction of the cardiac output is diverted to the placenta during pregnancy, with a corresponding reduction of physical working capacity. At the same time, the vigorous diaphragmatic movements necessary in maximal exercise are impeded by fetal growth. Venous return is impaired, and the reserve capacity of both the liver and the kidneys is severely taxed. In view of the fact that severe exercise leads to a reduction of visceral blood flow, there is some risk that the blood flow to the fetus will be curtailed by excessive exertion, and indeed, tape recordings of fetal heart rates have sometimes shown an exercise-induced slowing suggestive of oxygen lack. Excessive muscular efforts may also initiate abortion or premature labor. It is thus a wise precaution, particularly in the third trimester of pregnancy, to limit exercise to a moderate intensity. Nevertheless, occasional athletes continue to train quite hard, and a few have even competed within days of delivery, apparently without any harmful effects to the fetus.

There were once fears that vigorous exercise would complicate labor, but current opinion is that maintenance of good physical condition helps rather than hinders the birth process. One study of Hungarian athletes suggested that labor was shorter than average in 87 percent of competitors, and that cesarian sections were also less frequent in athletes than in sedentary subjects.

A graded return to physical activity, with specific exercises to restore the condition of the abdominal and pelvic muscles, is particularly helpful in the postpartum period. However, the energy requirements of lactation are substantial, and prolonged endurance activity should be avoided until after the child has been weaned. Noack reported that 10 to 15 German athletes returned to competition after pregnancy, eight making objective improvements over their previous best performances.

FURTHER READING

Albinson JG, Andrew GM. Child in sport and physical activity. Baltimore: University Park Press, 1976.

Baldwin KM. Muscle development: neonatal to adult. Exerc Sport Sci Rev 1984; 12:1–20.

Bar Or O. Pediatric sports medicine for the practitioner. New York: Springer Verlag, 1983.

Bauss R, Roth K. Motorische Entwicklung. Probleme und Ergbnisse von Langschnittuntersuchungen. Darmstadt: Institut für Sportwissenschaft, 1977.

Boileau RA. Advances in pediatric sports sciences, vol. 1. Champaign, Ill: Human Kinetics, 1984.

Borms J, Hebbelinck M. Pediatric work physiology. Basel: Karger, 1978.

Borms J, Hebbelinck M, Venerando A. Women in sport. Basel: Karger, 1980.

Borms J, Hebbelinck M. Venerando A, The female athlete. Basel: Karger, 1980

Brunner D, Jokl E. Physical activity and aging. Baltimore: University Park, 1970.

Caird FI, Dall JLC, Kennedy RD. Cardiology in old age. New York: Plenum, 1976.

Clarke HH. Physical and motor tests in the Medford boys' growth study. Englewood Cliffs, NJ: Prentice Hall, 1971.

Drinkwater B. Woman and exercise: physiological aspects. Exerc Sport Sci Rev 1984; 12:21–52.

Eston RG. The regular menstrual cycle and athletic performance. Sports Med 1984; 1:431–445.

Harris R, Frankel LJ. Guide to fitness after 50. New York: Plenum, 1977.

Ilmarinen J, Valimaki I. Children and sport. Berlin: Springer, 1984.

Kenney RA. Physiology of aging: a synopsis. Chicago: Year Book, 1982.

Klafs CE, Lyon MJ. The female athlete—a coach's guide to conditioning and training. 2nd Ed. St. Louis: CV Mosby, 1978.

Lavallée H, Shephard RJ. Frontiers of activity and child health. Québec City: Editions du Pélican, 1977.

Lavallée H, Shephard RJ. Child growth and development. Trois Rivières: University of Québec at Trois Rivières, 1981.

Malina RM. Secular changes in growth, maturation and physical performance. Exerc Sport Sci Rev 1979; 6:203–255.

Ostrow AC. Physical activity and the older adult. Psychological perspectives. Princetown, NJ: Princetown Book Company, 1984.

Ostyn M, Beunen G, Simons J. Kinanthropometry II. Baltimore: University Park Press, 1980.

Pate RR, Kriska A. Physiological basis of the sex difference in cardiorespiratory endurance. Sports Med 1984; 1:87–98.

Rarick GL. Physical activity. Human growth and development. New York: Academic Press, 1973.

Shephard RJ. Physical activity and aging. London: Croom Helm, 1978.

Shephard RJ. Physical activity and growth. Chicago: Year Book, 1982.

Shephard RJ. Physical activity and child health. Sports Med 1984; 1:205–233.

Shephard RJ,, Lavallée H. Physical fitness assessment. Springfield, Ill: CC Thomas, 1978.

Shephard RJ, Sidney KH. Exercise and aging. Exerc Sport Sci Rev 1979; 6:1–58.

Simri U. Physical exercise and activity for the aging. Natanya, Israel: Wingate Institute, 1975.

Smith EL, Serfass RC. Exercise and aging—the scientific basis. Hillsdale, NJ: Enslow Publishing, 1981.

Stager JM. The reversibility of amenorrhoea in athletes. Sports Med 1984; 1:337–340.

Wickstrom RL. Development and kinesiology: maturation of basic motor patterns. Exerc Sport Sci Rev 1975; 3:163–192.

Williams TF. Rehabilitation in the aging. New York: Raven Press, 1984.

ENVIRONMENT AND HEALTH

HIGH AND LOW AMBIENT PRESSURES

CHAPTER *11*

High ambient pressures are encountered in diving and underwater exploration; here, the main problems arise from the increase in overall gas pressure, and in the partial pressure of individual constituents. Commercial exploration may extend to substantial depths, but the recreational diver is normally content with quite shallow dives. Nevertheless, physiological problems can arise even in shallow water.

Low ambient pressures are met in some mining operations, in skiing, ballooning, and mountaineering. The altitudes of interest are somewhat lower than those considered by earlier generations of aviation physiologists and balloonists, but nevertheless the main problems still result from the reduced partial pressure of inspired oxygen.

HIGH AMBIENT PRESSURES

We shall first review briefly some of the technical problems encountered in free diving and in the use of self-contained underwater breathing systems and diving suits. We shall then consider in turn the physiological problems that arise during the increase of ambient pressure, during its maintenance, and during decompression.

Free Diving

During a breath-hold dive, the lungs are filled initially to their maximum volume. As the diver descends, there is a progressive compression of the intrathoracic gas volume, and when through a combination of circumstances this volume becomes less than the residual volume as measured at sea-level, there is a danger of a "thoracic squeeze," with rupture of the large intrathoracic veins into the chest cavity. Factors determining the extent and speed of onset of this danger include (1) the ratio of the external water pressure to the gas pressure when the lungs were filled, (2) the displacement of up to 1 liter of blood towards the thorax by a cooling of the limbs and by hydrostatic compression of the peripheral veins, (3) a reduction of intrathoracic gas volume owing to a respiratory quotient of less than unity, and (4) retention of carbon dioxide in the body fluids because of the high ambient pressure.

There is a further danger that consciousness may be lost underwater, due to a progressive decrease in the oxygen content of the lungs. The normal signal to end a breath-hold dive comes as a rising pressure of carbon dioxide in the blood and the cerebrospinal fluid stimulates the respiratory chemoreceptors. However, if there has been a period of hyperventilation prior to diving, the initial alveolar CO_2 pressure may be very low, and signals from a rising CO_2 pressure may be lost. The dive is then terminated only if symptoms of oxygen lack are perceived. Often, oxygen lack gives rise not to unpleasant symptoms, but rather to a euphoria that the diver allows to pass unnoticed. But even if ascent is begun as the oxygen pressure drops to a critical level, a figure of 8 kPa (which would be a marginal partial pressure of oxygen at a depth of 10 meters) necessarily becomes 4 kPa (probably insufficient to sustain consciousness) as the diver ascends towards the surface of the water. Remedies for this potentially fatal situation are (1) to avoid preliminary hyperventilation, and (2) to hold the supervisory (instructor to student) ratio to a sufficiently low level that any loss of consciousness while underwater is quickly perceived.

Underwater Breathing Systems

Recreational divers commonly use a snorkel, which enables them to breathe ambient air while the head and chest are underwater. In order to explore greater depths, open-circuit, self-contained underwater breathing apparatus (SCUBA) is worn. Typically, compressed air is supplied via a demand valve from a cylinder that is strapped to the back. Impending exhaustion of the cylinder is signalled by a second valve; this imposes a noticeable resistance to breathing when three-fourths of the available air supply has been used. In order to economize on gas, the diver can switch back to a snorkel arrangement when near the surface. The main limitation of the SCUBA system is that there is no substantial reserve of gas supply to accommodate a possible need for extended decompression.

A closed-circuit SCUBA system allows the rebreathing of gas after CO_2 absorption. This arrangement greatly extends the possible period of submersion. The diver also avoids making a tell-tale trail of expired gas bubbles—an important practical consideration in some military applications. A 1-kg canister of soda lime granules allows the absorption of about 200 liters of expired carbon dioxide. If pure oxygen is supplied to the system, there is a danger of oxygen poisoning at depths greater than 8 to 10 meters (as will be discussed). However, the range of operating depths can be greatly extended by respiring varying proportions of nitrogen and oxygen (for instance, 40 percent oxygen at a flow of 8 ℓ per minute is suitable at a depth of 43 meters, and 32.5 percent oxygen at a flow of 13 ℓ per minute is appropriate at a depth of 55 meters).

Diving Suits

Recreational diving suits are designed to provide thermal insulation, while protecting the skin against sharp coral reefs and wreckage. A rubberized suit tends to trap pockets of air at less than water pressure, allowing development of a subcutaneous "squeeze." Subcutaneous blood blisters form in the affected regions, in a manner analogous to the pulmonary squeeze discussed previously, because of a large pressure difference between the air pocket and the blood in the superficial veins.

Compression of the air space at depth largely destroys the thermal protection from a rubberized "dry" suit, since the extent of insulation varies with the thickness of the air film. Possible solutions to this difficulty include the use of a less readily compressed plastic fabric and a periodic reinflation of the rubber suit by a gas mixture with a low heat conducting capacity (e.g., a freon/CO_2 mixture).

A "wet" suit allows the entry of water at openings such as the neck, avoiding problems of subcutaneous squeeze. With this type of garment, a film of stationary water trapped beneath the suit is warmed by the body, providing some insulation against a cold environment. If a diver is working hard, the trapped water may indeed become too hot, and it is than necessary to open the suit, venting the warm water to its surroundings.

Problems During Increase of Ambient Pressure

During the increase of ambient pressure associated with a diver's descent, problems may arise from failure to equalize the respired gas pressure with pockets of trapped air in such sites as the middle ear (the condition known as baro-otitis), teeth which contain gas pockets (aerodontalgia), and the nasal sinuses (aerosinusitis). Often, gas trapping causes no more than pain in the affected region, but there may be hemorrhage into the low pressure part of the body. In the case of the middle ear there can be distortion with eventual rupture of the ear drum. A further possibility is collapse of the eustachian tube leading from the middle ear to the pharynx, with subsequent retraction of the tympanic membrane and persistent deafness. Prophylactic measures include (1) avoidance of deep diving when the entrances to the nasal sinuses and the eustachian tubes are narrowed by an upper-respiratory infection, and (2) regular dental inspection.

Submersion of the face and diving, (the "diving reflex"), together with an increase of arterial O_2 pressure, tend to cause a slowing of heart rate in a diver, but these responses are often attenuated by simultaneous isometric contraction of the major muscles and/or muscle vasodilatation associated with a defence ("fight or flight") reaction. Breath holding may restrict the cardiac output despite vigorous exercise, thus leading to a large rise of blood lactate that is seen after the dive is completed. If breathing is checked with a small volume of gas in the lungs during descent, there is also a danger that the thoracic contents may be compressed below residual volume, causing a thoracic squeeze to develop. A pressure differential may arise behind goggles, with a risk of conjunctival hemorrhage, bleeding into the eyelids and the fat pocket behind the eye (retroorbital fossa). A "squeeze" may also cause hemorrhage into folds and ridges of the skin beneath a dry suit, and if the ears are covered, blood blisters may develop in the external auditory meatus or on the outer surface of the tympanic membrane.

Problems Associated with Maintained Exposure to High Pressure

If exposure to a high ambient pressure is maintained, there are potential problems from oxygen toxicity, nitrogen narcosis, and respiratory exhaustion with CO_2 accumulation. If the water is cold, there is a risk of hypothermia, while difficulty in communication is also a common problem in the underwater environment.

Oxygen Poisoning. The breathing of pure oxygen produces harmful effects, even at sea level, after 6 to 12 hours of exposure. Potential problems include a depressed formation of the lipoprotein lining of the lungs (alveolar surfactant), pulmonary collapse, CO_2 retention, pulmonary congestion and/or vasoconstriction, and an increase of pulmonary vascular permeability with exudation of fluid into the air spaces of the lungs. The subject complains of cough and a pain in the chest, the vital capacity is reduced by the pulmonary changes, and cerebral toxicity of the high oxygen pressure is indicated by a circumscription of the visual field. If these findings are ignored, there may be a progression to other symptoms of disturbed brain function, including dizziness, nausea, euphoria, incoordination, confusion, and convulsions.

At rest, oxygen at a pressure of 2 atmospheres is tolerated for 6 hours and 3 atmospheres is tolerated for 3 hours, but during exercise the tolerance diminishes to 30 minutes at a pressure of 3 atmospheres. A common recommendation for the recreational diver is thus to limit exposure to 1 hour at a depth of 8 meters (Table 11-1). If ambient pressures exceed 3 to 4 atmospheres, even air has a high partial pressure of oxygen; similar problems may thus arise from the prolonged breathing of compressed air. The respiratory problems largely reflect a rapid blood-stream absorption of oxygen from closed-off segments of the lung, with collapse of the affected segments. The disturbed cerebral function, on the other hand, is mainly caused by an inhibition of vital enzymes by oxygen itself or by associated free radicals, with a reduction in brain levels of gamma amino butyric acid (GABA). Other contributory factors may be an oxidation of lipids in the cell membranes of the brain and narcosis from a substantial accumulation of carbon dioxide (since the high oxygen pressures depress ventilation and hamper the blood transport of carbon dioxide).

Nitrogen Narcosis. Accumulation of nitrogen has a narcotic effect on the brain. This becomes marked at the partial pressures of gas associated with water depths of more than 30 meters. The highest functions of the brain are first affected, thus giving a cheerful but dangerous euphoria (described by early investigators as "rapture of the deep"). There is usually an exaggeration of normal personality. Loss of reasoning ability, a slowing of reactions, and poor manual dex-

TABLE 11-1   Limiting Times Recommended to a
Diver Breathing Pure Oxygen

Depth (m)	Time (min)
3.0	240
4.5	150
6.1	110
7.6	75
9.1	45
10.7	25
12.2	10

Note: The tolerance of the recreational diver seems somewhat less than that observed with exercise in a deliberate chamber exposure to oxygen at increased ambient pressure.
Based on data of Duffner and Lanphier

terity are seen after 12 minutes at a pressure of 4 atmospheres. There are also changes of sensory perception, a feeling of impending black-out, and sometimes manic or depressive states. If these symptoms are ignored, gross incoordination and a total loss of consciousness follow.

Other inert gases have an even greater narcotic effect than nitrogen, their potency being proportional to their lipid solubility (Table 11-2). It is thus thought that the narcosis is caused by solution of the inert gas in the lipid phase of the cell membrane. One hypothesis is that this reaction displaces oxygen, thereby leading to a form of cellular oxygen lack (histotoxic hypoxia).

Any buildup of carbon dioxide within the body has a potentiating effect upon nitrogen narcosis, but symptoms are rapidly corrected by decompression of the diver to sea level conditions. If it is necessary to explore depths greater than 30 meters, it is usual to mix oxygen with gases that are much less toxic than nitrogen (e.g., the diver may inspire a mixture of oxygen and helium).

Respiratory Work Load. The increase in density of respired gas with the rise of ambient pressure increases the oxygen content of arterial blood (greater oxygen saturation of hemoglobin, and more oxygen in physical solution). Thus, there may be a small increase in maximum oxygen intake at moderate water depths. However, the work of breathing is also increased by the external resistance of the water and by an increase of turbulent resistance within the airway (the extent of turbulence being proportional to density of the respired gas). In consequence, there is a greater tendency for collapse of the airway during a vigorous expiration at depth than at sea level. Possible remedies for the diver are (1) to slow the rate of expiration at the expense of inspiration, (2) to increase the mean alveolar volume and thus increase the elastic forces guarding airway patency (a tactic opposed by water pressure), (3) to increase tidal volume and reduce the breathing rate (thereby re-expanding collapsed lung segments), and (4) to replace nitrogen by helium (which has a much lower density, and is thus less prone to develop turbulent flow).

Despite these various tactics, there is often a diminution of respiratory minute volume when a given power output is developed in deep water. In addition, there is a tendency to accumulation of carbon dioxide. Both problems are often exacerbated by the breathing equipment. A resistance that seems moderate with sea level gas densities becomes a heavy burden when it is increased several-fold by breathing underwater. When the diver is 30 meters underwater (4 atmospheres pressure), the maximum voluntary ventilation typically drops to only 50 percent of the sea level figure.

Other factors leading to CO_2 accumulation underwater include (1) inhibition of blood CO_2 transport by the high partial pressure of oxygen, (2) restriction of cerebral blood flow by the high oxygen pressure, (3) a depression of peripheral chemoreceptors by oxygen, (4) a depression of medullary respiratory centers by inert gases, (5) a long-term reduction in sensitivity of the respiratory centers, and (6) inefficiencies in the CO_2 absorbent canisters of SCUBA equipment (although an inspired CO_2 concentration of 0.25 percent is quite acceptable at sea level, it boosts alveolar P_{CO_2} by 1 kPa at a pressure of 4 atmospheres).

Hypothermia. Heat loss is substantial while swimming in cold water; indeed, because water conducts heat more readily than air, heat loss continues unless the water temperature is 33-34 °C. Unfortunately, the rate of heat loss is greatly increased if it is necessary to breath helium mixtures, since helium conducts heat more readily than the normal inspired gases. The

TABLE 11-2   Relationship of Narcotic Potency to Lipid Solubility of Gas

Gas	Narcotic Potency	Lipid Solubility
Xenon	25.0	1.700
Krypton	7.1	0.430
Argon	2.3	0.140
Nitrogen	1.0	0.067
Hydrogen	0.55	0.036
Neon	0.28	0.019
Helium	0.23	0.015

Based on data of Bennett (1969).

combination of an increased central blood volume (due to water pressure) and cold exposure usually provokes a marked urine formation (a "cold diuresis"). Body heat is best conserved by wearing either a "wet" or a "dry" suit, as discussed previously.

Communication Problems.   Vision while underwater is hampered by refractive distortions. These cause apparent changes in both the size and the distance of objects. A low overall level of illumination also leads to a blurring of the outlines of objects, with apparent changes in their colors.

Accurate perception of speech is made difficult by the increased gas pressures in the airway and by the breathing of abnormal gas mixtures, which alter the voice pitch. Further difficulties arise from resonance in breathing equipment, and extraneous noise (particularly hissing from gas cylinders). The intelligibility of speech is improved by talking more slowly, but this tactic carries the unfortunate penalty of reducing ventilation and thus the alveolar oxygen pressure.

Problems During Reduction of Pressure

During ascent from a dive, problems may arise from decompression sickness, expansion of trapped gas, and sudden loss of consciousness (see free diving).

Decompression Sickness.   Decompression sickness arises from a supersaturation of the tissues with an inert gas (commonly nitrogen). When a certain excess tissue pressure is reached relative to ambient values (commonly a ratio of about 1.75 to 1.00), bubbles begin to form intra- or extra-cellularly. Pain and injury result from (1) mechanical distortion and disruption of the tissues, (2) blockage of blood vessels by intra- or perivascular bubbles and lipid emboli, and (3) the after-effects of circulatory arrest.

Although symptoms cannot always be related closely to the location of periarticular gas bubbles as visualized by radiography or ultrasound, the disorder can be prevented by changing the composition of the respired gas from an oxygen–nitrogen mixture to pure oxygen. Symptoms during ascent are also avoided by use of tables based on the theory of nitrogen bubble formation, and if problems do arise they can be corrected by recompression of the diver. Gas bubbles are thus thought to be responsible for most of decompression sickness pathology. The commonest symptom is the "bends"—an ache or pain, felt near a major joint such as the knee. Other manifestations include skin rashes, respiratory symptoms (the "chokes"—a dry cough, shortness of breath, and a feeling of suffocation), migraine-like visual field defects, convulsive "epileptiform" attacks, spastic paralysis, and collapse. Collapse is sometimes secondary to the bends, but is more serious and potentially fatal if it arises as an unheralded primary episode, or is secondary to the chokes or neurologic symptoms. A pathological deterioration ("necrosis") of the heads of the long bones may also develop some months after exposure to the high pressure; this condition is particularly common with repeated exposure (as in commercial divers and tunneling workers).

Both the uptake of inert gas and its elimination follow a relatively slow, exponential time course, the rate of exchange between any given tissue and the environment depending on the ratio of local blood flow to tissue volume and gas solubility (Fig. 11-1). Exercise speeds elimination of the inert gas, and thus shortens the period of vulnerability to decompression sickness. However, vulnerability to decompression sickness is increased by exercise, heat, cold, oxygen lack, previous injury of a joint, infection, recent overindulgence in alcohol, recent previous exposure to an inert gas, and poor local circulation (whether due to lack of fitness, aging, or cardiovascular disease).

"Diving tables" are designed primarily to protect employees in industrial operations such as bridge and tunnel construction, where a fixed increase of ambient gas pressure is maintained throughout a working shift. It is much more difficult to specify a safe decompression schedule for the recreational diver, since the depth of submersion is continuously changing for the latter. One possible approach is for the diver to carry a small analogue computer that mimics blood flow, volume and lipid solubility for the various tissues of the body. Dangerous supersaturation of any one tissue can then be quickly detected, and the diver can slow the rate of ascent until this situation has been corrected.

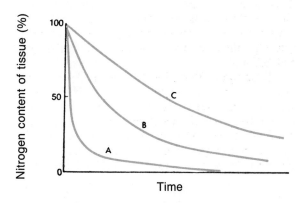

Figure 11–1   Clearance of nitrogen from three tissues during the breathing of 100 percent oxygen (or ascent from a dive). In tissue A, the ratio of local blood flow to the product of tissue volume and nitrogen solubility is large, so that clearance is rapid. In tissues B and C, the ratio of blood flow to (volume x solubility) is smaller, and elimination proceeds more slowly. In any given tissue, clearance can be replotted as a linear semilogarithmic relationship between nitrogen content and time. (After Shephard RJ. Physiology and biochemistry of exercise. New York: Praeger, 1982.)

Most forms of decompression sickness respond well to recompression. This reduces the size of the gas bubbles (with a rapid relief of symptoms), and it also favors their reabsorption. Oxygen administration is also a method of treatment recommended by some authors. Although in theory it speeds the rate of nitrogen elimination, in practice there may be an offsetting slowing of the circulation by the increased partial pressure of oxygen, and this would hamper nitrogen clearance. Once bubble formation has occurred, the affected joint remains vulnerable to a recurrence of the bends for several days. In an attempt to explain this finding, it has been postulated that a bubble–tissue complex with a very long half-life forms around the affected joints.

Gas Expansion. Gas expansion can damage the lungs if they are already well-filled with compressed gas while at depth and the breath is held by a closure of the glottis during a rapid ascent. The lungs may rupture into the mediastinum (filling this region with gas bubbles, the condition of surgical emphysema), into the pleura (giving an air-filling of the pleural space and collapse of the lungs, the condition of pneumothorax), or into a pulmonary vein (giving air emboli, which can cause a fatal blockage of the cerebral circulation).

In anesthetized dogs, the critical lung–water pressure differential for tearing of the lung tissues is about 10 to 11 kPa, but in humans, counter pressure is usually available from clothing and a voluntary tensing of the chest muscles; divers can thus withstand somewhat greater differential pressures than experimental animals.

Physical Aspects of Drowning

The physiological characteristics of a drowning person differ between fresh and salt water conditions. In fresh water, the plasma sodium ion concentration falls (because of a dilution of the blood by water that is absorbed in the lungs), while plasma potassium ion concentration rises (owing more to a leakage of potassium ions from hypoxic tissues than to a rupture of red cells into the hypo-osmotic plasma). These changes both predispose to the onset of ventricular fibrillation.

In salt water drowning, the high osmotic pressure of the water draws fluid from the blood into the lungs, thereby causing (1) a rise of plasma sodium ion concentration, (2) a general hemoconcentration, and (3) pulmonary edema.

With either type of drowning, inhaled water and vomitus irritate the bronchial tree, giving rise to both breath holding and bronchospasm. This, combined with the fluid inundation of the lungs, gives rise to hypoxia, hypercapnia, acidosis, a rise of blood pressure, and a vulnerability to cardiac dysrhythmias. If the patient remains untreated, blood pressure falls and hyperpnea gives place to terminal gasping.

After removal to a place of safety, the pulse of a drowning victim must be monitored to ensure the continued regularity of heart rhythm. Cardiac massage should be instituted if necessary. Obvious debris should be cleared from the mouth and the throat, and artificial respiration must be begun. Note that bronchospasm and a decrease of lung compliance both increase ventilatory impedance relative to a healthy person, so that quite high ventilatory pressures may be needed to develop an adequate tidal volume during resuscitation.

ACUTE RESPONSES TO LOW AMBIENT PRESSURES

The exercise physiologist is interested primarily in the responses of athletes to the hypoxia associated with quite moderate altitudes, such as those encountered in Mexico City (2,240 m). Ski resorts give occasional exposure to altitudes of 3,000 to 4,000 m, and occasional mining operations are found at altitudes as high as 6,000 m. However, few sports enthusiasts are exposed to the very high altitudes and the severe forms of oxygen lack encountered by early balloonists, aviators, and mountaineers.

The total ambient pressure decreases in logarithmic fashion with an increase of altitude, so that at 5,500 m the ambient pressure (and thus the partial pressure of oxygen) is approximately one-half of the sea level figure. Maximum oxygen transport is reduced, but on the other hand performance in some events is helped by a decrease of air resistance, a small reduction of gravitational acceleration, and a cooler environmental temperature.

Overall Oxygen Transport

Because of the sigmoid shape of the oxygen dissociation curve and some alteration of the 2:3 diphosphoglycerate-regulated affinity of hemoglobin for oxygen, a drop in the partial pressure of inspired oxygen does not produce a proportionate decrease of maximum oxygen intake (Fig. 11-2). Altitudes of up to 1,500 to 2,000 meters are tolerated with little change of maximum oxygen transport, but at higher elevations there is a progressive reduction of aerobic power and thus of endurance performance. This reflects not only a reduction of arterial oxygen saturation, but also a decrease of maximum heart rate. On some of the Everest expeditions, the maximum heart rate of young climbers had dropped as low as 135 beats per minute as they approached the summit.

During submaximal exercise, possible compensatory tactics for the decreased oxygen pressure include (1) a decrease of the inspired air-alveolar oxygen pressure gradient by hyperventilation, and (2) tachycardia with an increase of cardiac output at a given work-rate, so that a similar volume of oxygen is transported despite the drop in oxygen content of arterial blood.

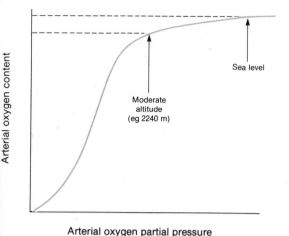

y-axis: Arterial oxygen content

Sea level

Moderate
altitude
(eg 2240 m)

x-axis: Arterial oxygen partial pressure

Figure 11–2 The effect of the normal sigmoid shape of the oxygen dissociation curve in maintaining the oxygen content of arterial blood at moderate altitudes.

Respiratory Adaptations

Hyperventilation is difficult to sustain, because it washes an excess of CO_2 out of the body. An arterial CO_2 pressure below 3.3 to 4.0 kPa also has an adverse effect on psychomotor function, because it reduces blood flow to the brain. In practice, the climber usually shows a small increase of ventilation relative to sea level conditions if the respired volume is measured at ambient pressure (BTPS), but if ventilation is expressed under standard dry gas conditions (STPD), the respiratory minute volume is diminished roughly in proportion to the decrease of maximum oxygen intake.

Intermittent breathing may develop at altitude, particularly when the subject is resting or at night. This reflects the phase lag between the immediate respiratory drive (oxygen lack acting on the carotid chemoreceptors) and the depressant effect of CO_2 washout upon the activity of the medullary respiratory control centers. The decrease of atmospheric density raises the critical velocity at which airflow in the bronchi becomes turbulent, and it also reduces the energy cost of inducing a given rate of turbulent airflow within the airways. The oxygen cost of a given BTPS ventilation is thus reduced, and the required STPD ventilation can be sustained with only a slight increase in the oxygen usage of the chest muscles relative to sea-level values.

Pulmonary Diffusion

The pulmonary diffusing capacity limits oxygen transport more at altitude than at sea level. We have seen that equilibration between alveolar gas and the pulmonary capillary blood varies as $D_L/\lambda Q$, where D_L is

the diffusing capacity, λ is a dimensionless factor describing the solubility of oxygen in the blood, and Q is the cardiac output (or more precisely, the pulmonary blood flow). The cardiac output at any given work-rate is not greatly changed at moderate altitudes, but since the reduction in arterial oxygen saturation now causes the subject to operate over the steep part of the oxygen dissociation curve, the solubility factor λ and thus the denominator in the equilibration calculation is increased. Moreover, for the purposes of our calculation D_L must be expressed per unit of concentration gradient (milliliter per minute per milliliter per liter) rather than in the usual units of milliliter per minute per mm Hg, and the value in millimeter per minute per milliliter per liter is substantially reduced at the altitudes of interest to athletes. Oxygen equilibration remains reasonably complete in the average alveolus, but saturation of the pulmonary venous blood becomes incomplete in those parts of the lung where the ratio of pulmonary diffusing capacity to blood flow is low and the capillary transit time is short. On the other hand, the impact upon arterial oxygen saturation of shunts that bypass the lungs becomes smaller at altitude, since there is a smaller disparity of oxygen content between pulmonary venous and mixed venous blood.

Cardiovascular Adjustments

Cardiac stroke volume both at rest and in moderate exercise may be reduced in the first few days at altitude. This reflects (1) fluid shifts and a resultant decrease of blood volume secondary to changes of acid–base balance, (2) water loss from hyperventilation in cold and dry mountain air, and (3) an effect of oxygen lack on the tissue capillary permeability, with an increased exudation of plasma into the tissues. Although blood volume is reduced by these several factors, there is a useful increase of hemoglobin concentration (and thus the amount of oxygen transported per liter of cardiac output) at the expense of some increase in the viscosity of the blood.

The maximum cardiac output is further reduced by a decline of maximum heart rate. Although the bradycardia can sometimes be reversed by the administration of oxygen, myocardial hypoxia is not the only cause of the low maximum heart rate. A reflex (vagally-mediated) slowing also seems to be involved, since normal values can often be restored by giving an injection of atropine.

Impact on Performance

The net result of the ventilatory and circulatory changes is a decrease in maximum oxygen intake of about 3.2 percent for each 300 meters of altitude in excess of 1,800 meters (Fig. 11-3). In the newcomer to altitude, the impact of the decrease in ambient pres-

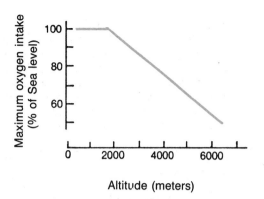

Figure 11–3 Influence of altitude on maximum oxygen intake. Note that because of such factors as the Sigmoid Phase of the oxygen dissociation curve, altitudes to 1,800 meters have little effect on oxygen transport, but at higher altitudes there is a decrease of a little over 1 percent per 100 meters of altitude. (After Shephard RJ. Physiology and biochemistry of exercise. New York: Praeger, 1982.)

sures upon physical performance may be greater than suggested by those figures, due to the adverse effects of an altered climate, loss of sleep, and (sometimes) gastrointestinal infections.

On the other hand, in the Mexico City Olympics new records were set in many types of competition. Performance in short-distance runs and in throwing events was helped by the diminished air resistance, while in longer endurance-type events, the performance handicap was less than the theoretical 7 to 8 percent because of (1) the progressive improvement of Olympic records from one competition to the next, (2) victories won by high-altitude natives such as the Kenyans, and (3) the substantial periods of altitude training and acclimatization that were adopted by many native sea-level athletes.

Anaerobic Work

At any given absolute work-rate, there is a greater accumulation of lactate at altitude than at sea level. However, anaerobic capacity and power are largely unchanged at altitude, unless there has been a major disturbance of tissue buffers (which can occur as a result of hyperventilation, elimination of carbon dioxide, and a compensatory reduction of bicarbonate reserves). The rate of lactate buildup in submaximal work is much as at sea level if the intensity of effort is expressed as a percent of the altitude-specific maximum oxygen intake.

High Altitudes

Simple compensatory mechanisms such as operation over the steep part of the oxygen dissociation curve no longer provide effective relief at the high altitudes reached by some mountaineers (5,000 to 8,000 meters).

Chest movements increase to the point where the oxygen cost of breathing accounts for a large fraction of the maximum oxygen intake, leaving little of the transported oxygen available for the needs of the leg muscles. Ascent then becomes a laborious process, and the climber must stop every few paces to allow oxidation of anaerobic metabolites.

ACCLIMATIZATION TO HIGH ALTITUDE

Respiratory Adaptations

While a "hunting" pattern of intermittent respiration (over-ventilation, followed by hypoventilation or a cessation of breathing, and then a further bout of hyperventilation) is characteristic of the newcomer to high altitude, this phenomenon is progressively lost over 3 to 6 weeks residence in the mountain environment. The first change, seen within 24 hours, is a decrease in the buffering capacity of the cerebrospinal fluid. This restores a normal pH in the immediate vicinity of the medullary chemoreceptors, facilitating central respiratory control. Over the next several weeks, the buffering capacity of arterial blood is also reduced. In consequence, the regulation of respiration is largely shifted back from the carotid chemoreceptors (where the signal is oxygen lack) to the medulla (which responds to CO_2 accumulation, but is little influenced by moderate changes in arterial oxygen pressure); in consequence, a sea level ventilation can be sustained without periodic problems of hypocapnia and interruption of breathing. Nevertheless, the increased discharge rate of the carotid chemoreceptors persists throughout exposure to low ambient pressures, and at very high altitudes the peripheral signal continues to play an important part in the regulation of ventilation. After acclimatization, the overall increase of respiratory minute volume that becomes possible is sufficient to boost alveolar oxygen pressures by the equivalent of a 1,000 meters decrease of altitude, with a 20 percent gain of maximum oxygen transport. The diminution of bicarbonate buffering in the adapted individual hampers CO_2 transport, but this disadvantage is offset at least in part by the increase of hemoglobin (since hemoglobin is also an important blood buffer).

The pulmonary diffusing capacity is augmented by the increase of hemoglobin concentration, and with long periods of residence, there may also be anatomic adaptations in lung structure (including an increase in the number of both alveoli and pulmonary capillaries).

Cardiovascular and Cellular Adaptations

The total blood volume is progressively restored toward the normal sea-level value if a person remains at altitude. The plasma volume remains subnormal, but there is an increase of red cell mass. New red cell production increases the red cell count at a rate of 1 to 2 percent per day. At first, large and immature red cells are seen, but once adaptation is complete, the cells have a normal hemoglobin content and a normal lifespan. Within the active muscle tissues, there is also an increase of myoglobin and of aerobic enzymes.

At rest and during moderate activity the heart rate, cardiac output, and regional blood flow all revert toward sea level values as the respiratory minute volume and hemoglobin concentration increase. However, the stroke volume remains low, suggesting a possible residual effect of hypoxia upon myocardial contractility. The maximum heart rate also remains lower than at sea level. At altitudes above 3,000 meters, residents show a high pulmonary arterial pressure. While this has the useful effect of increasing blood flow through the poorly perfused apical regions of the lungs (thus improving the matching of blood flow to ventilation), it eventually induces adverse reactions in the pulmonary vessels, particularly an increased muscularity of the arterioles, with a progressive increase of pulmonary arterial pressures and a reduction of pulmonary diffusing capacity.

Recommendation on Acclimatization

The ideal period of acclimatization for athletes who must compete at moderately high altitudes is still debated. Some authors favor several weeks of adjustment to the new environment, but this carries a number of disadvantages: (1) a slackening of the intensity of training, (2) a progressive loss of fluid from the circulation with a resultant decrease of stroke volume, and (3) adverse medical and psychological reactions to the unaccustomed environment. The optimum recommendation is probably a 3–day period of adaptation. This allows an adjustment of acid–base balance, a recovery from any "mountain sickness," an opportunity to learn an appropriate competitive pace for the new environment, and some increase of hemoglobin level without courting the various problems associated with a longer sojourn.

The Contribution of Genes

The relative importance of genes and environment to the adaptations seen in a high-altitude native remains uncertain. Typical features of the high-altitude native include a greater chest size, a larger pulmonary capillary bed, a greater cardiac volume, cardiac output, and hemoglobin level, and larger bone marrow. The carotid bodies are also of above average size, but they show a low sensitivity to both CO_2 and O_2 lack. Such peculiarities could reflect either colonization of mountainous regions by tribes with a favourable genetic endowment or childhood adaptations consequent upon exposure to low oxygen pressures from an early age.

ALTITUDE TRAINING CAMPS

Some athletes have had interest in the possibility that their sea-level performance might be enhanced by (1) a period of residence at high altitude, or (2) prolonged breathing of low-oxygen mixtures at sea level. At least one laboratory has advocated training while breathing through a long tube, an arrangement that assures exposure to both low oxygen and high CO_2 pressures.

Immediately after return to sea level from an altitude training camp, athletes show a tendency to hyperventilation. This reflects a deficiency of cerebrospinal buffers (particularly bicarbonate ions), a problem that is corrected within a few hours. The altitude-induced increase of red cell count is lost more slowly—for example, one-third of the increment seen after residence at 600 meters is still present after 17 days at sea level. In theory, there might thus be some gain of endurance performance for several days after return from an altitude training facility. However, in practice, any theoretical advantage from the greater hemoglobin concentration is largely offset by the learning of an incorrect pace and a lessening of training while at altitude. Thus most national teams no longer favor the use of altitude training camps.

PATHOLOGICAL REACTIONS TO HIGH ALTITUDE

Pathological reactions to high altitudes include "mountain sickness," high altitude deterioration, and high altitude edema.

Mountain Sickness

The normal threshold for the appearance of mountain sickness is thought to be exposure to an altitude of 3,000 to 3,500 meters, although with very vigorous training or participation in repeated athletic "heats," problems sometimes extend to more moderate altitudes.

Symptoms include loss of appetite, nausea, vomiting, and muscle weakness, with incoordination, lassitude or fatigue, irritability, headache, and loss of sleep. The condition develops progressively after a few hours at altitude, peaks at about 48 hours, and then regresses as the person becomes acclimatized to the new environment.

The physiological bases for the disturbance includes (1) the influence of low O_2 and CO_2 pressures on the tissue oxygen supply, and (2) disturbances of the intracellular fluid balance owing to either acid–base disturbances or anoxic failure of the sodium pump in cell membranes. Gastrointestinal symptoms seem related in part to alterations in both the volume and composition of pancreatic secretions. Immediate complaints are reduced by administration of the carbonic anhydrase inhibitor acetazolamide, although it is not clear whether this drug acts by increasing CO_2 retention (thus allowing a rise in bicarbonate stores), or whether it promotes diuresis (thus correcting fluid retention). Irrespective of mechanisms, the long-term value of carbonic anhydrase inhibition is debatable, since the adaptive diminution of plasma bicarbonate is slowed by the use of this drug, while the decrease of plasma volume is exacerbated, and the deterioration of psychomotor performance is not always corrected.

High-Altitude Deterioration

While exceptional individuals such as the Sherpa, Tensing, have conquered Mount Everest without breathing cylinder mixtures of oxygen, 5,500 meters seems about the limit of adaptation for the average person without some supplementation of the oxygen supply.

At very high altitudes, some climbers show a progressive worsening of condition ("high altitude deterioration"). Sleep is lost, appetite becomes poor, body mass and physical working capacity diminish, and the affected individual becomes gradually more lethargic over the course of several weeks.

One major feature of high-altitude deterioration is a severe water loss, due to changes of the acid–base balance, hyperventilation in cold, dry air, and vigorous sweating induced by a combination of hard physical work and solar radiation. A daily fluid intake of 3 liters or more, while needed for equilibrium, may be difficult to sustain when the low barometric pressure restricts the preparation of attractive hot beverages (for instance, water cannot be boiled to a hot enough temperature to brew a good cup of tea). The diet of the mountaineer may also be poor and unpalatable, since only limited rations are carried, and it is difficult to cook in a small tent. The energy intake may drop far below the daily energy expenditure. Problems in maintaining fluid and energy balance are frequently compounded by illness, intense mental and physical stress, severe cold exposure, and sleep loss. Hyperventilation may divert much of the maximum oxygen intake to the respiratory muscles, so that even a bowel movement creates an excessive ventilatory demand. Finally, the heat loss of saturating expired gas with water vapor may exceed the body's potential heat production, with a resultant progressive drop in core temperature.

High altitude deterioration is best prevented by insisting on an adequate intake of food and fluid. Once the condition is established, the only practical remedy is rapid evacuation to a lower altitude.

High-Altitude Edema

An intense waterlogging of the lungs (pulmonary edema) is sometimes seen 9 to 36 hours after climbing to an altitude over 3,000 meters. Clinical features include an acute shortness of breath, a blood-stained and watery phlegm, chest discomfort, cough, nausea, and vomiting. Examination discloses breath sounds typical of an alveolar exudate, with an ECG tracing that is typical of right heart strain and intense pulmonary vascular congestion on a posteroanterior chest film. Attacks seem most common in young men who return to vigorous work immediately on reaching high altitude following a period of residence at sea level. Often there is a history of an associated respiratory infection.

Factors contributing to the pulmonary edema include (1) an increase of central blood volume secondary to CO_2 washout and peripheral vasoconstriction, (2) pulmonary venous constriction caused by the low alveolar oxygen tension, (3) an increase of total blood volume following earlier exposure to altitude, (4) an increase of cardiac output (induced by the combination of heavy physical work and oxygen lack), (5) a hypoxic reduction of myocardial contractility, and (6) an increase in permeability of the pulmonary vessels due to a combination of hypoxia and respiratory infection.

Attacks are generally avoided by an appropriate period of acclimatization. Established cases require hospital treatment, including bed rest, oxygen, and an administration of antibiotics to avoid secondary infection.

FURTHER READING

Bennett PB. The aetiology of compressed air intoxication and inert gas narcosis. Oxford: Pergamon Press, 1966.

Bennett PB, Elliott DH. The physiology and medicine of diving and compressed air work. London: Baillière, Tindall & Cassell, 1969.

Brendel W, Zink RA. High altitude physiology and medicine. New York: Springer Verlag, 1982.

Empleton BE, Lanphier EH, Young JE, Goff LG. The new science of skin and scuba diving (3rd Ed.). New York: Association Press, 1970.

Gillies JA. A textbook of aviation physiology. Oxford: Pergamon Press, 1965.

Goddard R. International symposium on the effects of altitude on physical performance. Chicago: Athletic Institute, 1967.

Houston CS. High altitude physiology study—collected papers. Calgary, Alberta: Arctic Institute of North America, 1980.

Jokl E, Jokl P. Exercise and altitude. Basel: Karger, 1968.

Lambertsen CJ. Underwater physiology. Baltimore: Williams & Wilkins, 1967.

Lambertsen CJ. Underwater physiology. Proceedings of the IVth Symposium on Underwater Physiology. New York: Academic Press, 1971.

Margaria R. Exercise at altitude. Amsterdam: Excerpta Medica, 1967.

Miles S. Underwater medicine. London: Staples Press, 1962.

Porter R, Knight J. High altitude physiology: Cardiac and respiratory aspects. Edinburgh: Churchill-Livingstone, 1971.

Rahn H, Yokoyama T. Physiology of breath-hold diving and the ama of Japan. Washington, DC: National Academy of Sciences, 1965.

Sutton JR, Coates G. Pathophysiology of high altitude illnesses. Exerc Sport Sci Rev 1983; 11:210–231.

Sutton JS, Houston CS, Jones NL. Hypoxia, exercise and altitude. New York: Liss, 1983.

West JH, Lahiri S. High altitude and man. Bethesda, Md: American Physiological Society, 1984.

Woods JD, Lythgoe JN. Underwater science. An introduction to experiments by divers. Oxford: Oxford University Press, 1971.

EXTREMES OF AMBIENT TEMPERATURE

CHAPTER *12*

THE CONCEPT OF BODY TEMPERATURE

Extent of Homiothermy

Humans are homeotherms—that is, they regulate body temperatures within a fairly close range, even when faced by a major disturbance of heat flux due to vigorous activity or a severe environment. However, it is useful to note at the outset of this chapter that thermal regulation is incomplete. Core temperature increases by 0.5⁰ C from early morning to afternoon or evening (a circadian rhythm) and from the first to the second half of the menstrual cycle. In a marathon runner, the body temperature may also rise by 4⁰ C over the course of a race, and a swim across the English channel or Lake Ontario can depress body temperature by 2⁰ C or more.

Likewise, there are substantial variations of temperature from one part of the body to another. The limbs are usually cooler than more central regions, although after a hard bout of running the legs may be warmer than the body core. The mean body temperature is often calculated as 65 percent of the core reading plus 35 percent of skin readings averaged over 8 to 12 sites.

Measuring Body Temperature

The core reading may be estimated using a clinical thermometer inserted into the rectum, a fine wire thermocouple resting lightly on the eardrum or in the esophagus, or a radio-transmitting "thermal pill," which is swallowed and retained in the gastrointestinal tract. The sublingual temperature, although commonly used by clinicians to detect a fever, is not a suitable index of body temperature after exercising, since the tongue is cooled several degrees by mouth-breathing in cold air. Sometimes the rectal temperature is also in error, falsely high readings being obtained because of a current of hot blood returning from the exercising legs.

Skin temperatures are generally measured by taping thermocouples to representative areas of the body surface. Various weighting factors have been proposed when calculating an average skin temperature—for example, Hardy and DuBois proposed taking 7 percent of the head reading, with 14 percent from the arms, 5 percent from the hands, 7 percent from the feet, 13 percent from the legs, 19 percent from the thighs, and 35 percent from the trunk.

Acceptable Limits of Core Temperature

The highest core temperature compatible with a full subsequent recovery of cerebral function is 42⁰ C, although terminal readings of 43.5⁰ C have been recorded just before death of the affected individual.

Those working in hot environments such as deep mines are usually held to a pace that keeps core temperatures below 39.2⁰ C, to give some margin of protection against heat illnesses. However, much higher temperatures than this are frequent when endurance competitions are held during the summer months.

Body function is also impaired if core temperatures drop below 36⁰ C, and consciousness is usually clouded with a reading of less than 35⁰ C, although some swimmers have concluded their participation in distance events such as a Lake Ontario swim with final temperatures as low as 34.0 to 34.5⁰ C. The shivering mechanism fails below 34⁰ C, and at 32⁰ C, vasodilatation of the skin gives a rapid and dangerous heat loss.

Comfort and Thermal Neutrality

A person feels comfortable in a thermally neutral environment (when the body is neither losing nor gaining heat). While 23 to 25⁰ C is an appropriate thermally neutral air temperature for a lightly clothed and sedentary office-worker, 19 to 21⁰ C is more comfortable if moderate physical activity is required.

When assessing room temperature, signals from the skin (particularly over the limbs) are interpreted relative to the intensity of activity, skin blood flow, and the intensity of sweating or shivering. The target temperature for the skin seems to be in the range of 32.0 to 32.5⁰ C. Water conducts heat away from the body more readily than air, so that a comfortable thermally-neutral water temperature is 20 to 30⁰ C for a vigorous swimmer, and 35 to 37⁰ C for an instructor who is merely standing in a pool.

MECHANISMS OF HEAT EXCHANGE

Temperature and Energy Balance

The body, like other machines, is not 100 percent efficient (Chapter 1). Exchange of heat with the environment is thus essential to continued metabolism. The quantity of heat to be dissipated is equal to the metabolic rate (M) minus the useful external work that is performed (W).

If the subject is to be in thermal equilibrium, heat production must be matched by heat exchanged through conduction (C), convection (K), radiation (R), and evaporation (E). Under unstable conditions, there are also changes in body heat stores (S). The total equation for thermal balance thus becomes:

$$(M - W) = E \pm C \pm K \pm R \pm S$$

Heat Stores

The body can be regarded as storing heat, because its temperature is normally higher than that of the environment. The size of the heat store depends on the temperature differential between the body and its immediate environment, the body mass, and the specific heat of the tissues (the last, being the amount of heat needed to raise the tissue temperature by 1^0 C, is about 3.48 kJ per gram).

The maximum safe heating of the body is about 4^0 C, or (assuming a uniform heat distribution) 835 kJ in a 60-kg woman ($4 \times 60 \times 3.48 = 835$ kJ). If the subject is working with a mechanical efficiency of 25 percent, and the metabolic rate is 60 kJ per minute, the potential heat store could thus be filled within 835/45, or 18.6 minutes. Acceptable cooling of 2^0 C in a 60-kg subject might be thought to imply a heat loss of no more than 418 kJ, or in a situation where the heat loss is 2 kJ per minute (for example, a subject who is wearing arctic clothing and sitting in still air at -40^0 C) some 200 minutes of cold exposure. In fact, peripheral cooling is usually much greater than that of the core, so the possible period of exposure is increased several fold.

A corollary of the heat storage concept is that any loss of fluid inevitably raises body temperature. If a young woman weighing 60 kg has a body temperature of 37^0 C while exercising on a track heated to an air temperature of 20^0 C, her initial heat store is $17 \times 60 \times 3.48 = 3550$ kJ. After she has lost 2 ℓ of sweat, body mass is only 58 kg, so that (other factors being equal), the stored heat must be accommodated by increasing the average body temperature to 37.6^0 C ($17.6 \times 58 \times 3.48 = 3550$ kJ). In practice, of course, much of the sweat is evaporated, and the latent heat of vaporization provides compensatory cooling.

Conduction

Conduction normally accounts for only a small fraction of total heat transfer. However, appreciable conduction of heat to the body occurs when walking barefoot on hot sand, while heat is lost from the body when wearing inadequately insulated boots in snow, or when immersed in cold water.

Convection

Convection involves a forced transfer of heat, whether caused by the movement of gas or fluid. The quantity of heat that is exchanged depends on the temperature gradient, the thermal conductivity of the gas or fluid, and the volume flow per unit area at the exchanging surface. The three main barriers to convective heat loss from the body are (1) a thin film of stationary air or water in immediate contact with the outer surface of the skin or clothing, (2) air trapped inside the clothing, and (3) the layer of subcutaneous fat.

The first of these barriers is generally the most important. In animals (but to a much lesser extent in humans) the thickness of the air film can be increased by piloerection (making the hair or fur stand on end). Heat loss is greatly increased if movement over the surface of the skin and/or clothing is augmented by (1) a stiff breeze or water current, (2) movement of the limbs (e.g., running or swimming), and (3) passive movement of the body (e.g., downhill skiing or snowmobiling). At high altitudes, the decrease of gas density reduces the extent of convection, while underwater gas convection of heat is increased by both the increase of gas density and the breathing of gases with a high thermal conductivity (such as helium). The combined heat transfer by conduction and convection proceeds about 20 times as fast in water as in air.

Radiation

Objects radiate energy at a rate dependent on the nature of their surface and their absolute temperature (which is measured in degrees Kelvin, 0^0 K $= -273^0$ C). At body temperature (310^0 K), radiation proceeds much as would be expected for a black surface (that is, with little reflection of heat). Solar radiation obviously comes from a source of much higher temperature than the body. Radiation from the body into space is then negligible relative to energy received from the sun. The wavelength of solar heating is also shorter than the radiation emitted by the body. Thus, there is an appreciable reflection of the sun's rays from skin and light-colored clothing. In a hot and dry climate, a light colored suit can halve the radiant heat load. This would otherwise amount to perhaps 15 kJ per minute during the afternoon, when the sun is fairly low and the ground is warm; however, at midday, when the sun is immediately overhead, the body presents a smaller total surface to the sun, and the radiant load is only about 6 kJ per minute.

Evaporation

The evaporation of 1 g of water dissipates 2.43 kJ of energy (due to the latent heat of vaporization of water). The maximum rate of sweat secretion is about 30 mℓ per minute, and once the skin has been fully wetted by the sweat, some 40 to 50 percent of this volume is evaporated (the rest merely rolls to the ground). The corresponding heat dissipation averages 29 to 36 kJ per minute (although this figure can be influenced by air speed and the water deficit of ambient air—the difference between the observed water content and that needed for 100 percent saturation, measured at skin temperature).

In addition to sweating, there is a small "insensible perspiration" of about 0.35 mℓ per minute, which always occurs at the skin surface (thermal cost 0.8 to 0.9 kJ per minute), and a respiratory water loss (as expired air becomes saturated with water vapor). The latter loss may rise to 300 mℓ per hour (5 mℓ per minute) in a cold dry climate, thus giving rise to a heat dissipation of 13 kJ per minute.

MEASURING CLIMATE

Climate may be assessed in physical or in subjective terms. Physical data to be considered include wet and dry bulb temperatures, air speed, and globe thermometer readings. Subjective scales equate sweat rate relative to the comfort of partially-clothed industrial workers.

Minard Index

Minard developed a wet bulb, globe thermometer index (WBGT) for marine recruits training both indoors and outdoors:

WBGT indoors = 0.7 (T_W) + 0.3 (T_D)
WBGT outdoors = 0.7 (T_W) + 0.2 (T_G) + 0.1 (T_D)

The wet bulb thermometer (T_W) has a wick, moistened with distilled water—evaporative cooling is produced by whirling the bulb of the thermometer in a "sling psychrometer" or by using a small fan to draw a steady air current over the wick. The globe temperature (T_G) is measured from a thermometer whose bulb is suspended inside a black globe. In order to adjust for reflection of radiation at the skin surface and postural effects (the projected area of the body relative to the angle of solar radiation), the globe can be painted an appropriate shade of grey rather than black. The dry bulb temperature is obtained from a standard thermometer that is kept away from radiant heat sources.

Minard suggested caution was necessary when exercising if the WBGT exceeded 28° C, and that the training of unacclimatized recruits should be restricted if the WBGT was higher than 29.5° C. More recently, the United States National Institute of Occupational Safety and Health proposed a limiting WBGT of 30° C for light work (14 kJ per minute), 27.8° C for moderate work (14 to 21 kJ per minute), and 26.1° C for heavy work (>21 kJ per minute). The American College of Sports Medicine has recommended cancelling a road race if the WBGT exceeds 28° C. A figure of 23 to 28° C implies a high risk that some of the contestants in a distance event will develop heat stress. If the starting temperature is between 18 and 23° C, some caution is still needed as air temperature, humidity, and radiation may all increase over the day. Below 18° C, the risks are much lower, although it is still possible for sensitive individuals to develop some degree of heat stress.

Effective Temperature

The effective temperature is a temperature that would provide a level of comfort equivalent to the observed conditions if the ambient air were still and saturated with water vapor (Fig. 12–1). The original nomogram for the calculation of effective temperature was based on the comfort of young men stripped to the waist and engaged in moderate activity. Some adjustment of values is necessary when performing more vigorous exercise while wearing different amounts of clothing.

Predicted 4-Hour Sweat Rate

The predicted 4-hour sweat rate (P4SR, Fig. 12–2) is also calculated by means of a nomogram. The P4SR is designed to integrate the heat stress imposed by a given combination of environment, clothing, and physical activity. The point of entry to the wet bulb scale on the nomogram is adjusted upwards by Δ_t if the globe temperature (T_G) exceeds the dry bulb temperature (T_D) ($\Delta_t = 0.4 [T_G - T_D]$), if the metabolic rate exceeds 3.8 kJ per minute per m^2 of body surface area,

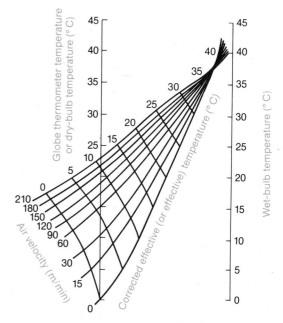

Figure 12–1 Nomogram for the calculation of effective temperature (equivalent comfort of men stripped to the waist and performing moderate exercise) at selected air velocities. If the "corrected effective temperature" is calculated, the globe temperature is used in place of the dry bulb reading (based on a chart published by the American Society of Heating, Refrigerating and Air Conditioning Engineers, 1967).

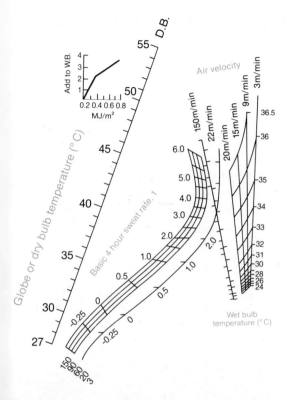

Figure 12–2 A nomogram for the prediction of 4-hour sweat rate of men wearing shorts. Note that the wet bulb temperature used to predict thermal stress is increased by a factor Δ_t under the following circumstances: (1) if the globe temperature (T_G) exceeds the dry bulb temperature (T_D), $\Delta_t = 0.4\,(T_G - T_D)$, (2) if the metabolic rate exceeds the energy cost of sitting, the wet bulb temperature is augmented, and (3) if the men are wearing industrial clothing such as overalls, the wet bulb temperature is increased by 1° C. (Modified from Kerslake).

or if the clothing assembly provides more insulation than army shorts.

THERMOREGULATION

The main temperature regulating centers are in the hypothalamus. Acute adjustment to heat is achieved by a combination of cutaneous vasodilatation and sweating, and in cold the options include (1) vasoconstriction, (2) increased physical activity, (3) the wearing of additional clothing, (4) shivering, and (5) at least in some species "non-shivering" thermogenesis (through an increased heat production in brown fat).

Heat Exposure

Circulatory Adjustments. Skin blood flow is increased by a release of sympathetic vasoconstrictor tone in the hands and feet, active vasodilatation over the trunk and proximal parts of the limbs, a release of

bradykinin from the sweat glands, and a direct effect of temperature on the vessels. In light activity, cutaneous blood flow can reach 9 to 10 ℓ per minute, adding substantially to the cardiac cost of a given level of physical activity. With more vigorous and sustained exercise, much of the skin flow is redirected to muscle (increasing the risk of heat stress). The exercise-induced reduction of visceral blood flow is also exaggerated in the heat, but nevertheless the total circulatory demand is greater than under temperate conditions.

The veins share in the peripheral vasodilatation, so that as core temperature rises, their capacity is enhanced for a given distending pressure. The resultant reduction of central blood flow is enhanced by a rapid exudation of fluid into the active tissues, reflecting an increase of (1) capillary pressure, (2) capillary permeability, and (3) extravascular leakage of protein. At any given power output, stroke volume thus decreases and heart rate rises if exercise is sustained in the heat. The decline in overall circulatory function causes a progressive diminution in flow to the viscera as exercise continues, with a danger of ischemia in the liver (shown by a decreased elimination of substances such as sulfobromophthalein and an escape of hepatic enzymes into the blood stream), in the kidneys (seen as renal failure and an accumulation of urea in the blood stream), and in the adrenal glands (the condition of heat shock, with an impaired secretion of adrenal cortical hormones).

Little oxygen is extracted from blood that is directed to the skin. The mean arteriovenous oxygen difference at a given power output is thus reduced in the heat. There is also less rise of systemic blood pressure. The resulting decrease of muscle blood flow leads to (1) a greater usage of glycogen reserves, and (2) a greater accumulation of lactate in submaximal exercise. In a hot environment, the heart rate at an oxygen intake of 22 mℓ per kilogram per minute is increased by 17 to 18 beats per minute, while at an oxygen intake of 32 mℓ per kilogram per minute it is increased by 7 to 8 beats per minute. Over short periods of heat stress, there is little reduction of maximum oxygen intake, but aerobic power is diminished if heat exposure or exercise lasts long enough to cause a peripheral sequestration of fluid.

Sweat Production. Sweating is stimulated mainly by an increase of core and skin temperatures, but other sources of input to the thermo-regulatory centers of the hypothalamus are the venous thermoreceptors, neuromuscular reflexes, and the osmoreceptors of the plasma. The maximum sweat rate (about 2 ℓ per hour) is sufficiently large that physical activity is often limited by the ability to evaporate sweat rather than the ability to produce it. Until the skin is completely wetted, the rate of evaporation depends on the area of the sweat film. Sweat usually begins to drip from the body when production reaches about one-third of the maximum sweat rate. Swimming in warm water is poorly tolerated, since sweating then depletes the blood volume without contributing anything to the cooling of the body. Local overactivity of the sweat glands may occur in parts of the body that are excessively clothed. With prolonged exposure to a combination of heat, high humidity, and excessive clothing, the skin becomes macerated, and this is probably the main reason why sweat production declines over the course of 3 to 4 hours of heat stress, even if body fluid volumes are well maintained.

At any given rate of working, a person who is acclimatized to a hot environment sweats earlier and in greater quantities than a person who is accustomed to temperate conditions. Trained subjects sweat less at a given absolute power output. However, they produce as much sweat as an untrained individual at a lower rectal temperature, and they can probably produce more sweat than an untrained person during maximum effort. There is a considerable degree of interaction between heat acclimatization and endurance training.

While heat stress alone tends to deplete the plasma volume, exercise in a warm environment also decreases the volume of tissue fluid. Repeated bouts of exercise in a hot climate can cause cumulative disturbances of both fluid and mineral balance.

Cold Exposure

Circulatory Adjustments. Cold exposure causes cutaneous vasoconstriction, with increases of peripheral vascular resistance, systemic blood pressure, and afterloading of the heart. The effective insulation of the fat is increased if blood is no longer flowing through it, and a reduction of blood flow to the muscles of the limbs has a similar insulating effect.

In extreme cold, paralysis of the smooth muscle in the walls of the arterioles may cause a paradoxical vasodilatation and a "hunting" reaction (where wide dilatation of the vessels alternates with periods of intense vasoconstriction). Venous return from the limbs is diverted from the superficial vessels to the venae comitantes, vessels that run on either side of the main arterial supply. With this arrangement, heat is exchanged between arterial and venous blood, and peripheral cooling is minimized.

Voluntary Activity. If vasoconstriction is not enough to counteract body cooling, the subject can increase metabolic heat production by exercising. However, this is a less helpful tactic than might be imagined, since the accompanying movements of the limbs displace the film of stationary air or water on the surface of the clothing, and unless the garments are well-closed at the neck and around the hands and feet, cold air or water may also be pumped underneath them. In cold air, a metabolic activity as large as 15 kJ per minute must be produced by exercising in order to counter a heat loss of 2 kJ per minute observed while sitting at rest. Likewise, if a sailor is tipped into cold

water by the capsizing of a boat, attempts at swimming pump cold water over and under clothing; it is thus a better tactic to huddle in a fetal position (which minimizes the effective body surface) than to swim (unless the shore is close at hand).

Assessing Clothing. The insulating value of clothing is commonly assessed in CLO or TOG units. Originally, 1 CLO corresponded to the insulation provided by standard British indoor clothing such as a business suit. As the unit became more standardized, it was regarded as sufficient covering to assure comfort at a temperature of 21° C, with an air velocity of 10.2 cm per second and a relative humidity of less than 50 percent. More recently, this somewhat arbitrary index has been translated into precise Standard International units of heat transfer; 1 CLO offers a thermal gradient of 2.58° C for a heat flux of 1 kJ per minute per m² of surface. The military clothing that is worn in the arctic provides 4 CLO of insulation, and the double layer of caribou skin chosen by the Inuit during the coldest months of their winter hunting offers as much as 11 CLO of protection. Given a 4 CLO assembly, an exercising subject with a metabolic heat production of 15 kJ per minute can remain in thermal equilibrium in still air at −40° C (Fig. 12–3).

For most activities, the insulation provided by clothing should be variable. If garments are allowed to become soaked with sweat during bouts of hard work, much of their insulation is destroyed. Mist or rain has an equally disastrous impact upon insulating properties, and if the ambient temperature is above

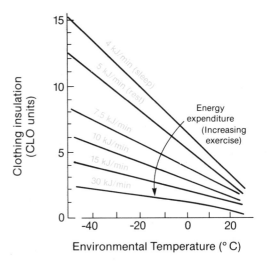

Figure 12–3 Insulating value of clothing needed for thermal equilibrium at various environmental temperatures and various rates of exercise. Note that for equilibrium, the activity must more than make good the resting heat loss. For example, in still air at −40° C, the rate of cooling is −2 kJ per minute, but an energy expenditure of 15 kJ per minute is needed to restore equilibrium.

freezing it is important to provide an outer, waterproof layer. In some respects, it is more difficult to protect subjects against cold, driving rain than against snow (which falls off the surface of the clothing). In the arctic, the best simple type of clothing assembly is a tightly woven outer sailcloth (to protect against the wind) and an inner blanket, (which traps air warmed by body heat).

Effects of Grease. In cold water, additional protection is sometimes sought by applying a layer of lanolin or Vaseline to the skin. The insulation is similar to that provided by body fat—a 1 mm layer generates a thermal gradient of 0.14 to 0.17° C at rest, but 1.4 to 1.7° C if there is a tenfold increase of metabolism as during distance swimming.

Effects of Shivering. The final recourse of the cold-exposed subject is an increase of metabolism. While cold exposure may induce some changes of metabolism without visible shivering ("nonshivering thermogenesis"—for example, a leakage of protons at the mitochondrial membranes of brown fat), the main method of boosting heat production is shivering. This involves an increase of muscle tone with a periodic, simultaneous contraction of agonists and antagonists that causes a violent oscillation of the limbs.

Unless activity is in itself vigorous enough to sustain core temperature, the energy cost of exercise in the cold is increased by shivering (Fig. 12–4). The peak energy usage during violent shivering is equivalent to about five times basal metabolism, or 22 to 25 kJ per minute. Since there is less limb displacement during shivering than during many types of exercise, it may be more effective than vigorous activity as a method of restoring core temperature. It remains uncertain whether the prime stimulus to shivering comes from the cutaneous cold receptors or from a general decrease in the peripheral heat content of the body.

Effects on Neural Function. The velocity of nerve conduction, and thus the speed of reflex responses, decreases as local temperature falls. Nerve block is complete at 8 to 10° C. Discomfort and a deterioration of skilled psychomotor performance is seen with a heat loss of 170 kJ per m² of body surface, and the maximum safe heat loss is about 340 kJ per m².

ACCLIMATIZATION TO HEAT AND COLD

Terminology

Physiologists have attempted to distinguish three rather similar words—acclimation, acclimatization, and adaptation—when discussing reactions to a harsh environment such as extreme heat or cold. Acclimation was originally conceived as the process of becoming habituated to a new environment, although some authors have also used this term to describe physiolog-

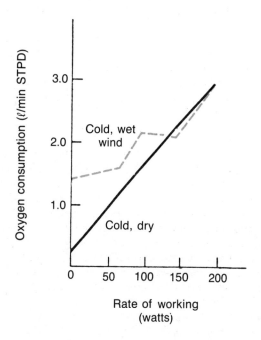

Figure 12–4 To illustrate how the energy cost of walking under cold dry conditions is boosted by shivering when the subject is drenched and exposed to a strong wind (based on experiments of Pugh, 1972).

ical adjustments to heat or cold that develop under controlled experiments such as a hot or a cold environmental chamber. Acclimatization is the normal term for the functional compensations made over several days or weeks of exposure to the totality of a new environment (for example, the Canadian who flies from a Winnipeg winter to the unaccustomed milieu of South India). Adaptation reflects more long-term adjustments—including genetic changes—which fit the individual to life in a specific environment. In the context of climate, acclimation is well-recognized by the subject; after a few days of exposure, extremes of both heat and cold become much more bearable. There is also obvious physiological evidence of acclimatization to extremes of heat, but proof of the occurrence of physiological acclimatization to cold is more sketchy, and there is relatively little evidence of long-term anatomical adaptations to either extreme of temperature.

Heat Acclimatization

The primary physiological change during heat acclimatization is an earlier and a greater production of sweat for a given rise of core temperature. In a well-acclimatized subject, sweat production may be as much as doubled.

Because of the increased sweating, the skin temperature is lower when in a hot environment, and more heat is carried to the skin per unit of blood flow. If heat dissipation was previously inadequate, the acclimatized person may show an increased blood flow to the skin, but more usually, acclimatization allows a part of the superficial blood flow to be redirected from the skin to the viscera and to the working muscles. These changes, together with an increase in tone of the venous capacity vessels and some expansion of plasma volume, account for a lower heart rate and an increased stroke volume when an acclimatized individual exercises at any given power output.

Acclimatized subjects also show an increased secretion of the hormone aldosterone. This reduces the sodium content of sweat and urine, while increasing the excretion of potassium ions. There may also be a reduced secretion of thyroid hormone with prolonged heat exposure. Such a change of endocrine activity would link carbohydrate metabolism more closely to the resynthesis of phosphagen, thus allowing a reduction of basal metabolism. Finally, there are adjustments of behavior—an acclimatized person learns to move economically and to keep away from sources of intense heat.

The rate of acclimatization depends more upon the intensity than the frequency or duration of heat exposure. The process is exponential in nature, with much of the adjustment occurring in the first 3 days; adjustments have largely been completed after approximately 2 weeks. Individuals who are initially in good physical condition adapt more readily than obese and sedentary subjects; indeed, there is some cross-adaptation between cardiorespiratory training and heat exposure, and for the fullest adjustment a person should undertake hard physical work in the heat.

On leaving the tropics, adaptations persist for only a few weeks, but acclimatization is apparently restored at an accelerated pace if the subject returns to a hot climate.

Cold Acclimatization

While some smaller species show obvious long-term metabolic adaptations to cold, debate continues on the extent of general cold acclimatization in humans. The Korean pearl divers who were historically exposed to very cold water, reputedly developed an increase of resting metabolism in response to this stress. More recently, they have equipped themselves with wet suits, and the stimulation of resting metabolism during winter diving is no longer observed.

In addition to an increase of thyroxine secretion, some animals show a hypertrophy of brown fat. This tissue can generate large quantities of heat through a "futile cycle" of fat breakdown and resynthesis, as protons leak across the mitochondrial membranes in this tissue. The adult human apparently does not have any significant quantity of brown fat, although some investigators have suggested that a similar "futile cycle" can be initiated in normal fat depots, and several recent

reports have shown that exercise in the cold helps to reduce body fat, at least in male subjects.

The main adjustment of humans to cold seems to be insulative rather than metabolic. The core temperature at which shivering occurs is decreased, blood flow to the extremities is reduced, and the subject feels more comfortable in the cold. Adjustments of behavior, including alterations in movement patterns and a more appropriate choice of clothing, also reduce the cold stress in any given climate; indeed, compensation may be so efficient that the personal microclimate of an arctic traveller differs little from that found when the same individual is living under temperate conditions.

Occupational groups such as fisherfolk suffer repeated local exposure of the hands to cold water. The immediate reaction is a typical "cold pressor response," with an increase of both heart rate and blood pressure (Fig. 12–5). However, with repeated exposure to cold water, the pressor reaction diminishes, and blood flow to the hands remains sufficient to conserve dexterity while working under very cold conditions. It is less clear whether this is an example of local cold acclimation or of cold acclimatization, since attenuation of the cold pressor response is not observed in subjects with an injury of the prefrontal cortex (the part of the brain involved in habituation).

PATHOLOGICAL REACTIONS TO HEAT AND COLD

Heat Syncope

Syncope reflects an inadequate venous return to the heart and a resultant fall of systemic blood pres-

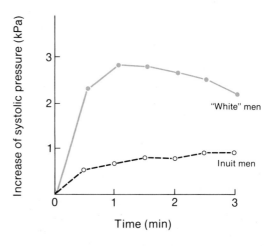

Figure 12–5 Cold pressor response in "white" men and Inuit men frequently exposed to severe cold. The hands of each group were immersed in water at 4° C, starting at time zero. (Based on experiments of LeBlanc and associates)

sure. This often triggers a vasovagal attack with muscle vasodilatation and a slowing of heart rate. Factors contributing to syncope in a hot environment include: (1) fluid loss in sweat (water exhaustion), (2) peripheral pooling of blood in veins that are relaxed by the heat, (3) peripheral exudation of fluid (a heat edema developing in dependent parts of the body), and (4) a large skin blood flow.

Prevention is by provision of adequate fluids. When exercising hard, thirst does not give an appropriate indication of the body's water needs. Competitors should thus be encouraged to drink the maximum volume that can be absorbed from the gastrointestinal tract while exercising, (the equivalent of about 150 mℓ every 15 minutes). Proprietary drinks contain various combinations of minerals and carbohydrates, but if the objective is fluid replacement, they offer no advantage over pure water. Indeed, if a drink contains more than 5 percent glucose, the resultant osmotic pressure of the solution slows the emptying of the stomach. The advantage of flavor claimed by manufacturers of some proprietary drinks is illusory, since taste perception is altered by vigorous effort. The minerals provided are also inappropriate. Sweat is a dilute solution relative to the plasma, and in consequence both plasma sodium and plasma potassium concentrations rise rather than fall during vigorous exercise. Finally, the energy content of a 5 percent glucose solution (30 g per hour, equivalent to about 8 kJ per minute) could make only a small contribution to the metabolic demands of activity (although this contribution can be increased if a low osmotic pressure glucose polymer solution is substituted for the normal form of glucose).

Treatment of syncope includes: (1) lying down with the legs elevated, (2) tepid sponging (sponging with cold water would cause cutaneous vasoconstriction, increasing the heat stress), and (3) oral administration of fluids. Hot blankets increase the circulatory load and should be avoided.

Heat Exhaustion

Heat exhaustion generally reflects a moderate fluid depletion that has developed over a day of vigorous exercise in the heat. In addition to symptoms of fatigue, irritability, and loss of performance, there is a deterioration of mechanical efficiency and an increased liability to accidents.

Given a series of athletic heats or tournaments in a hot climate, a progressive salt depletion may develop over several days or weeks; there is an associated chronic decrease of blood volume (salt-deficiency exhaustion). This causes the competitor to show a progressive loss of initiative and energy, with complaints of dizziness and blackouts (heat neurasthenia). When a person is exposed to unusual amounts of heat, a daily record of body mass should be kept. If body mass appears to be decreasing, the urine should be tested to check its salt content.

Normally, addition of extra salt to salads and vegetables provides an adequate means of maintaining sodium balance while living in a hot environment. Provision of salt tablets is not recommended. The tablets are liable to cause gastric irritation and can pass through the bowel without absorption. They also tend to enter the blood stream as a highly concentrated "slug" that merely exacerbates fluid loss from the kidneys.

Heat Stroke

Heat stroke is one symptom of a potentially fatal failure of thermoregulation. A rectal temperature of over 40^{0} C is a warning of impending heat stroke, and for this reason the safe working limit for acclimatized miners has been set at 39.2^{0} C. The risk to summer athletes is substantial relative to this standard. Many marathon runners, distance cyclists, and North American football players reach higher temperatures than this, rectal readings of 41^{0} C being not uncommon in the height of summer.

A progressive rise of core temperature in the stroke victim is compounded by dehydration, a falling output of sweat (anhidrotic heat exhaustion), a diminished blood flow to the skin, and general circulatory failure. An inadequate blood flow to the brain may cause hallucinations, coma, and irreversible brain damage. There may also be damage to poorly perfused kidneys (heat anuria, renal failure) and adrenal glands ("heat shock" with a sustained drop of blood pressure). Biochemical findings include massive increases in plasma enzymes (CPK, LDH, SGOT), hematuria, proteinuria, and a rise of blood urea.

Useful preventive measures are (1) a scheduling of races at cool times of the day, (2) cancelling events if the environmental stress is excessive, (3) avoiding the wearing of uniforms that are impermeable to sweat, (4) avoiding drugs such as amphetamines (which reduce skin blood flow), and (5) careful monitoring of body temperature in exhausted competitors (oral temperature readings must be avoided since the tongue is cooled by hyperventilation).

Treatment includes rapid cooling by tepid sponging, administration of fluids, and early admission to hospital (for restoration of electrolyte balance, with subsequent monitoring of renal and adrenal function).

Heat Cramps

A person who is sweating hard loses up to 2 g of salt per hour from a total body pool of 175 g. There is a parallel loss of other minerals such as potassium, magnesium, and calcium. The resultant acute disturbance of electrolyte balance may cause painful cramps ("Stoker's cramps", so called because they were commonplace in the furnace rooms of coal-fired ships).

Cramps are particularly common on first reaching the tropics, partly because the subject has not learned to increase salt intake, and partly because the increased secretion of aldosterone has yet to develop.

Heat Rash

Excessive sweating and a maceration of the skin may cause a blockage of the sweat ducts (heat rash). This situation is often compounded by secondary fungal or bacterial infection of the skin.

Frostbite

If local cooling is sufficient to freeze intracellular fluid, the cells may suffer irreversible damage (frostbite). Because the freezing point is depressed by dissolved minerals, the critical local temperature is -1 to -2° C.

Cold-Induced Angina and Bronchospasm

Exposure to cold air or water causes cutaneous vasoconstriction and an increase of systemic blood pressure, increasing both the pre- and afterloading of the heart. The oxygen cost of exercise is also increased by shivering, and there is thus an increase of cardiac work-rate.

The impact of cold dry air on the airways initiates a bronchospasm, particularly in asthmatic patients. This increases the work of breathing. There may also be a reflex narrowing of the coronary vessels (Bezold - Jarisch reflex).

These various factors provoke angina in some postcoronary patients when they attempt to exercise in the cold. One obvious solution is to preheat the inspired air by use of a rebreathing tube or heat exchanger.

Cold Hyperventilation

On plunging into cold water, intensive stimulation of the cutaneous cold receptors may cause an uncontrollable reflex hyperventilation (with inhalation of water and choking). Occasionally, it may also provoke cardiac arrest or ventricular fibrillation.

Cold Hypothermia

General body cooling by hill-walking in rain and mist or cold-water immersion can be fatal. Factors predisposing to disaster have included: (1) inadequate provision of clothing, (2) loss of insulation in clothing due to drenching by mist, rain, sweat, or water immersion, (3) misjudging the extent of cooling on the hills (there is a loss of radiant heating due to mist, an increase of windspeed on the hilltops, and a decrease of temperature with ascent), (4) inadequate physical activity (due to injury, mismatching of fitness between members of a climbing party, or exhaustion after becoming lost in the mist), and (5) confusion due to the ingestion of alcohol, a low blood sugar (hypoglycemia), or the accumulation of ketone bodies in the blood (ketonemia).

Cold exposure increases the mobilization of body fat from the adipose tissue depots, and this tendency is exaggerated by a combination of exhausting exercise and lack of food. The accumulation of ketone bodies leads to confusion of the subject and an increased risk of injury. These changes are compounded by a slowing of muscular contraction and a malfunction of the sensory receptors. Cold exhaustion, a drop in blood pressure (postural hypotension), and collapse lead to a progressive and potentially fatal decrease of core temperature.

Complications of hypothermia include depression of respiration, metabolic acidosis, circulatory failure, and renal failure. Paradoxical vasodilatation of the skin vessels may cause a misleading sensation of warmth, and a confused subject may thus remove clothing, giving to the rescuer the superficial appearance that there has been a sexual assault rather than a cold-induced accident.

Preventive measures include (1) insistence on the provision of clothing that is adequate for the anticipated environment, (2) development of plans to rewarm and feed individuals who cannot remain active due to injuries, (3) matching of parties in terms of fitness and skill, and (4) carriage of adequate food, supplies, and emergency shelter in case a mountain path is lost in the mist.

Immediate treatment of the hypothermia victim includes rewarming plus cardiac or respiratory resuscitation as necessary. Early evacuation to hospital is desirable, since potential complications include such emergencies as cardiac fibrillation, circulatory failure, and renal failure.

FURTHER READING

Adolph EF. Origins of physiological regulation. New York: Academic Press, 1968.

Buskirk ER. Temperature regulation with exercise. Exerc Sport Sci Rev 1979; 5:45–88.

Cumming GR, Snidal D, Taylor AW. Environmental effects on work performance. Ottawa: Canadian Association of Sports Sciences, 1972.

Edholm OG, Gunderson EKE. Polar human biology. London: William Heinemann, 1973.

Folk GE. Introduction to environmental physiology. Philadelphia: Lea & Febiger, 1966.

Harvald B, Hart Hansen JP. Circumpolar health 1981. Copenhagen: Nordic Council for Arctic Medical Research. Report Series 33, 1981.

Hensel H. Thermoreception and temperature regulation. New York: Academic Press, 1981.

Horvath SM. Exercise in a cold environment. Exerc Sport Sci Rev 1982; 9:221–264.

Horvath SM, Yousef MK. Environmental physiology: aging, heat and altitude. New York: Elsevier, 1981.

Houdas Y, Ring EFJ. Human body temperature. Its measurement and regulation. New York: Plenum Press, 1982.

Itoh S. Physiology of cold adapted man. Hokkaido: Hokkaido University, 1974.

Johnson SC, Ruhling RO. Aspirin in exercise-induced hyperthermia. Sports Med 1985; 2:1–7.

Kerslake D McK. The stress of hot environments. London: Cambridge University Press, 1972.

LeBlanc J. Man in the cold. Springfield, Ill: CC Thomas, 1975.

Leithead CS, Lind AR. Heat stress and heat disorders. London: Cassell, 1964.

Milan FA. The human biology of circumpolar populations. London: Cambridge University Press, 1980.

Mount LE. Adaptation to thermal environment. Baltimore: University Park Press, 1979.

Nadel ER. Problems with temperature regulation during exercise. New York: Academic Press, 1977.

Renbourn ET. Materials and clothing in health and disease. London: HK Lewis, 1972.

Robertshaw D. Environmental physiology. London: Butterworths, 1974.

Robertshaw D. Environmental physiology III. Baltimore: University Park Press, 1979.

Shephard RJ. Adaptation to exercise in the cold. Sports Med 1985; 2:59–71.

Shephard RJ, Itoh S. Circumpolar health. Toronto: University of Toronto Press, 1976.

Yoshimura H, Kobayashi S. Physiological adaptability and nutritional status of the Japanese. A. Thermal adaptability of the Japanese and physiology of the Ama. JIBP Synthesis Vol. 3. Tokyo: University of Tokyo Press, 1975.

Yousef MK, Horvath SM, Bullard RW. Physiological adaptations: desert and mountain. New York: Academic Press, 1972.

FITNESS AND HEALTH

This chapter examines the potential impact of habitual exercise upon the course of cardiovascular and other diseases, discusses the design of rehabilitation programs, and considers potentially harmful acute effects of vigorous exercise.

PATHOLOGICAL CONSIDERATIONS

A program of graded exercise training could improve performance in certain forms of congenital heart disease. However, exercise is more commonly prescribed in the prevention and treatment of ischemic heart disease. Ischemic heart disease covers a variety of pathologies, including not only myocardial infarction, but also sudden "electrical" death (a failure in the normal electrical activation of the heart), chronic myocardial degeneration, angina, and coronary atherosclerosis or arteriosclerosis.

Myocardial Infarction

A myocardial infarct develops whenever a sector of the myocardium becomes ischemic for sufficient time to cause its death. The term means, literally, "stuffed with blood," and this description aptly reflects the vascular congestion that is seen as the sector of dead muscle is replaced by scar tissue.

There are at least four possible causes of ischemia: (1) a plaque of fatty tissue (Fig. 13–1) may break free from the wall of a coronary artery to cause a blockage of the coronary circulation by lodging at a more peripheral site, (2) hemorrhage may occur into a plaque from the high pressure, upstream side, causing it to swell and block the vessel concerned, (3) clotting may occur on the surface of a plaque, particularly if it is calcified, thereby gradually narrowing the corresponding vessel until occlusion is complete, and (4) a relative oxygen lack may result from a high rate-pressure product, even in the absence of frank occlusion. This last situation is particularly likely if the blood pressure is increased by anger or isometric exercise.

The extent of the infarct depends in part on the degree of anastomosis between the major coronary vessels beyond the site of vascular obstruction. Some animal experiments have shown a substantial development of collateral anastomoses in response to endurance training, but it is less clear whether humans can be protected against future heart attacks in this way. The size of the infarct can often be gauged from the increase of serum enzyme levels, such as creatine kinase, following the acute incident. Enzyme readings peak 1 to 3 days after infarction. If much tissue dies, myocardial function is impaired by a segment of ventricular wall that is either inert or moves in a "paradoxical" fashion (expanding as the ventricle contracts). An exercise test performed within a few weeks of infarction thus provides a useful guide to prognosis.

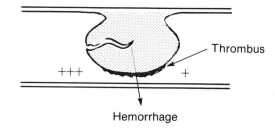

Hemorrhage

Figure 13–1 The problems that may arise from an atherosclerotic plaque in the coronary vessels are: (a) the vessel is narrowed, restricting flow, and giving relative ischemia in the myocardium distal to the plaque; (b) a pressure gradient is created across the plaque, particularly when coronary flow is increased by exercise. Hemorrhage may occur into the plaque from a high to a low pressure region, causing it to swell; (c) the plaque may be enlarged by the deposition of thrombus on its surface; (d) the plaque may become dislodged and obstruct a more distal vessel.

About one-third of patients survive the acute episode (the proportion being higher in young rather than in older people), and there is a 20 to 25 percent chance that infarction may recur over the next 5 years. The main causes of death in the early postinfarction period are cardiac failure and ventricular fibrillation. Occasionally, the scarred myocardium may develop into an aneurysm that may rupture into the pericardium; as blood accumulates in the pericardial sac, the ventricle is stopped by external compression (the condition of cardiac tamponade).

The clinical picture that is associated with myocardial infarction depends greatly on the severity of the attack. Some incidents are indeed mistaken for something quite benign, such as a touch of arthritis in the shoulder or an attack of indigestion. More typically, there is a severe, vise-like pain in the midline, lasting at least 2 minutes (and often 20 to 30 minutes), and the patient shows signs of collapse (pallor, sweating, nausea, and a weak pulse). If a heart attack is suspected, an ambulance should be summoned and the pulse monitored for the possible onset of ventricular fibrillation or asystole. Assuming that the observer has the necessary training, cardiac massage should be applied if the heart stops.

Many forms of exercise can apparently provoke both fatal (Table 13–1) and nonfatal cardiac incidents. About 25 percent of younger patients who are recovering from myocardial infarction give a history of vigorous and unaccustomed exercise immediately prior to their attack (about five to ten times the expected frequency of vigorous activity in a North American community). Although it is difficult to rule out the possibility that the apparent frequency of antecedent exercise may have been boosted by pondering on "causes" of the incident, a 24-hour plot of the timing of episodes certainly shows a deficiency of cardiac emergencies both during sleep and during the hours of normal work.

TABLE 13–1   Activities Undertaken by 174 Athletes who Sustained Cardiovascular Deaths While Exercising

Activity	No. of Deaths	Activity	No. of Deaths
Baseball	1	Judo	3
Basketball	17	Pentathlon	1
Bowls	2	Quoits	1
Boxing	2	Riding	1
Climbing	2	Running	57
Cricket	2	Shot-put	4
Curling	4	Skiing—downhill & Nordic	13
Cycling	4	Skipping	1
Dancing	4	Softball	1
Football (rugby, soccer&US)	25	Squash	1
		Swimming	8
Golf	4	Wrestling	3
Gymnastics	3	Weight lifting	1
Hockey	1	Yachting	2

From Shephard RJ. Ischaemic heart disease and exercise. London: Croom Helm, 1981.

Certainly, in terms of pathology, vigorous exercise seems likely to provoke the breaking away of an embolus, hemorrhage into a plaque, and (if there is a rise of blood pressure) a relative ischemia of the myocardium. The impact of exercise upon clotting mechanisms is complex, some aspects being accelerated and others slowed. Nevertheless, complete blockage of a coronary vessel by thrombosis seems more likely to occur when blood flow is limited by sleep.

Angina

Angina is a symptom caused by a short duration (and thus reversible) bout of myocardial ischemia. The pain (which is thought to reflect a local stimulation of pain receptors by the metabolic byproducts of ischemia) is again located in the midline, but (perhaps because discomfort is less severe), a radiation of the sensation to the inner aspect of the left arm, the neck, the jaw, or the ear is often reported. Symptoms are typically precipitated by vigorous exercise (e.g., hurrying up a hill), cold exposure, or emotion. The pain usually lasts for less than 2 minutes, and it is readily relieved by either rest or trinitrin tablets (glyceryl trinitrate). The latter reduce blood pressure by dilating venous reservoirs, thus diminishing the cardiac work-rate.

Atherosclerosis

Atherosclerosis is a partial blockage of major arteries by subendothelial fat. There is an increase of mucopolysaccharides and an accumulation of lipids (particularly cholesterol) immediately beneath the vascular endothelium. Subsequently, individual plaques become enlarged by inflammation, hemorrhage, and calcification, with deposition of thrombi on the ulcerated, exposed surfaces.

Atherosclerosis affects not only the coronary arteries, but also the other major arterial vessels. It has been described as a childhood illness, since fatty streaking of the aorta can be seen in quite young North American children. Postmortem examination of United States soldiers who died in Korea showed that relatively advanced atherosclerosis was already present in many of the sample.

Progressive atherosclerosis can be slowed by an increase of HDL cholesterol. The HDL apoprotein serves as a scavenger, clearing excess cholesterol from the bloodstream and returning it to the liver.

Arteriosclerosis

Arteriosclerosis may coexist with atherosclerosis. It is a manifestation of aging, loss of elasticity in the vessel walls being associated with a deterioration in their collagen fibers and a progressive calcification, until some vessels have the texture of a small concrete pipe.

In a young adult, a large part of the stroke volume is accommodated by an expansion of the aorta and major arteries. However, this cannot occur once the vessels become calcified and rigid. In consequence, there is an increase of systolic pressure, and the pulse wave assumes a collapsing form, with pressures dropping steeply after closure of the aortic valve (Fig. 13–2). Arteriosclerotic calcification may involve the cardiac

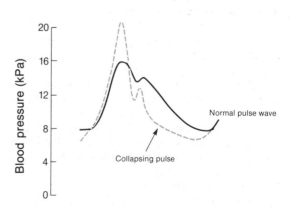

Figure 13–2 Comparison of arterial pulse wave between healthy young individual and older patient with arteriosclerosis. Note that because of a stiffening of the arterial wall the arteriosclerotic individual has a high peak systolic pressure in the early phase of cardiac ejection, but this pressure is poorly sustained.

valves, causing a narrowing of their apertures (e.g., aortic stenosis) or a diastolic leakage (e.g., aortic regurgitation). Weakness of the vessel wall may give rise to an aortic or large vessel aneurysm, which on occasion can rupture into the thorax.

If arteriosclerosis develops in the more peripheral arteries, it may limit blood flow to a specific muscle group such as the gastrocnemius. Endurance exercise may then cause ischemic pain in the muscle concerned (the syndrome of intermittent claudication).

THE "EPIDEMIC" OF ISCHEMIC HEART DISEASE

There has been a substantial "epidemic" of ischemic heart disease over the present century (Fig. 13–3), with a 2½-fold increase in the recorded frequency of ischemic heart disease deaths from 1931 to 1951. Fatal incidents apparently plateaued in the mid 1960s, and in North America the incidence of cardiac deaths has subsequently dropped by about 30 percent.

Risk Factors

A substantial list of risk factors has been identified as increasing an individual's chances of developing ischemic heart disease. The three prime candidates are cigarette smoking, a systemic blood pressure greater than 21.3/12.7 kPa (160/95 mm Hg), and a serum cholesterol greater than 7 mmol per liter (270 mg per deciliter with a low HDL-LDL cholesterol ratio. Other factors increasing risk are male sex, a family history of heart attacks, lack of exercise, poor glucose tolerance or frank diabetes, and the use of contraceptive drugs (in women). The impact of mesomorphy, a "Type A" personality, and a high serum uric acid is less well established. Obesity was once thought to be an important risk factor, but is now said to have little adverse effect after allowance has been made for its correlation with two other major risk factors (hypertension and an adverse blood lipid profile). However, the argument is partly semantic, since the correction of obesity still reduces the likelihood of a heart attack (because it reduces hypertension and corrects an adverse lipid profile).

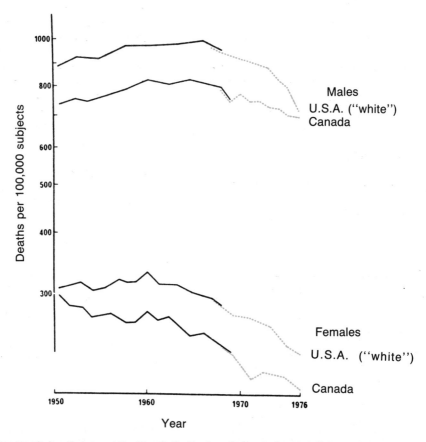

Figure 13–3 Course of "epidemic" of ischemic heart disease. Data as analysed by TW Anderson for Canadian and U.S. "white" subjects aged 55-64 years, adjusted to allow for a change in the method of classifying ischemic heart disease (1968, USA; 1969, Canada), as shown by the interrupted lines.

Changes in Lifestyle and the Cardiac Epidemic

Many aspects of lifestyle changed coincident with the onset of the ischemic heart disease epidemic—physical activity was curtailed by automation and the availability of private cars, the consumption of refined carbohydrates, such as sugar, increased enormously, and the use of cigarettes became widespread between the two World Wars.

Likewise, there are many factors claiming a causal role in the stemming of the cardiac epidemic. There has been a substantial improvement in survival prospects because of advances in medical treatment (particularly in use of beta-blocking drugs to reduce the chances of subsequent ventricular fibrillation). Exercise has also become popular since the early 1970s, and, at least among men, there has been a substantial decrease in the number of habitual cigarette smokers. Finally, many North Americans have made a conscious attempt to reduce their intake of saturated animal fat. Probably all of these factors have made some contribution to the observed improvement in risk, although the decrease in cigarette consumption seems the prime reason for the advance in cardiac health.

EXERCISE AND THE PREVENTION OF ISCHEMIC HEART DISEASE

There are abundant physiological reasons why an increase of habitual physical activity might be helpful in avoiding clinical ischemic heart disease. However, it remains difficult to obtain unequivocal proof of a preventive role for endurance exercise.

Physiological Changes

The physiological changes that might influence the risk of a heart attack can be grouped in terms of their energy costs (Table 13–2).

Some potential responses are purely a consequence of participation in a group program. Equal benefit might then be anticipated from an alternative type of group activity (such as hypnotherapy). Camaraderie is found in the group environment, with encouragement and support from other patients facing similar problems. Regular advice is also obtained from the class leader, including admonitions to stop smoking, to lead a less stressful type of existence, and to improve overall lifestyle.

Other responses require a substantial energy expenditure, but the intensity of activity is of only secondary importance. In this category, we may note the correction of obesity, the reduction of serum cholesterol and triglycerides, the increase of the HDL-LDL cholesterol ratio, and the improvement of glucose tolerance.

The majority of potential exercise-induced changes are associated with moderate, endurance-type training. The cardiac work-rate is decreased as exercise heart rate and blood pressure fall. Red cell mass and blood volume are often increased and the clotting tendency is diminished (although the lysis of clots is increased). There may also be an increase of heart volume. The output of growth hormone is increased (possibly to mobilize fat, possibly to preserve tissue protein in the face of vigorous catabolism). The blood concentration of thyroid hormone is also increased or at least normalized by physical activity.

Intense training may serve to habituate the participant to the symptoms associated with all-out exercise. Catecholamine output also seems to drop. Finally, at least in animal experiments, involvement in an intensive exercise training plan increases both the dimensions of the coronary arterial tree and the extent of collateral anastomoses.

Historical Evidence

Attempts have been made to draw a parallel between the ischemic heart disease epidemic and vari-

TABLE 13–2   Some of the Possible Mechanisms Whereby an Exercise Prescription Might Reduce the Risk of Ischemic Heart Disease

Light Activity	Moderate Activity	Intense Activity	Increased Energy Consumption
Prudent living Camaraderie Joie de vivre Relaxation Correction of "stress"	Reduced cardiac workload, heart rate, blood pressure, increased myocardial efficiency Improved O_2 transport, red cell mass, arterial O_2 content, blood volume, blood flow distribution, tissue enzyme activity Hormonal changes, neurohormonal balance, catecholamine secretion, growth hormone, thyroid hormone Blood coagulability, fibrinolysis, platelet "stickiness" improved	Coronary artery size enlarged Collateral vessels developed Habituation	Adipose tissue decreased Serum cholesterol reduced Serum triglycerides reduced Glucose tolerance improved

Based on a schema of S. M. Fox, but classified in terms of the pattern of exercise required.

ous indices of physical activity such as the per capita consumption of fossil fuels, or the per capita food consumption. There is substantial evidence suggesting that there was a decline of habitual activity from 1900 to the mid 1960s, and (at least in the upper socioeconomic groups) there has subsequently been a revived interest in leisure activity. However, the data is not sufficiently precise to establish a causal link between these changes and the cardiac epidemic.

"Primitive" Societies

Some "primitive" societies apparently show a low incidence of ischemic heart disease. This has been attributed to the need for a high daily energy expenditure. One study of the Inuit found that the men in a northern settlement who were following a traditional lifestyle as hunters used 15 to 16 MJ of energy per day, as much as "white" workers engaged in the heaviest types of industry such as forestry and mining (Table 13-3). Certain African populations such as the Masai can apparently consume a diet rich in blood, milk, and other sources of fat with impunity because they also have a high daily energy expenditure. Bang has demonstrated that traditional Greenland Eskimos have a very favorable lipid profile. Unfortunately, civilization is now robbing most of these ethnic populations of their traditional active pursuits. As a result they have shown an accumulation of body fat, a deterioration of lipid profile, and an increase of blood pressure. It seems probable that over the next few years the incidence of ischemic heart disease will also increase toward the levels encountered in "white" society.

Occupational Comparisons

A number of studies have compared the cardiac health of employees in supposedly active and inactive occupations (Table 13-4)—for example, London bus drivers versus conductors who climbed periodically to

TABLE 13-3 Energy Expenditures of Male Inuit Pursuing Various Types of Traditional Hunting and Fishing

Activity	Energy Expenditure (MJ/day)
Summer fishing	18.6
Winter fishing	16.9
Summer caribou hunt	16.3
Winter caribou hunt	16.1
Sealing at ice hole	14.6
in boat	14.4
at floe edge	10.6
Walrus hunt	15.4
Average (8 types of hunt)	15.4

Data of Shephard, standardized to a body mass of 65 kg.

TABLE 13-4 The Influence of Regular Occupational Activity Upon Various Indices of Ischemic Heart Disease

Index of Ischemic Heart Disease	Mean Ratio Active/Inactive	Range	Number of Studies
Myocardial infarction	0.56	0.33–0.98	9
Coronary heart disease			
Attack rate	0.60	0.17–1.03	16
Mortality	0.66	0.28–1.22	21
Myocardial pain	0.48	0.21–0.68	8
Vascular pathology	0.76	0.51–1.00	7
Angina pectoris	1.36	0.65–1.98	7

Based on data accumulated by Fox and Haskell, expressed as ratio of incidence in active versus inactive population.

the upper deck of the bus to collect fares, switchmen in the railyards versus ticket clerks, postal carriers versus clerks, longshoremen versus tally clerks, and field versus office workers in the Jewish kibbutzim. In general, the "heavy" workers had about 4 MJ per day greater energy expenditure than the sedentary comparison groups, this difference being associated with up to a 50 percent lower incidence of fatal myocardial infarction. In a few studies where a lower cardiac mortality was not seen in the supposedly active group (Los Angeles civil servants, Chicago gas workers), it has been argued that the level of occupational activity was insufficient to confer protection and that there were substantial ethnic and cultural differences between occupationally inactive white- and occupationally active blue-collar employees.

Most occupational comparisons suffer the limitation of self selection; for example, Morris showed that bus drivers wore larger uniforms than the conductors when they were first recruited by London Transport—the drivers were an inherently fatter population and thus had a greater initial risk of ischemic heart disease. Kellerman has claimed that in the typical Kibbutz, work is assigned by a committee without regard to the preference of the individual, and that in this situation all employees share a common diet. Nevertheless, the Kibbutz study shows the largest (70 percent) reduction of ischemic heart disease in the active population. Paffenbarger has also shown that in longshoremen the cardiac benefit persists after adjustment of the data for risk factors such as smoking habits, hypertension, and excessive body mass (Table 13-5).

One puzzling feature of the London bus study was that there was little difference in angina or postmortem cardiac scarring between drivers and conductors—possibly, the high activity levels of the conductors brought any myocardial ischemia to light, but it remained "silent" in the drivers.

TABLE 13-5   Influence of Low Energy Output, Cigarette Consumption, and Systolic Blood Pressure Upon Relative Risk of Fatal Heart Attack, Adjusted for Age and Two Other Major Risk Factors

Type of Death	Low Energy Output	Cigarettes (<1 pack/day)	Systolic Blood Pressure (<mean)
Sudden	3.3	1.6	2.7
Delayed	1.6	2.1	1.4
Unspecified	1.7	2.5	2.2
All	2.0	2.1	2.1

Based on data of Paffenbarger for Californian longshoremen.

TABLE 13-6   Protection Against a First Heart Attack With an Additional Weekly Leisure Energy Expenditure of 800 kJ

Secondary Risk Factor	Protection Against First Heart Attack	
	Secondary Risk Factor Present	Secondary Risk Factor Absent
Cigarette smoking	0.45	0.65
Systolic pressure >130 mm Hg	0.54	0.65
Diastolic pressure >80 mm Hg	0.74	0.54
Quetelet index >34	0.63	0.62
Parent dead	0.61	0.57
No varsity sport	0.63	0.61

Data of Paffenbarger for Harvard Alumni, expressed as ratio of risk for active versus inactive individuals.

Leisure Habits

Given increasing industrial automation, it is argued that any future epidemiological studies will of necessity consider leisure habits rather than work patterns. There is currently a large socioeconomic gradient of leisure activity in most developed countries, with professional workers adopting much more active recreational pursuits than blue collar groups. While community studies such as those conducted in Framingham and Tecumseh show about a twofold advantage of cardiac death rate to active inhabitants, comparisons are better restricted to a single socioeconomic category.

Morris carried out such a prospective study of 17,000 executive-grade civil servants and found significant protection against ischemic heart disease from various daily leisure activities—for instance, 20 minutes or more of "vigorous getting about" (apparently rapid walking), 5 minutes of near-maximal activity, or the climbing of 450 stairs per day. Paffenbarger followed up a large population of Harvard Alumni, and he also saw a linkage between leisure-time physical activity and protection against ischemic heart disease. This protection persisted after adjustment of the data for other risk factors (Table 13-6). The criticism of self-selection could not be categorically answered; nevertheless, there was no benefit among those who were active at college but subsequently stopped exercising, but benefit was seen in those who began exercising after leaving university. The threshold energy expenditure for cardiac protection was an additional expenditure of 2 MJ per week, and maximum benefit was seen with an added expenditure of about 8 MJ per week.

Longevity of Athletes

Athletes often engage in a much greater volume of training for a longer period than does the general public. However, in general they are a highly selected population.

Some early comparisons of university-class athletes showed an advantage of longevity of up to 2 years relative to the general insured population. However, such comparisons ignored the privileged position of university graduates in that era. A comparison of athletes with others attending the same university showed no advantage. Indeed, relative to "intellectuals" who obtained academic honors, there was a 2-year disadvantage in the athletes. Montoye pointed out that some people who were athletes at university become less active than their contemporaries by the time they reach the "coronary-prone" years. They may also have a higher body mass and are more likely to be heavy smokers with a high alcohol consumption. Other problems of studying athletes are (1) the death of a well-known player may more likely be given media prominence than the death of an intellectual, (2) sports enthusiasts have a high death rate for various noncardiac conditions, including vehicle accidents and death in military combat, (3) sometimes "control" alumni are physically active, although they failed to gain an "athletic letter" while at university, and (4) some major league sports attract participants who have an adverse body build that increases their vulnerability to death from ischemic heart disease.

One group of competitors who remain active until an advanced age are cross-country skiers. Karvonen found that Finnish champions had a 4 to 5 year advantage of longevity over their contemporaries. However, he was careful to point out that this might reflect an associated healthy lifestyle—particularly a lifelong abstinence from cigarettes.

Prospects for Experimental Studies

It might seem a simple matter to resolve the extent of protection obtained from physical activity by randomly allocating subjects to a vigorous exercise and a control regimen. Let us suppose we wished to demonstrate a 50 percent reduction of cardiac episodes, with a 90 percent chance of showing an effect at the 0.05 level of probability. Given further an attack rate of about 2 per 1,000 per year in an initially healthy middle-aged population, a simple application of statistics shows that for such proof the control group must have 56 incidents, and the active group 28 incidents. There would thus be a need for 28,000 person-years in each of two groups—for example, a total population of 14,000 followed for 4 years.

This calculation assumes an absence of dropouts. However, in practice, as many as 50 percent of the residual sample defect from an exercise group every 6 months, while a substantial number of the control population become "contaminated" with an interest in exercise. Thus, a much larger sample than 14,000 must be recruited to accumulate 56,000 person-years of exercise experience. Moreover, the final sample becomes highly atypical of the population from which it is drawn. In 1962, Taylor estimated the cost of a definitive trial at U.S. $31 million. The Multiple Risk Factor Intervention Trial (MRFIT) recruited 12,000 experimental and 12,000 control subjects, but made only a casual exercise intervention towards the midpoint of the trial. An expenditure of some U.S. $120 million yielded rather limited and inconclusive evidence on the benefits of exercise and other types of lifestyle change.

It is unlikely that there will be further attempts to examine the cardiac benefits of exercise in the general population. The chances of arranging a manageable trial can of course be improved if the incident rate is increased—by using a high-risk population or those who have already sustained a heart attack, but the applicability of the findings is then correspondingly limited.

EXERCISE FOR POSTCORONARY PATIENTS

Proof of Benefit

Even in postcoronary patients, proof of benefit from exercise is tantalizingly elusive. The Southern Ontario multicenter trial was initiated with the hope that conclusive evidence might be obtained from a sample of 750 patients, divided in a stratified random fashion between a program of high-intensity exercise and a low-intensity, homeopathic control program. However, a decisive answer was not obtained because (1) the dropout rate from the exercise program was at least 10 percent each 6 months, as opposed to the predicted 35 percent cumulative loss over a 4-year trial, (2) a substantial proportion of the control group became interested in exercise, (3) the recurrence rate among patients referred to the exercise rehabilitation trial was substantially less than in the general "postcoronary" population, (4) training had a slow onset, so that many patients were lost to the trial before there was any scope for benefit, and (5) the frequency of fatal recurrences was heavily influenced by a small subpopulation with deep ST segmental depression (who should probably have been identified as a separate stratum, demanding a

different pattern of treatment). Considering only the groups to which patients were initially assigned, the Southern Ontario trial showed no significant benefit from exercise (or perhaps more correctly, the confidence limits ranged widely from a positive to a negative effect). Considering the actual behavior of the patients as assessed from gains of oxygen transport (an approach that is anathema to a statistician), there was about a 30 percent gain of prognosis among those who assumed a more active lifestyle.

Several other trials have been organized around the world. None has been as large as that conducted in Southern Ontario, and most have been plagued by similar problems. Considered individually, all have been inconclusive, but if data from the various investigations is pooled, a statistically significant benefit of exercise of between 20 and 30 percent is seen (Table 13–7). This decrease in mortality is therapeutically useful, and is indeed larger than that induced by drastic cholestyramine treatment in the much publicized Lipid Research Trial.

Optimum Training Plan

Given the number of nonfatal coronary episodes (at least 150,000 per year in the United States alone), it is not feasible to contemplate providing medically supervised exercise programs for cardiac patients over any extended period. A tapered plan of supervised training is thus recommended.

During the first 3 months after infarction, the patient begins exercising two to three times per week, under close medical observation. Exercise is prescribed on the basis of a laboratory stress test, and reactions to the prescription are observed carefully in the gymnasium. If there are unusual symptoms, their nature is explored by telemetry.

Over the next year, the patient is transferred to a program of once weekly gymnasium classes, supplemented by a home prescription. The gymnasium sessions begin with an informal class discussion of problems with the class leader. There is then a warm-up of approximately 10 minutes, which includes slow walking and calisthenics, with an emphasis upon im-

TABLE 13–7   Benefit of Exercise Following Myocardial Infarction

| | Cumulative Survival | | |
Interval (years)	Exercise (%)	Control (%)	Significance of Difference*
0–1	95.6	93.2	0.031
1–2	93.3	89.7	0.011
2–3	91.1	87.5	0.024
3–4	87.9	84.0	0.075

* Based on a 1 – tailed t test for each individual comparison. Pooled data from Wilhelmsen, Hakkila and Shaw.

proving flexibility. At least 30 minutes is devoted to personally prescribed endurance activity (alternating slow walking with fast walking or jogging). There follows a brief (10 to 15 minutes) ballgame for fun, and then a gradual cooldown of slow walking (5 to 10 minutes duration). The gymnasium sessions provide an opportunity to observe reactions to the home prescription, and to monitor home activities through weekly diary sheets.

The home prescription specifies a limiting pulse rate, a distance to be covered in a specified time, and any symptoms that signal a need to moderate activity (e.g., R 4 km in 40 minutes, pulse <130 beats per minute, stop if extrasystoles detected; repeat prescription five times per week).

In the second and subsequent years, the frequency of attendance at the rehabilitation center is cut to once in 4 or even 8 weeks. This holds class size within manageable bounds and gives the program director an opportunity to monitor progress, at the same time providing the individual patient with continuing motivation.

Over the first 10 years of the Toronto Rehabilitation Centre program there have been four cardiac incidents, three on the premises and one in the fifth mile of a run. Two were successfully resuscitated. Pointers to future planning were (1) an unreported attack of influenza in one of the four incidents, and (2) prolonged standing in a hot and humid shower area after exercise in two of the remaining three cases.

EXERCISE IN OTHER CONDITIONS

Obesity

If a longterm (6 to 12 months) approach is acceptable, exercise provides a successful method of treating moderate obesity. It has the important advantages of (1) being positive advice, and (2) lightening the depression that often accompanies severe dieting. A gradual approach to fat loss allows establishment of a new lifestyle and improvement of body image, with a lessened risk of recidivism. In contrast to diet alone, an exercise regimen ensures that protein is not lost along with the unwanted fat. Sustained, moderate-intensity activity is more effective in correcting obesity than is a brief burst of high-intensity exercise, in part because more energy is expended, and in part because a higher proportion of this energy is fat. The high body mass places a heavy stress on the various major joints during exercise, and for this reason walking is preferred to jogging. The fat also impedes heat elimination, and particular care is thus necessary when exercising in hot weather.

Diabetes

An increase of physical activity is helpful in the treatment of maturity-onset (Type II) diabetes, but it is less clearly advantageous in the Type I diabetes of the child and young adult. In Type II diabetes, the blood sugar is decreased and the need for insulin is lessened by exercising. This reflects in part the correction of any associated obesity, and in part the greater glucose hunger of active muscles. Particularly in athletes, care must be taken that during an exercise bout an excess of injected insulin is not absorbed from subcutaneous depots.

Chronic Pulmonary Disease

Several authors have now described subjective benefit when patients with chronic obstructive pulmonary disease participate in regular endurance exercise programs. However, there is little evidence that the increased physical activity augments scores on standard tests of respiratory function—indeed, it is difficult to conceive how exercise could restore destroyed pulmonary tissue.

Part of the benefit may be psychological. Some training of the respiratory muscles, with adoption of a more economical pattern of breathing, may lessen respiratory distress during exercise. Subjects may also overcome their fears of physical activity and walk on the treadmill in a mechanically more efficient manner, while a strengthening of the active muscles may decrease exercise-induced lactate formation and thus dyspnea. Probably the most important basis of improvement is a breaking of the vicious circle of fear, inactivity, muscle weakness, and ever-increasing dyspnea.

Unfortunately it is quite difficult to motivate chronic obstructive pulmonary disease patients to become regular program participants. Initially, there is no critical incident such as an infarction to stir their enthusiasm, and in the later stages of the disease severe dyspnea makes even mild exercise unpleasant. Oxygen administration may be helpful in overcoming severe symptoms in the early stages of the rehabilitation process.

Intermittent Claudication

Peripheral arteriosclerosis and intermittent claudication respond favorably to progressive exercise. Generally, increased activity seems to stimulate the development of alternative vascular pathways around areas of arterial vascular obstruction. The best plan for such patients seems a modified interval-type of training, short recovery intervals being allowed each time claudicant pain is sensed.

Mental Disorders

Many subjects explain that the main reason they exercise is to "feel better." There is thus logic in prescribing exercise both for depressive mental disorders, and for reactive depressions induced by conditions such as myocardial infarction. Our observations on postcoronary patients support the view that physical activity helps to correct what is sometimes a severe postinfarction depression.

General Health

A subject's perceived health status normally moves along a continuum between health and disease. The expense of medical visits and brief periods of hospitalization often reflects a mood-induced displacement of status rather than the onset of organic disease. We were thus not surprised to find that initiation of an employee fitness program improved perceived health to the point that individual workers were subsequently using about 0.5 less hospital bed-days per year and were also making three fewer visits to their doctors per year.

SAFETY OF EXERCISE

Concerns are raised periodically about the safety of vigorous exercise. A report from Orange County, California noted that eight men had died while jogging in a single year, and it was queried whether this was more than a chance of phenomenon. Other reports were more reassuring; a survey of 500,000 participants in long-distance skiing events in Sweden revealed only two deaths, and there had been only 10 deaths during 12 million person-hours of skiing in Finland.

Typical Pathologies

Jokl provided case histories from 76 episodes of sudden death during or immediately following exercise. Postmortem examination generally revealed some cardiopulmonary abnormality (although it is less clear how frequently similar findings might have been noted in others dying from causes such as car accidents). Narrowing or occlusion of the coronary arteries was seen in 34 cases, rupture of a major blood vessel in 22 cases, heart failure in 17 cases, chronic myocardial degeneration in eight cases, acute infarction in five cases, and congenital or degenerative valvular problems in four cases.

Risks of Active Leisure

Several recent studies have provided precise estimates of risk. Thompson examined all reports of sudden deaths during jogging for the Rhode Island population from 1975 through 1983; 7.4 percent of men aged 30 to 64 years reported jogging at least twice per week, and from this figure a risk of one death per 7,620 jogger-years, or one death per 396,000 person-hours of jogging, was established. A 5-year study of YMCAs conducted by Vander found a somewhat similar figure of one cardiovascular incident (fatal or nonfatal) per 486,000 participant-hours. Vuori examined autopsied adults in Finland, and in keeping with the other two surveys just described, he found a several-fold increase in the risk of sudden cardiovascular death during physical activity (2.5- to 3.6-fold in nonstrenuous exercise, and 5.3- to 13.1-fold in strenuous exercise). Relatively speaking, 40- to 49-year-old subjects were at greater risk than 50 to 69 year olds during exercise; possibly, the middle-aged subjects were less willing to rest if they encountered symptoms.

Stress Testing

Bruce set the risks of exercise stress testing at one incident in 3,000 maximum tests, and one incident in 15,000 submaximum tests. His population apparently included a mixture of cardiac patients and ostensibly healthy, middle-aged individuals. Rochmis and Blackburn collected data from laboratories across North America. Sixteen cardiovascular emergencies developed in 170,000 tests, 13 within an hour of exercise, and the remaining three over the next 23 hours. A further 40 patients were hospitalized for chest pain or dysrhythmia. All of these incidents were in subjects known to have cardiovascular disease.

Postcoronary Exercise Classes

Haskell examined the risks associated with the operation of postcoronary exercise classes. He obtained data on 949,568 hours of exercise from 86 clubs and found one incident of cardiac arrest per 29,674 hours of exercise. Restricting his analysis to more recent data, in which techniques of patient screening and monitoring had undoubtedly improved, the risk dropped to one episode in 268,922 hours of exercise.

The experience of the Toronto Rehabilitation Centre accords well with these statistics. In a practice limited to patients seen relatively early after myocardial infarction, exercise testing carried a risk of about one cardiovascular emergency in 10,000 tests; there was one cardiac incident for every 114,000 hours of exercise (the rate being about three times higher when the patients were unsupervised than when they were exercising at the Centre).

Program Implications

Several practical lessons can be drawn from this data: (1) the attack rate is very low even for a postcoronary population; it is thus not an economical proposition to provide medically-supervised exercise in perpetuity for such patients, (2) a more effective basis of continuing care is to train the general public in methods of cardiopulmonary resuscitation, and (3) although the risks of an attack are increased three to sevenfold during vigorous exercise, this disadvantage is more than offset by an improved prognosis between bouts of physical activity.

There are few pointers to the avoidance of cardiac incidents. Exercise prescriptions should be reduced during extremes of hot and cold weather or if the patient is under emotional pressure. It is also helpful to teach the patient the symptoms associated with premature ventricular contractions and anginal pain. Unaccustomed exercise without an adequate warmup, over-hot showers, and prolonged standing in a humid changing area are to be avoided. Finally, at least in a statistical sence, the risk of an incident is increased about twofold by the observation of ST segmental depression during an exercise test.

FURTHER READING

Amsterdam EA, Wilmore JH, de Maria AN. Exercise in cardiovascular health and disease. New York: Yorke Books, 1977.

Bjorntorp P. Physiological and clinical aspects of exercise in obese persons. Exerc Sport Sci Rev 1983; 11:159–180.

Blackburn H. Measurement in exercise electrocardiography. Springfield, Ill: CC Thomas, 1969.

Blocker WP, Cardus D. Rehabilitation in ischemic heart disease. New York: Spectrum Publications, 1983.

Brunner D. Studies in preventive cardiology. Tel Aviv: Tel Aviv University, 1973.

Cohen LS, Mock MB, Ringqvist I. Physical conditioning and cardiovascular rehabilitation. New York: Wiley, 1981.

Dawber TR. The Framingham study. The epidemiology of atherosclerotic heart disease. Cambridge, Mass: Harvard University Press, 1980.

Ellestad MH. Stress testing—principles and practice. Philadelphia: FA Davis, 1975.

Evang K, Andersen KL. Physical activity in health and disease. Baltimore: Williams & Wilkins, 1966.

Evered D, Whalen J. The value of preventive medicine. London: Pitman, 1985.

Franklin BA, Rubenfine M. Clinics in sports medicine: cardiac rehabilitation. Philadelphia: WB Saunders, 1984.

Froelicher VF. Exercise testing and training. Chicago: Year Book, 1984.

Hanninen O, Kukkonen K, Vuori I. Physical training in health promotion and medical care. Ann Clin Res 1982; 14: Suppl. 34: 1–172.

Hollmann W. Korperliches Training als Pravention. Stuttgart: Hippokrates Verlag, 1965.

James WE, Amsterdam EA. Coronary heart disease, exercise testing and exercise rehabilitation. Miami, Fla: Symposia Specialists, 1977.

Karvonen MJ, Barry AJ. Physical activity and the heart. Springfield, Ill: CC Thomas, 1967.

Kellermann JJ. Comprehensive cardiac rehabilitation. Basel: Karger, 1982.

Kellermann JJ, Denolin H. Critical evaluation of cardiac rehabilitation. Basel: Karger, 1977.

Kenney WL, Zambraski EJ. Physical activity in human hypertension. A mechanisms approach. Sports Med 1984; 1:459–473.

Keys A. Seven countries. A multivariate analysis of death and coronary heart disease. Cambridge, Mass: Harvard University Press, 1980.

Larson OA, Malmborg RO. Coronary heart disease and physical fitness. Baltimore: University Park Press, 1971.

Long C. Prevention and rehabilitation in ischemic heart disease. Baltimore: Williams & Wilkins, 1980.

Lubich T, Venerando A. Sports cardiology. Bologna: Aulo Gaggi, 1980.

Mason JO, Powell KE. Symposium on public health aspects of physical activity and exercise. Public Health Reports 1985; 100:113–224.

Montoye HJ. Physical activity and health. An epidemiologic study of an entire community. Englewood Cliffs, NJ: Prentice Hall, 1975.

Naughton JP, Hellerstein HK. Exercise testing and exercise training in coronary heart disease. New York: Academic Press, 1973.

Northcote RJ, Ballantyne D. Sudden death and sport. Sports Med 1984; 1:181–186.

Oscai LB. The role of exercise in weight control. Exerc Sport Sci Rev 1973; 1:103–125.

Podell RN, Stewart MM. Primary prevention of coronary heart disease: a practical guide for the clinician. Reading, Mass: Addison Wesley, 1983.

Polednak A. The longevity of athletes. Springfield, Ill: CC Thomas, 1979.

Pollock ML, Schmidt DH. Heart disease and rehabilitation. Boston: Houghton Mifflin, 1979.

Pollock ML, Wilmore JH, Fox E. Exercise in health and disease. Evaluation and prescription for prevention and rehabilitation. Philadelphia: WB Saunders, 1984.

Roskamm H, Reindell H, König K. Körperliche Aktivität und Herz- und Kreislauferkrankungen. Munchen: Johann Ambrosius Barth, 1966.

Shephard RJ, ed. International symposium on physical activity and cardiovascular health. Can Med Assoc J 1967; 96:695–915.

Shephard RJ. Exercise and chronic obstructive lung disease. Exerc Sport Sci Rev 1976; 4:263–296.

Shephard RJ. Ischaemic heart disease and exercise. London: Croom Helm, 1981.

Slutsky R, Froelicher VF. The electrocardiographic response to dynamic exercise. Exerc Sport Sci Rev 1979; 6:105–124.

Thompson PD. Cardiovascular hazards of physical activity. Exerc Sport Sci Rev 1982; 10:208–235.

Tipton CM. Exercise training and hypertension. Exerc Sport Sci Rev 1984; 12:245–306.

Verstappen F, Van den Hoogenband CR, Greep JM. International congress on sports and health. Int J Sports Med 1984; 5, Suppl:1–118.

Vyden JK. Post myocardial infarction management and re-habilitation. New York: Dekker, 1983.

Wenger NK. Exercise and the heart. (2nd Ed.). Philadelphia: FA Davis, 1985.

Wilson PK. Adult fitness testing and cardiac rehabilitation. Baltimore: University Park Press, 1975.

Zohman LF, Tobis JS. Cardiac rehabilitation. New York: Grune & Stratton, 1970.

MISCELLANEOUS TOPICS

CHAPTER *14*

EFFECTS OF ERGOGENIC AIDS

A wide variety of approaches have been tried by the occasional unsporting athlete in an attempt to gain an "edge" over other competitors. This chapter considers certain abuses that are currently prevalent, including the administration of "alkalis," caffeine, anabolic steroids, sympathomimetic amines, beta-blocking agents, "blood doping," and "nerve doping."

Alkalis

Since sprint activity is halted by the fall of intramuscular pH, it seems probable that performance could be improved if the intravascular and intracellular buffering of hydrogen ions were to be increased. Early attempts to administer bicarbonate apparently had little effect upon performance, possibly because the drug was administered too long before competition. Body buffers and pH levels are normally adjusted quite quickly by changes in respiratory minute volume and the urinary excretion of bicarbonate, so that the body might well compensate completely for a premature alkalosis.

It is also possible that by altering the sensitivity of the respiratory controller or shifting the O_2 dissociation curve to the left, an alteration of buffering capacity may have an adverse impact upon more sustained performance. Nevertheless, Gledhill and his associates have recently shown that an appropriately timed dose of sodium bicarbonate can yield an advantage of almost 3 seconds in times for an 800 meter track event. The main action of the bicarbonate appears to be a speeding of lactate transport out of the active muscles, thus facilitating repeated bouts of heavy work. The optimum pH in their experiments lay in the range of 7.4 to 7.5, greater degrees of alkalosis having an adverse impact upon performance. Since bicarbonate is a natural body constituent, there is no simple method whereby doping control agencies can regulate this particular abuse.

Caffeine

For a number of years, long-distance cyclists have taken substantial amounts of caffeine in attempts to boost their performances. Given the prevalence of tea and coffee drinking, an outright ban upon caffeine ingestion is hardly practical. However, urinary caffeine concentrations of more than 15 g per milliliter are now proscribed for international competitors. A paper by Berglund and Hemmingsen noted a 1.7 percent gain in the performance of caffeine-treated cross-country skiers. Possible explanations include (1) central stimulation (with a shortening of reaction time and a lessening of fatigue), (2) inhibition of the normal breakdown of 3–5 cyclic AMP with a mobilization of depot fat, and (3) a potentiation of calcium ion release from the sarcoplasmic reticulum.

Excessive amounts of either coffee or caffeine cause irritability, tremors, palpitations, an irregular pulse, gastrointestinal disturbances, and sleeplessness. Two other potent xanthine constituents are found in tea. Theophylline is a coronary vasodilator and diuretic, and theobromine increases muscle force, presumably again by an action on calcium release from the sarcoplasmic reticulum.

Anabolic Steroids

Athletes involved in power competitions have believed for many years that massive doses of anabolic steroids would increase muscle strength, and some observers have pointed to a sudden surge in world records coincident with the widespread availability of these compounds.

Human experimentation has been difficult, because while many athletes take 100 to 300 mg of a synthetic androgen methandrostenolone (Danabol) per day, the ethical dose is only 10 mg per day. Perhaps because of this discrepancy in dosage, physiologists have argued that (1) androgens did not increase the normal response to hard training shown by an athlete eating a good quality, high protein diet, (2) if there was some additional increase of body mass with androgens, this reflected an increase of body water rather than lean tissue, (3) if there was an increase of lean tissue, this reflected the belief of the athlete in the efficacy of androgens, psychological effects of the androgens, or a stimulation of appetite, and (4) even if there was an increase of lean tissue, there was no gain of muscle strength relative to athletes who had avoided this abuse. However, dispassionate review of the evidence now suggests that massive, sustained dosages of androgen can increase both lean mass and strength. An individual's sense of wellbeing may also be improved, and competitiveness is increased. Clinical doses have little effect, because of the inhibition of pituitary gonadotrophin secretion as androgen levels rise. However, massive doses of androgen increase the stimulus to muscle hypertrophy at the price of a total inhibition of testosterone secretion by the interstitial cells of the testes.

The synthetic androgens are designed to sustain the protein anabolic effects of testosterone, while minimizing masculinizing effects. Nevertheless, prolonged administration of androgens to female competitors leads to a progressive development of male secondary sex characteristics. Modern methods of urine analysis (a combination of gas chromatography and mass spectrometry) are fairly successful in detecting steroid doping, although chemical proof of drug abuse can be made more difficult by alkalizing the urine. Some athletes who have been anxious to avoid penalties for doping have reputedly ceased taking steroids 6 weeks prior to competition. A second ruse has been to stimulate natural androgen production by the administration of pituitary growth hormone.

One suggested remedy for all forms of steroid abuse is to keep a weight register of athletes involved in power sports. Any competitors who show a sudden, unexpected increase of lean mass can then be investigated very closely.

Various dangers of androgens have been cited, particularly premature closure of the epiphyses in children of both sexes, and masculinization of female competitors. In males there is at least a temporary suppression of testosterone secretion and spermatogenesis; there have also been reports of baldness, hypertension, diabetes, disturbed liver function, hepatic carcinogenesis, and prostate tumors.

Sympathomimetic Amines

At one time, sympathomimetic compounds such as the amphetamines were taken by some endurance athletes in order to improve mood, to lessen the sense of fatigue, and to constrict the skin blood vessels. On occasion, this unwise practice contributed to death from heat stress. The amines in question have only a short period of action, and they are easily detected by modern doping controls. However, problems continue to arise because athletes take such drugs unknowingly in proprietary cold and hay fever remedies. If an athlete suffers from exercise-induced bronchospasm, it is permissible to administer the mast-cell stabilizing substance sodium cromoglycate; the rules of some competitions also permit the use of bronchial-specific dilator amines.

Beta-Blocking Agents

Beta-blocking agents such as propranolol have reportedly been taken by competitors in ski jumping and shooting events as a means of reducing undesired responses to catecholamine release such as tachycardia and tremor. One competitor at the Commonwealth Games in Brisbane claimed to be taking propranolol for medical reasons, but a careful urine analysis showed that the dose taken had been at least 20 times that required for any legitimate therapeutic purpose!

"Blood Doping"

The concept of blood-doping is simple. A sample of 250 to 500 ml of blood is withdrawn from an athlete and is stored for a period of about a month. During this time, the blood volume and hemoglobin of the competitor are restored by natural regenerative processes. The blood sample is then reinfused, increasing both blood volume and total hemoglobin. United States cycling competitors admitted adopting this tactic in the 1984 Olympic Games. Not all early experiments demonstrated an advantage from reinfusion, but Gledhill and his associates have suggested that in experiments where there was a seeming lack of response, the reinfused blood had deteriorated during storage.

With modern methods of preserving blood, reinfusion gives an increase of maximum cardiac output and oxygen transport that is almost directly proportional to the expansion of blood volume. Particularly in female subjects, additional blood does not bring the red cell count and hematocrit to the theoretical ceiling where maximum cardiac output would be limited by an increase of blood viscosity. Indeed, in Gledhill's experiments, the maximum cardiac output was increased after reinfusion, possibly because of a better perfusion of the myocardium.

The only available method of testing athletes for this abuse is to look at the rate of red cell metabolism. Values for the reinfused cells are substantially less than the normal average figure.

"Nerve Doping"

Some athletes have apparently attempted to modify their inherited muscle fiber characteristics, using appropriately selected patterns of electrical stimulation of their motor nerves. While there is some possibility of converting Type IIb to Type IIa fibers by selective patterns of electrical stimulation, the response thus induced is no greater than that which could be elicited by vigorous training. Moreover, there seems no possibility for the conversion of Type IIa to Type I fibers other than by the drastic process of neural transplantation (Chapter 5).

EXPOSURE TO AIR POLLUTANTS

The reputation of Los Angeles for intense episodes of urban air pollution renewed scientific interest in the effect of atmospheric pollutants upon athletic performance as preparations began for the 1984 Olympic Games. Fortunately, the weather proved favorable to the dispersal of pollutants during the period of competition. The recorded ambient levels of substances such as ozone and nitrogen oxides were quite low, and no specific complaints relating to air pollution were registered by athletes.

Environmental engineers recognize two main categories of air pollution—oxidant smog and reducing smog. The oxidant smog is produced largely from vehicle exhaust and is prevalent in the Los Angeles basin. The reducing smog is a byproduct of the combustion of fossil fuels such as coal and oil and is encountered in European cities where homes are heated by burning soft coal.

Oxidant Smog

The main toxic constituents of oxidant smog are carbon monoxide, nitrogen oxides, and unburned hydrocarbons. The last two classes of compound interact in the sunshine of the upper atmosphere to yield ozone.

Carbon monoxide blocks oxygen transport because of its high affinity for hemoglobin (200 to 250 times that for oxygen-hemoglobin bonding). Carbon monoxide also causes a leftward shift in the oxygen dissociation curve, thus making it more difficult for oxygen to diffuse from hemoglobin to myoglobin as blood perfuses the active tissues. The blood of the rural non-smoker contains about 0.5 percent carboxyhemoglobin, formed by the hemolysis of red cells, but the carbon monoxide burden rises to 1.0 to 1.5 percent in the nonsmoking city dweller and to 5 to 10 percent in a heavy cigarette smoker. A person jogging beside a busy highway has a substantial local exposure to carbon monoxide, and carboxyhemoglobin figures as high as 5 percent have been reported even in nonsmokers. Apart from the immediate effects on oxygen transport, there have been suggestions that a carboxyhemoglobin level of more than 3 percent (1) impairs psychomotor performance (Table 14–1), (2) shortens the time to the onset of anginal pain in a patient with myocardial ischemia, and (3) increases the risk of a myocardial infarct in a middle-aged adult with some impairment of the coronary circulation.

The main effect of the other constituents of oxidant smog is upon the eyes. Itching, conjunctival congestion, and lacrimation could all impair performance in events where visual skills were important.

Because of the large respiratory minute volumes developed by the endurance athlete, and the bypassing of the normal filtration mechanisms of the nose, the threshold concentration of ozone required for the appearance of respiratory effects is reduced from 0.37 to

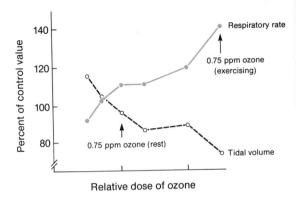

Figure 14–1 Influence of ozone exposure on respiratory pattern adopted when exercising at 75 percent of maximum oxygen intake. Based on data of Folinsbee, Silverman, and Shephard.

about 0.2 ppm in a vigorously exercising subject. Symptoms of substernal distress and soreness are accompanied by a reduction of lung volumes and adoption of a rapid, shallow pattern of breathing (Fig. 14–1).

The levels of oxidant pollutants show a marked diurnal rhythm, peaking after about an hour of bright sunshine. The simplest preventive measure is thus to schedule competitions when levels of pollution are low. There have also been suggestions that protection against the adverse effects of ozone might be obtained from administration of antioxidants such as vitamin C or vitamin E.

Reducing Smog

The burning of fossil fuels generates sulphur dioxide and soot particles and, particularly if absorbed on soot, dust or salt, the SO_2 tends to be converted to the more toxic sulphur trioxide (SO_3). In England, during the early 1950s, concentrations during two severe episodes of pollution were sufficient to cause several thousand excess deaths relative to the anticipated mortality rate; young children, the elderly, and those with chronic chest disease were particularly affected. The situation has since been alleviated somewhat in most countries by the building of taller smokestacks (which disperse the smoke and oxides of sulphur over distances of several hundred kilometers) and by the fitting of precipitators (which remove much of the particulate matter, and thus avoid the conversion of SO_2 to the more toxic SO_3).

While there have not been any specific reports that reducing smog has caused problems in athletes, again, for any given concentration of pollutant, the combination of mouth-breathing and a large respiratory minute volume put the endurance athlete at an increased risk relative to a sedentary individual. One effect of the sulphur oxides is to induce a progressive paralysis of the tracheal ciliae, thereby leaving the individual who

TABLE 14–1 Some Reported Effects of Carbon Monoxide Upon Central Nervous Function, With the Corresponding Critical Blood Carboxyhemoglobin Readings

Function	Critical Blood Carboxyhemoglobin (%)
Vigilance task	1.8–3.1
Error of time estimation	1.8
Auditory duration discrimination	2.5–4.0
Visual intensity discrimination	3.0
Tracking task	3.0
Choice reaction time	3.5–4.0
Visual acuity	4.5
Vigilance	5.0
Mental performance and finger dexterity	7.2

has been exposed to such gases more vulnerable to small particles, including bacteria. Given that athletes are commonly affected by upper respiratory infections, this may be an important consideration.

The best tactic for the athlete is to avoid training or competition when pollution levels are high. A gauze mask over the face may clear the air of larger particles, but an effective gas filter has too high an airflow resistance to be acceptable to most sports enthusiasts.

CIGARETTE SMOKING

Medical Hazards of Cigarette Smoking

There is a long list of medical reasons for abstinence from cigarette smoking. Smokers have an increased risk of various types of cancer, including tumors of the lungs, larynx, bladder and urinary tract, the breasts (in women), and the mouth and lips (particularly in pipe smokers). Other hazards include chronic bronchitis and emphysema, coronary vascular disease, and thromboangiitis obliterans. Pregnant women are more liable to premature delivery, and they show an increased perinatal mortality. There have also been reports of an increased incidence of cirrhosis and gastric ulcer in smokers, although this may reflect an association between alcoholism and heavy cigarette consumption. Upper respiratory infections have a longer duration in the smoker. Minor illnesses also lead to longer periods of restricted activity, absence from work, and bed rest.

At the age of 25 years, a 40 cigarette per day addiction shortens the lifespan by 8 years, and even 10 cigarettes per day shorten life by 5 years. After smoking withdrawal, there is a gradual return to normal health in the next 10 years.

Physiological Consequences of Smoking

From the physiological point of view, the main handicaps of the smoker are an increase of blood carboxyhemoglobin, ciliary paralysis, airway irritation, and bronchospasm.

Carbon Monoxide.   While concern is expressed about ambient carbon monoxide levels of 35 to 40 ppm, the smoke inhaled from a cigarette contains 40,000 ppm of carbon monoxide. It is thus common to find carboxyhemoglobin figures of 5 to 10 percent in a heavy smoker, and a rebreathing estimate of blood carbon monoxide provides a helpful check on the success of smoking withdrawal (the strength of addiction is such that as many as 10 percent of smokers will tell physicians they have stopped smoking when objective measurements show this to be untrue). The carbon monoxide readily traverses the placental barrier, and is one reason for the low birth weight, retarded development, and

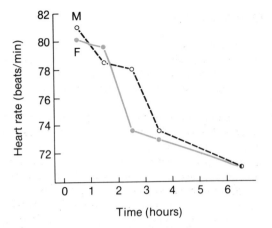

Figure 14–2 Resting heart rate in relation to time since last cigarette (based on data from Rode, Ross, and Shephard).

perinatal mortality of children born to smoking mothers. The immediate effect of the carboxyhemoglobin plus the nicotine on the adult is a small increase of heart rate (5 to 10 beats per minute), more obvious during rest than during sub-maximum exercise (Fig. 14–2). A longer term reaction is a compensatory polycythemia (with an associated increase in the risk of various types of intravascular thrombosis). The carbon monoxide is eliminated from the body with a half-time of 3 to 4 hours; thus, the blood carboxyhemoglobin of the smoker drops to more normal levels over a night of sleep.

Irritant Chemicals and Particles.   The various irritant chemicals in the smoke first stimulate but soon paralyse the tracheal ciliae. In consequence, particles are retained in the airway. This in turn increases liability not only to respiratory infections but also to various industrial pneumoconioses.

Irritation of the bronchial mucosa gives rise to edema, an increase of mucus secretion, and hypertrophy of the mucus glands. These conditions may cause a tendency to airway collapse, with a further increase in the risk of respiratory infection.

The combination of inert particles and irritant chemicals found in tobacco smoke gives rise to a rapid reflex bronchospasm. A 30 percent increase of airway resistance can be detected within 15 seconds, and the effect persists for at least 1 hour after smoking. Whereas a healthy young adult uses perhaps 5 percent of maximum oxygen transport in the respiratory muscles, this figure can rise to 10 to 15 percent in a heavy smoker. In a young smoker, where there is simply an acute bronchospasm, the effect is reversed with 1 to 2 days of abstinence from cigarettes, but in an older person where there are secondary mucosal changes, the smoking-related increase of airway resistance is much more permanent. Many smokers are unaware that they have become short of breath as a consequence of their addiction, and a simple exercise test with demonstration of dyspnea can be a useful aid to a smoking withdrawal program.

Cardiovascular endurance is adversely affected by the dyspnea, and partly for this reason very few competitors in endurance sports are smokers.

Nicotine. The nicotine content of cigarette smoke tends to provoke coronary vascular spasm and premature ventricular contractions. The exercise stress test of a heavy smoker may also show deep ST segmental depression of the electrocardiogram—a further adverse feature of the addiction that can be exploited in smoking withdrawal programs.

The Manufacturers' Quest for "Safe" Smoking Material

Will there ever be a "safe" form of tobacco use? While habitual cigar and pipe smokers rarely inhale the smoke, and thus have a lower incidence of most forms of cancer than a cigarette smoker, a cigarette smoker who switches to a pipe or a cigar continues to inhale the smoke, and because cigar and pipe tobacco smoke contains more irritants, the final state may be worse than the first. Likewise, if "low tar" cigarettes are used, they (usually) have a low nicotine content. The smoker thus consumes a greater number of cigarettes to maintain the habitual dose of nicotine, so that the inhaled dose of tar remains unchanged, while the amount of carbon monoxide that is inhaled may actually be increased.

Effects of Smoking Withdrawal

After smoking withdrawal, there may not be any major increase of maximum oxygen intake as measured by conventional techniques. Nevertheless, as airway resistance becomes normalized, an increased proportion of the aerobic power is available to the working muscles.

Body mass may increase by 2 to 5 kg in the first year after smoking withdrawal. Reasons include the absence of nicotine suppression of appetite, a restoration of normal taste sensation, and a wish for alternative indulgences to cigarettes. Some women become sufficiently discouraged by the temporary accumulation of body fat that they revert to smoking, and it is thus important to combine advice on diet and exercise with a smoking withdrawal program. However, from a health point of view, 5 kg of fat has a much smaller impact on longevity than an uncorrected cigarette habit.

Passive Smoking

In recent years, there has been much discussion of the risks of "passive smoking." The smoker exposes bystanders to two main types of smoke: mainstream smoke (partially filtered by the cigarette and the lungs of the smoker) and the much more toxic sidestream smoke from a smoldering cigarette. The density of the smoke within a closed space such as an office or restaurant depends not only on the number of smokers who are present, but also on ventilation. In an attempt to save on heating and refrigeration costs, many commercial buildings recirculate air, adding only a minimum of fresh air at each ventilation cycle.

Under the worst likely conditions, a passive smoker may receive as much as one-twentieth of the dose of tobacco smoke inhaled by the smoker. When a small European car is driven with the windows closed, smoking by the occupants can push carbon monoxide concentrations within the vehicle to 80 to 100 ppm. The carboxyhemoglobin level thus rises appreciably in nonsmoking fellow passengers. Other evidence of passive smoke exposure includes the urinary excretion of nicotine and cotinine, substances that could only have come from cigarette smoke.

The immediate physiological responses to passive smoking include (1) eye irritation and lacrimation, with a reduction in stability of the tear film (changes that impair vision and increase the chance of an eye infection), (2) an increase of nasal airway resistance, with an augmentation of nasal secretions, and (3) annoyance by the odor (although nasal receptors quickly adapt to the smell).

Small changes of respiratory function are seen with heavy exposures, particularly in subjects with sensitive airways. In young children, passive exposure to cigarette smoke also seems to increase the risk of respiratory infections (possibly because infants have little potential to escape from their smoking mothers); older adults who have lived for many years with a smoking partner apparently have an increased risk of carcinoma of the lungs (Table 14–2).

ALCOHOL

This brief section considers the physiological effects of alcohol and their interaction with physical performance, leaving to other texts a discussion of psychosocial problems and alcohol addiction.

TABLE 14–2 Mortality of Nonsmoking Wives From Various Conditions, Expressed as Ratio to Values Observed When Husband is a Nonsmoker

Cause of Death	Risk Ratio if Husband is Current or Former Smoker	
	1–19 cigs/day	≥20 cigs/day
Lung cancer	1.61	2.08
Emphysema and asthma	1.29	1.49
Cancer of cervix	1.15	1.14
Cancer of stomach	1.02	0.99
Ischemic heart disease	0.97	1.03

Based on data of Hirayama.

Alcohol Absorption

Alcohol is absorbed relatively quickly from the stomach, thereby reaching peak concentrations 30 to 45 minutes after ingestion. It is cleared from the blood stream by oxidation in the liver, the enzyme alcohol dehydrogenase reducing the concentration by 10 to 20 mg per deciliter per hour. Those who have a substantial habitual intake of alcohol reputedly increase their clearance rate through an increased alcohol dehydrogenase activity.

The blood level observed after a given alcohol ingestion depends on the speed of drinking, the nature of accompanying food, the type of beverage, body size, and the amount of body fat. Most countries have designed traffic legislation on the basis that there is a threshold concentration for intoxication, although there is unfortunately a wide inter-individual variation of the threshold (if such exists). Approximately 10 percent of the population are clinically intoxicated, with an unsteady gait, slurred speech, and irresponsible behavior, at blood levels as low as 10 to 50 mg per deciliter, and two-thirds of the population are obviously intoxicated at a concentration of 100 to 150 mg per deciliter. Partly for political rather than physiological reasons, the legal blood level is set at 50 to 80 mg per deciliter in different countries. The 80 mg standard corresponds to the ingestion of four whiskies or two pints of beer by a large man, but a woman may reach this ceiling with only two standard drinks.

Physiological Effects

Although alcohol is popularly considered as a stimulant, in reality it depresses the brain, beginning with the highest functions such as judgment, self-control, and self-criticism. The typical response to drinking is an exaggeration of normal personality—for example, an extrovert continues to drive at the same speed, but with diminished accuracy, while introverts maintain their accuracy at the expense of speed. Athletes such as pistol shooters who sense their performance is impaired by overarousal have sometimes deliberately taken alcohol as a depressant drug.

In most forms of activity, alcohol hampers rather than improves performance. Vision is impaired and reaction times are slowed at blood levels of 40 to 80 mg per deciliter. Over the range 30 to 100 mg per deciliter there is a progressive deterioration of psychomotor function, with an increase of body sway, a loss of arm steadiness, and finally, difficulty in the coordination of walking. Hearing is also impaired at blood levels of 100 to 150 mg per deciliter.

A lessening of central inhibition may decrease the sense of fatigue and increase muscle force. Cutaneous vasodilatation gives a misleading impression of body warmth (rather, alcohol intoxication causes an increased heat loss and a vulnerability to hypothermia). In submaximum exercise, the heart rate is increased and the blood pressure is usually lower. The maximum oxygen intake, measured over a brief period, is unchanged, but there may be a decrease of endurance due to the cutaneous vasodilatation. In addition to the effects of vasodilatation, there is diuresis that is provoked not only by the volume of fluid ingested but also by inhibition of the pituitary antidiuretic hormones.

Effects on Long-Term Health

From the long-term health perspective, it has been suggested that moderate doses of alcohol increase HDL levels and are thus of medical value. This is a seductive argument, but in fact other adverse features of alcohol overshadow any small benefit from the increase of HDL cholesterol.

The sedative effect of alcohol plus the associated ingestion of excess energy frequently cause the heavy drinker to become obese. Moreover, alcohol forms an increasingly large fraction of total energy intake at the expense of necessary vitamins and proteins, this being a major factor in the development of cirrhosis of the liver. Finally, periodic major binges seem to have a specific toxic effect on both skeletal and cardiac muscle, because myoglobin and muscle enzymes are liberated into the blood stream.

FURTHER READING

Gledhill N. Bicarbonate ingestion and anaerobic performance. Sports Med 1984; 1:177–180.

Horvath SM. Impact of air quality on exercise performance. Exerc Sport Sci Rev 1982; 9:265–296.

Hultman E, Sahlin K. Acid-base balance during exercise. Exerc Sport Sci Rev 1981; 8:41–128.

Kochakian CD. Anabolic-androgenic steroids. Berlin: Springer Verlag, 1976.

McCafferty WB. Air pollution and athletic performance. Springfield, Ill: CC Thomas, 1981.

Morgan WP. Ergogenic aids and muscular performance. New York: Academic Press, 1972.

Shephard RJ. The risks of passive smoking. London: Croom Helm, 1982.

United States Department of Health, Education and Welfare:
    Smoking and health: a report of the surgeon general (1979)
    The health consequences of smoking for women (1980)
    The changing cigarette (1981)
    The health consequences of smoking: cancer (1982)
    The health consequences of smoking: cardiovascular disease (1983)
    The health consequences of smoking: chronic obstructive disease (1984)
    Rockville, Md.: US Dept of Health & Human Services.

Williams MH. Drugs and athletic performance. Springfield, Ill: CC Thomas, 1974.

Wynder EL, Hoffman D. Tobacco and tobacco smoke. New York: Academic Press, 1967.

INDEX

A

Acclimatization
  to cold, 178
  to heat, 177–178
  to high altitudes, 166–167
Acid-base balance, 106–107
Activity. *See* Habitual activity; Physical activity
Activity duration, 111
Adenosine diphosphate. *See* ADP
Adenosine triphosphate. *See* ATP
Adjustment. *See* Acclimatization
ADP (adenosine diphosphate)
  as energy source, 5
  and tissue respiration, 105
Adrenal cortex, 41–42
Adrenocorticotrophic hormone (ACTH), 40
Aerobic power
  of child, 148–149
  field tests of, 118
  measurement of, direct, 114–115
  prediction procedures, submaximum, 115–118
Afferent information, 63
Aging
  and blood pressure, 151
  and body fat, 152
  and cardiovascular system, 151
  and ECG, 151–152
  and employment potential, 153
  and exercise, 154
  and fitness, 111
  functional loss with, 149–150
  interpretation of data on, 150
  and muscle, 152
  and oxygen transport, 150–152
  and performance, 153
  and respiratory system, 150
  and sensory systems, 152–153
  and skeletal support system, 152
  theories of, 149–150
  and training, 153–154
Agonists, 51
Air pollutants, 197–199
Alcohol
  absorption, 201
  as energy source, 7
  on long-term health, 201
  physiological effects of, 201
Aldosterone, 41–42
Alkalis, 196
Alveolar pressures, 87
Alveolar ventilation, 96–97
Ambient pressures. *See* High altitudes; High ambient pressures; Low ambient pressures
Ambient temperature. *See* Body temperature; Climate temperature
Amenorrhea, 46
Amines, sympathomimetic, 197
Anabolic steroids, 196–197
Anaerobic capacity, 113
Anaerobic power, 112–113
Anaerobic work, 166
Androgens, 44–46
Angina, 180, 185
Animals, 2–3
Anorexia nervosa, 35
Antagonists, 51, 59–60
Anxiety, 3
Arteriosclerosis, 185–186
Arteriovenous oxygen difference, 132
Astrand nomogram, 115–116
Atherosclerosis, 185
ATP (adenosine triphosphate)
  and anaerobic glycolysis, 5–6
  and cardiac muscle, 78–79
  as energy source, 5
  and energy yield, 22–24
  and tissue respiration, 105
  and transfer of energy, 55–56
Automatic movement, 57–58, 63

B

Balance, 64
Bed rest, 127
Beta-blocking agents, 197
Biochemical correlates, 18
Biological age, 150
Blood doping, 197
Blood flow distribution
  muscle, 84–85
  to other organs, 87–88
  pulmonary, 87
  skin, 85–86
  visceral, 87
Blood glucose, 121–122
Blood lipid profile, 33, 35, 134
Blood pressure
  and aging, 151
  and cardiac output, increasing, 79
  and cardiac work rate, 78–79
  and exercise, 77–78
  and hypotension, 77
  and pulse pressure, 77
  resting, 76–77
  and training, 132
Body fat. *See also* Fat; Obesity
  and aging, 152
  and epidemiological indices, 31
  estimates of, 31–32
  and fitness, 119
  and injury, 123
  percentage of, ideal, in athlete, 29
  and skinfold predictions, 31
  and training, 133–134
Body mass, 29–31
Body temperature. *See also* Cold; Heat
  and circulatory adjustments, 175–176
  and climate, 174–175
  and clothing, 176–177
  and conduction, 173
  and convection, 173
  and core temperature, acceptable limits of, 172
  and energy balance, 172
  and evaporation, 173–174
  and exercise, 123
  and grease, 177
  and heat stores, 173
  and homiothermy, 172
  measuring, 172
  and neural function, 177
  and radiation, 173
  and shivering, 177
  and sweat production, 175–176
  and thermal neutrality, 172
  and thermoregulation, 175–177
  and voluntary activity, 176
  and warmup, 56–57
Bone. *See also* Skeletal support system
  blood flow to, 88
  injury, 147–148
  in skeletal support system, 69
  and training, 133
Brain
  blood flow to, 87–88
  and movement skills, 63
Breathing. *See also* Aerobic power; Respiratory system
  and high ambient pressures, 162
  regulation of, 107
  work of
    elastic, 101–102
    inertial, 103
    and muscles, accessory, 104–105
    overall, 103–104
    resistive, 102–103
Bronchospasm, 180

C

Caffeine, 196
Calisthenics, 137
Carbohydrate reserves, 22